D0038934

Handbook of
Postoperative
Complications

Handbook of Postoperative Complications

D.J. Leaper
*Professor of Surgery and
Honorary Consultant Surgeon,
University of Newcastle upon Tyne,
University Hospital of North Tees*

and

A.L.G. Peel
*Consultant Surgeon,
University Hospital of North Tees*

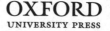

OXFORD
UNIVERSITY PRESS

OXFORD
UNIVERSITY PRESS

Great Clarendon Street, Oxford OX2 6DP

Oxford University Press is a department of the University of Oxford.
It furthers the University's objective of excellence in research, scholarship,
and education by publishing worldwide in

Oxford New York

Auckland Bangkok Buenos Aires Cape Town Chennai
Dar es Salaam Delhi Hong Kong Istanbul Karachi Kolkata
Kuala Lumpur Madrid Melbourne Mexico City Mumbai Nairobi
São Paulo Shanghai Taipei Tokyo Toronto

Oxford is a registered trade mark of Oxford University Press
in the UK and in certain other countries

Published in the United States
by Oxford University Press Inc., New York

© Oxford University Press, 2003

A catalogue record for this title is available from the British Library

Library of Congress Cataloging in Publication Data
(Data available)

ISBN 0 19 263070 9 (flexicover)

10 9 8 7 6 5 4 3 2 1

Typeset by Cepha Imaging Private Ltd
Printed in Italy
on acid-free paper by Giunti Industrie Grafiche

Preface

Complications after surgery have been minimized through improved knowledge of surgical physiology and preoperative preparation. Research has led to a greater understanding of the response to surgery and anaesthesia, and has been complemented by clinical trials which have laid down principles and guidelines; venous thromboembolic and antibiotic-wound infection prophylaxis are examples. If a complication is to be avoided then it becomes critical, for audit and research purposes, to accurately define what the complication is. Ideally, complications should be registered by an unbiased, trained observer. In the United Kingdom, comparison of the incidence of complications between health trusts, regions, and foreign countries would be totally invalid if definitions of outcomes (performance indicators) were inadequate.

Seromas after mastectomy are so common that they might not be regarded as a complication. No surgical manoeuvre can clearly reduce their incidence nor, in some instances, the need for multiple repeated aspirations. It would be inappropriate, however, not to discuss this when obtaining consent for mastectomy—failure to do so may be regarded as a complication! Wound infection after surgery is a complication that may have dire consequences, such as secondary haemorrhage when a wound infection involves a vascular graft, but it must be carefully defined. Infection after clean-wound surgery has been recorded as being as high as 15%. It is controversial, but it seems that prophylactic antibiotics have little effect. To compare wound infection rates between surgeons or hospitals not only are the definitions important, using the detailed ASEPSIS or Southampton scoring systems, but also an in-depth surveillance is required (with a blinded trained observer) for at least 30 days postoperatively. Other complications have an incidence simply based on how hard the investigator looks. Anastomotic leak after low anterior resection is such an example. The incidence based on clinical definition is between 5 and 10% (faecal peritonitis, fistula, or an otherwise unexplained postoperative pyrexia), but if digital, endoscopic, and gastrograffin enema criteria are all used then the incidence has been shown to be as high as 70%, although not all are clinically significant.

Complications are clearly important and are increasingly used as measurable, clinical-performance indicators. Surgeons, as a consequence, are vulnerable. The principal consequences of postoperative complications are:

1. To the patient; and to their relatives, work, and lifestyle. Patients expect a very high standard, and complications cause discomfort, a delay in return to normal duty, and occasionally may lead to their death.

2. Complications, particularly when major, also often cause a feeling of failure to the operating surgeon even when they cannot in any way be ascribed to a failure of care. For trainees (and trainers for that matter) this is precisely what tutors and supervisors are for: to share this within open audit sessions.

3. A complaint or litigation relating to an alleged lack of care or negligence. Good communication may reduce this, but staff must be prepared for this outcome and need to learn how to cope with it.

4. The incidence and nature of complications must be openly and accurately collected and discussed in regular audit meetings of structure, process, and outcome. If guidelines are not modified and revisited in 'audit loops', clinical governance and league tables will take the responsibility away and dictate strategy.

5. Complications cause an increase in hospital stay. The increased costs have been highlighted by HMOs in countries such as the United States of America where private healthcare is more prevalent. Operating costs are increased and subscriptions to medical defence organizations may also be increased.

Anticipation of complications: achieving the lowest rates

Some operations are known to have a higher rate of complications, the consequences of which may be life-threatening. Oesophagogastric cancer surgery is an example. Regular ward rounds should anticipate and recognize a complication at a stage when it is potentially reversible. An anastomotic leak may present with a low-grade pyrexia at 7–8 days and must be excluded before it progresses to an abdominal abscess, mediastinitis, or peritonitis, when redo, or second-look, surgery has less chance of salvaging a life-threatening situation. Remember: **anticipate**, **recognize** early signs, and **act**.

Perioperative prophylaxis is not entirely reliable. The use of prophylactic antibiotics may have reduced the wound infection rate to under 5% for clean-contaminated (e.g. open cholecystectomy) operations, but these 5% will have the consequences of a wound infection. Again this needs to be discussed with the patient when taking consent, and subsequently needs accurate audit. If local infection rates rise then protocols must to be reviewed. An added risk of infection or attendant sepsis may be anticipated prior to cholecystectomy if, for example, the patient is jaundiced, particularly one with common bile duct stones, and when an open operation is undertaken.

Evidence-based medicine

There is little practice in surgery which is based on scientifically proven trial results. Examples of surgical practice that is based on appropriate randomized clinical trials (RCTs) include bowel preparation before colorectal surgery, antibiotic prophylaxis in clean-contaminated and contaminated elective surgery, and prophylaxis of venous thromboembolism. Clinical governance will insist that guidelines, written following systematic Cochrane-style reviews or meta-analysis, are followed to the letter when this type of evidence is available. Many of these reviews are rather preliminary, are open to interpretation, and may not indicate with any clarity where randomized prospective clinical trials are needed, but they do emphasize the weaknesses of many trials. Further guidance and protocols may come from the National Institute of Clinical Excellence (NICE) or the Centre for Health Improvement (CHImp), but most surgery will continue to be undertaken on established principles, passed on through publications, continuing medical education, or training programmes.

Operative surgery has been traditionally learnt through an apprenticeship, but the amount of experience gained in training is bound to fall with the introduction of Calman training reforms, and the reduction of working hours in particular. To partly compensate for this, surgery should be undertaken on a team-basis, which involves anaesthetists and intensivists, nursing staff, and professions allied to medicine, such as pharmacy and physiotherapy. All this raises the expectations and success of surgery.

Postoperative complications

In this book, postoperative complications have been covered as general complications or those encountered after specific types of surgery. It is aimed at undergraduates and those undertaking early postgraduate training in surgery (basic surgical training up to MRCS), and even beyond this (higher surgical training up to the Intercollegiate Fellowship). The book may be useful to theatre staff (scrub team, operating department assistants (ODAs), and recovery-room nurses) and surgical ward staff.

D.J.L.   February 2003

Contents

Contributors

Gordon Carlson Consultant Surgeon/Senior Lecturer, Hope Hospital, Salford, Manchester

Mark Carpenter SpR Intensive Medicine, Northern Deanery, Newcastle upon Tyne

Edwin Clark Research Fellow, Hope Hospital, Salford, Manchester

Philip Dean Head of Pharmacy Services, University Hospital of North Tees, Stockton-on-Tees

Andrew Dickenson Research Fellow, University Hospitals of Leicester

Roger Finney Consultant Haematologist (retired), University Hospital of North Tees, Stockton-on-Tees

Rafael Guerrero SpR in Cardiothoracic Surgery, The General Infirmary, Leeds

Lynne Harris Pharmacist, Clinical Pharmacy Team Leader, Bishop Auckland General Hospital

Maurice Hawthorne Consultant Surgeon, North Riding Infirmary, Middlesbrough

Dalvi Humzah Consultant Plastic Surgeon, The Radcliffe Infirmary, Oxford

David Leaper Professor of Surgery/Honorary Consultant Surgeon, University Hospital of North Tees, Stockton-on-Tees

Iona Macloed Consultant Gynaecologist, University Hospital of North Tees, Stockton-on-Tees

Chris Munsch Consultant Cardiothoracic Surgeon, The General Infirmary, Leeds

Duncan Parry Vascular Research Fellow, St James's University Hospital, Leeds

Anthony Peel Consultant Surgeon (retired), University Hospital of North Tees, Stockton-on-Tees

Amar Rangan Consultant Orthopaedic Surgeon, James Cook University Hospital

Laurence Rosenberg Consultant Surgeon, University Hospital of North Tees, Stockton-on-Tees

Peter Royle Consultant Anaesthetist, University Hospital of North Tees, Stockton-on-Tees

Eileen Scott Research & Development Co-ordinator, University Hospital of North Tees, Stockton-on-Tees

Julian Scott Consultant Vascular Surgeon/Reader in Surgery, St James's University Hospital, Leeds

Rajesh Shah SpR in Cardiothoracic Surgery, The General Infirmary, Leeds

Andreas Skolarikos SpR in Urology, Freeman Hospital, Newcastle upon Tyne.

Abbreviations

AAA	abdominal aortic aneurysmectomy
ABC	airways, breathing, circulation
ABCDE	airways, breathing, circulation, disability, exposure (in trauma patients)
ABPI	ankle brachial-pressure index
ACE	angiotensin-converting enzyme
ACL	anterior cruciate ligament
ADH	antidiuretic hormone
ADR	adverse drug reaction
AKA	above-knee amputation
ALT	alanine aminotransferase
AMI	acute myocardial infarction
A/P	abdominoperineal
APACHE	Acute Physiology and Chronic Health Evaluation (severity of illness score)
APTT	activated partial thromboplastin time
ARDS	acute respiratory distress syndrome
ARF	acute renal failure
ASA	American Society of Anesthesiologists
ASB	assisted spontaneous breathing
ASEPSIS	Additional treatment, the presence of Serous discharge, Erythema, Purulent exudate, Separation of deep tissues, Isolation of bacteria, and the duration of inpatient Stay
AST	aspartate aminotransferase
ATIII	antithrombin III
ATN	acute tubular necrosis
AV	arteriovenous
BIPAP	biphasic positive airway pressure
BKA	below-knee amputation
BMI	body mass index
BP	blood pressure

BT	bleeding time
CAD	coronary artery disease
CARS	compensatory anti-inflammatory response syndrome
CBF	coronary blood flow
CCU	coronary care unit
CFV	common femoral vein
CHImp	Centre for Health Improvement
CI	cardiac index
CK-MB	creatine kinase membrane-bound
CMV	cytomegalovirus
CO	cardiac output
COAD	chronic obstructive airways disease
COPD	chronic obstructive pulmonary disease
CP	cerebellopontine
CPAP	continuous positive airway pressure
CRP	C-reactive protein
CSU	catheter-specimen urine
CT	computed tomography
CVC	central venous catheter
CVP	central venous pressure
Da	dalton
DIC	disseminated intravascular coagulation
DO_2	oxygen delivery
DTPA	diethylenetriaminepentaacetic acid
DVT	deep vein thromboses
EMRSA	epidemic methicillin-resistant *Staphylococcus aureus*
ERCP	endoscopic retrograde cholangiopancreatography
ES	endoscopic sphincterotomy
ESR	erythrocyte sedimentation rate
ESWL	extracorporeal shock-wave lithotripsy
ET	endotracheal
EVAR	endovascular aneurysm repair
FBC	full blood count
FES	fat embolism syndrome
FEV_1	forced expiratory volume in 1 second
FiO_2	fractional concentration of oxygen in inspired gas

FNAC	fine-needle aspiration cytology
FRC	functional residual capacity
FTSG	full-thickness skin graft
GMC	General Medical Council
GTN	glyceryl trinitrate
GvHD	graft versus host disease
HAS	human albumin solution
HBV	hepatitis B virus
HCV	hepatitis C virus
HDU	high-dependency unit
HES	hydroxyethyl starch
HIV	human immunodeficiency virus
HMO	health maintenance organization
HRT	hormone replacement therapy
IABP	intra-aortic balloon pump
iaDSA	intra-arterial digital subtraction angiography/arteriography
ICA	internal carotid artery
ICP	intracompartmental pressure
ICU	intensive care unit
IHD	ischaemic heart disease
IL	interleukin
IMA	inferior mesenteric artery
In	indium
INR	international normalized ratio
IPPV	intermittent positive-pressure ventilation
ITU	intensive therapy unit
IV	intravenous
IVC	inferior vena cava
ivDSA	intravenous digital subtraction angiography
IVU	intravenous urography
JVP	jugular vein pressure
kPa	kiloPascal
LFT	liver function tests
LMWH	low molecular-weight heparin
LSV	long saphenous vein
LV	left ventricle

MAOI	monoamine oxidase inhibitor
MH	malignant hyperthermia
MI	myocardial infarction
MODS	multiorgan dysfunction syndrome
MRCNS	multiply resistant, coagulase-negative staphylococcus
MRI	magnetic resonance imaging
MRSA	methicillin-resistant *Staphylococcus aureus*
MSA	multiple stab avulsions
MSOF	multiple system organ failure
MSU	midstream urine
NBM	nil by mouth
NICE	National Institute for Clinical Excellence
NSAID	non-steroidal anti-inflammatory drug
NSGC	non-seminomatous germ-cell
nvCJD	new variant Creutzfeldt–Jakob disease
NYHA	New York Heart Association
ODA	operating department assistant
PA	pulmonary artery
PaO_2	partial pressure of oxygen in arterial blood
$PaCO_2$	partial pressure of carbon dioxide in arterial blood
PAF	platelet activating factor
PAFC	pulmonary artery flotation catheter
PAWP	pulmonary arterial wedge pressure
PCA	patient-controlled analgesia
PCAS	patient-controlled analgesia system
PCNL	percutaneous nephrostolithotomy
PE	pulmonary embolism
PEEP	positive end-expiratory pressure
PEG	percutaneous endoscopic gastrostomy
PEJ	percutaneous endoscopic (transgastric) jejunostomy
PEM	protein-energy malnutrition
PIA	platelet impedance aggregation
PMN	polymorphonuclear neutrophil
PONV	postoperative nausea and vomiting
PPI	polyphosphoinositide
PPN	peripheral parenteral nutrition

PRN	*pro re nata* (i.e. when required)
PT	prothrombin time
PTA	percutaneous transluminal angioplasty
PTCA	percutaneous transluminal coronary recanalization
PTFE	polytetrafluoroethylene
PTP	post-transfusion purpura
PUJ	pelviureteric junction
PVD	peripheral vascular disease
PVR	pulmonary vascular resistance
RCOG	Royal College of Obstetricians and Gynaecologists
RCT	randomized controlled trial
REM	rapid eye movement
RIMA	reversible inhibitor of monoamine type A
RSD	reflex sympathetic dystrophy
RTI	respiratory tract infection
rtPA	recombinant tissue plasminogen activator
RSTL	relaxed skin tension lines
RV	right ventricle
SDD	selective decontamination of the digestive tract
SFJ	saphenofemoral junction
SHOT	Serious Hazards of Transfusion Scheme
SIA	subintimal angioplasty
SIMV	synchronized intermittent mandatory ventilation
SIRS	systemic inflammatory response syndrome
SLE	systemic lupus erythematosus
SMAS	superficial musculoaponeurotic system flaps
SNP	sodium nitroprusside
SPJ	saphenopopliteal junction
SSG	split-thickness skin graft
SSI	surgical site (wound) infection
SSV	short saphenous vein
SVR	systemic vascular resistance
TAA	thoracoabdominal aneurysms
Tc	technetium
TED	thromboembolic deterrent
TIA	transient ischaemic attack

TNF	tumour necrosis factor
TOS	thoracic outlet syndrome
TPA	tissue plasminogen activator
TPN	total parenteral nutrition
TRALI	transfusion-related acute lung injury
TRISS	Trauma and Injury Severity Score
TUR	transurethral resection
TURP	transurethral resection of the prostate
UFH	unfractionated heparin
UTI	urinary tract infection
VF	ventricular fibrillation
VGS	vein graft stenosis
VO_2	oxygen uptake (i.e. volume of oxygen utilization)
VQ	ventilation–perfusion scan
VRE	vancomycin-resistant enterococci
VSD	ventricular septal defect
VTE	venous thromboembolism

Part 1
General complications

Chapter 1
Infective complications of surgery in general

Postoperative pyrexia

Patients with a postoperative pyrexia will be seen on every ward round in general surgery; it is a common complication which should neither be ignored nor be treated blindly with antibiotics. The most likely cause is best considered by reference to a postoperative time-scale (see table below).

Likely causes of postoperative pyrexia

Days 1–3	Metabolic response to trauma
	Atelectasis
	Systemic or local inflammatory response
	Pre-existing disease
	SIRS or extensive local dissection/haematoma
	Drug reactions
	IV fluids (pyrogens; incompatibility)
	IV-line infection
	Instrumentation of urinary tract
	Endoscopy (ERCP)
Days 4–6	Spreading wound infection (*Strep. pyogenes*)
	Chest infection (early)
	Urinary infection
	IV-line (peripheral and central) infection
Days 7–10	Suppurative wound infection
	Chest infection
	Urinary infection (if catheter still in place)
	Deep venous thrombosis
	Deep abscess

ERCP, endoscopic retrograde cholangiopancreatography

Early (days 1–3)

As part of the metabolic response to trauma and inflammatory response, the release of cytokines, and other mediators, may cause a low-grade early pyrexia. Atelectasis is a more common cause of pyrexia, particularly when there is inadequate pulmonary effort related to pain or pre-existing disease. Atelectasis means there is an absence of gas in the lungs—examination may reveal poor basal air entry with retained secretion and dullness to percussion. Poor gas exchange may give hypoxia and poor saturation on oximetry.

Treatment is adequate physiotherapy with humidified oxygen to prevent secondary infection. Antibiotics are unnecessary.

Local inflammation related to extensive dissection or haematoma may add to the metabolic response. Systemic inflammation, expressed as SIRS (systemic inflammatory response syndrome), may relate to pre-existing disease. For example, a patient who had an appendicectomy for a gangrenous perforated appendix the day or night previously may well still have a temperature, although hopefully settling.

Drugs may cause a pyrexia, as may any IV fluids which are not pyrogen-free or are contaminated. Remember that blood or blood products may cause pyrexia and also need to be discontinued to avoid incompatibility complications.

Peripheral IV lines may also cause a local inflammatory reaction, particularly if the same line is being used 2–3 days after surgery. Central lines put in as an emergency for therapy or monitoring may also be a source of pyrexia. Treatment is removal or replacement and, in the case of central catheters, culture of the catheter tip and high-dose antibiotics.

Instrumentation or endoscopy of a viscus may cause a marked pyrexia relating to a transient bacteraemia. Cystoscopy in an infected urinary tract is an example. Persisting pyrexia should not be ignored—antibiotics alone may not be sufficient, particularly if there is a perforation.

Intermediate (days 4–6)

Spreading wound infection caused by β-haemolytic streptococci, or one of the synergistic gangrenous infections (or very rarely *Clostridium perfringens*) may be seen as early as this. There are often systemic signs of infection (hyperdynamic circulation and SIRS) as well as local signs of crepitus, cellulitis, or lymphangitis. In subdermal gangrene this may not be so obvious.

By this time specific chest infections (other than atelectasis) may be apparent. Patients with pre-existing pulmonary disease are most at risk: chronic bronchitis and emphysema, chronic obstruction pulmonary disease, reduced respiratory reserve, and of course smokers. Specific pathogens such as *Haemophilus influenzae* or *Streptococcus pneumoniae* may be the cause in pneumonias. Aerobic Gram-negative bacilli are usually the cause of pneumonias in surgical patients being ventilated on intensive care units (ITUs); after aspiration pneumonitis (patients with small-bowel intestinal obstruction are at risk unless decompressed by nasogastric aspiration) a 'soup' of organisms may be expected, but *Staphylococcus aureus* relates to lung abscess.

There are clinical features of inadequate ventilation and hypoxia with SIRS, together with cough and sputum (and occasionally haemoptysis). Chest X-ray may show diffuse changes (as in aspiration) or bilateral basal bronchopneumonia or a lobar pneumonia with a pleural effusion. Progression to empyema or lung abscess occurs later. Respiratory failure may supervene.

Treatment is urgent with humidified oxygen, physiotherapy, and monitoring. Although sputum (from expectoration or aspiration) needs to be sent for microbiology, the empirical use of antibiotics should be started early. If aspiration is possible, early bronchoscopy and lavage may be life-saving.

Urinary tract infections are common if a urinary catheter has been in place for more than a few hours, particularly in female patients. Catheter care is an important aspect of prevention. Symptomatic patients, once a catheter is removed, justify treatment with fluids and urinary antiseptics. Antibiotic therapy should be reserved for those patients who have a midstream urine/catheter-specimen urine (MSU/CSU) report which shows >10^5 bacteria/ml or a white cell count of >50 or red cell count (in the absence of surgery or trauma) of >100 cells/high-power field on microscopy. Culture and sensitivities may confirm that the empirical choice of antibiotic (e.g. trimethoprim) is justified or indicate that a change is needed if the clinical response is unsatisfactory. The treatment of sterile pyuria is controversial. The removal of a urinary catheter should be undertaken as soon as possible.

Later (days 7–10+)

Wound infections are more likely in this period and are of suppurative type. The commonest pathogen is *Staph. aureus* (clean surgery), but other offending organisms usually relate to contaminated surgery (e.g. the synergy of a coliform with *Bacteroides* spp. after colorectal surgery). The median time to presentation of this type of wound infection is 9 days, which is less likely to be associated with systemic signs (such as SIRS).

Deep-seated abscesses usually have a predisposing cause such as peritonitis or following an anastomotic leak. They are associated with the classical 'church spire' swinging temperature. These abscesses can be imaged using ultrasound, computed tomography (CT), magnetic resonance imaging (MRI), or occasionally isotope scans. Because such abscesses tend to 'point' they may be safely drained by interventional techniques.

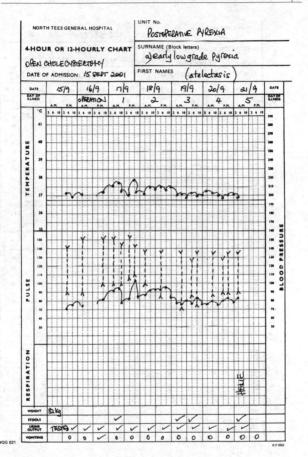

Postoperative patterns of pyrexia. (a) Early low-grade pyrexia (e.g. atelectasis).

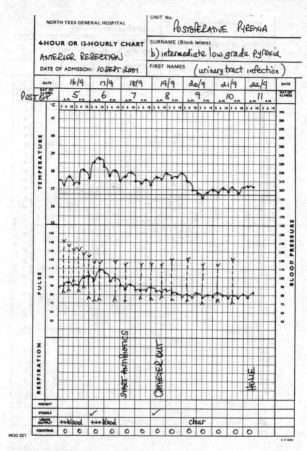

Postoperative patterns of pyrexia. (b) intermediate low-grade pyrexia (e.g. wound infection, UTI, RTI).

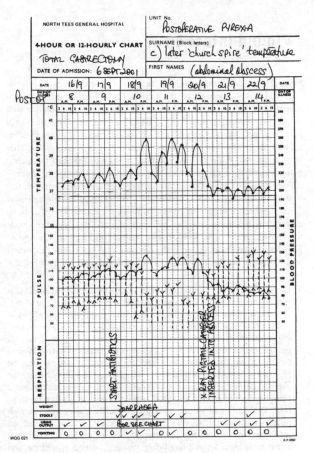

Postoperative patterns of pyrexia. (c) later 'church spire' temperature of abdominal abscess.

Wound infection

Wound infection is a common complication of surgery. With the increasing trend to day-case or short-stay surgical it is unusual to see it in hospital practice. Careful definition, assessed by a blinded trained observer with an adequate follow-up period (e.g. 6 weeks) is the only way to be sure of infection rates. The median time to a wound infection is 9 days: spreading cellulitis caused by β-haemolytic streptococci may be seen 3–4 days after surgery, whereas some staphylococcal infections may manifest themselves 5–6 weeks' postoperatively. Recognition and treatment of superficial surgical site (wound) infections (SSIs) is therefore transferred to primary healthcare, where recognition may be delayed and inappropriate treatment given (antibiotics instead of suture removal, for example). SSIs can be expensive to healthcare services—estimates of £100–1000 have been made for the treatment of a postoperative wound infection in the United Kingdom. Surveillance of wound infection rates is clearly important and the following definition and classification should be used for this purpose:

• **Definition of wound infection**—For audit purposes it is critical that wounds are assessed by a trained unbiased observer using adequate definitions. A wound infection may be described as the discharge of pus or fluid from which a pathogen can be cultured, sometimes with spreading erythema. A 30-day surveillance should be used for best accuracy, a period advocated by the American Centers for Disease Control. Wound infections are superficial SSIs. Intra-abdominal infections must be reported as deep SSIs. A minor wound infection should not delay the planned date of return home, but a major one may do so with systemic complications of pyrexia and SIRS (see later) and with wound disruption. The grading of wound infection is usually reserved for research purposes—a useful scheme being the ASEPSIS score based on Additional treatment, the presence of Serous discharge, Erythema, Purulent exudate, Separation of deep tissues, Isolation of bacteria, and the duration of inpatient Stay. The cause of infection can be related to the time of bacterial exposure—exogenous from an external source (e.g. poor theatre or ward disciplines) or endogenous from the patients' own flora (e.g. organisms from their own skin or bowel).

• **Classification of wound infection**—This was traditionally related to the theoretical risk of contamination (see Table: *Categories of wound infection*), although there is evidence to show that these classes do work. It has been estimated that contamination with 10^6 potential pathogens/gram of tissue is required to lead to a wound infection, but this is exponentially lower, as few as 100–1000 organisms, in the presence of ischaemia or foreign bodies (such as silk sutures or prosthetic grafts). Antibiotic prophylaxis is given empirically to cover the spectrum of anticipated organisms (e.g. flucloxacillin in clean prosthetic surgery against staphylococci; or cefuroxime and metronidazole in elective colonic surgery to cover aerobes such as *Escherichia coli* and anaerobes such as *Bacteroides* spp. in addition, of course, to effective bowel preparation).

Categories of wound contamination

Ia	Clean (e.g. hernia, varicose veins, breast)	Hollow viscus not opened No inflammatory process encountered
Ib	Clean prosthetic surgery (e.g. vascular grafts, joint prosthesis)	No break in aseptic ritual
II	Clean-contaminated (e.g. elective open cholecystectomy)	GIT, RT or UGT opened without significant spillage
III	Contaminated (e.g. appendicectomy or elective colorectal surgery)	Acute inflammation encountered without pus Gross spillage from an open viscus or major break in asepsis
IV	Dirty (e.g. abscess or faecal peritonitis)	Pus or perforated viscus encountered

GIT, gastrointestinal tract; RT, respiratory tract; UGT, urogenital tract.

Rational antibiotic prophylaxis has been associated with falls in wound infection from 20–30% to <10% in clean contaminated operations; 60% to 15–20% in contaminated surgery, and over 60% to <40% in dirty surgery. There is currently some controversy surrounding wound infection rates after non-prosthetic, clean-wound surgery, particularly for breast surgery, where rates of >15% have been reported when in-depth surveillance has been used. The use of prophylactic antibiotics is also controversial but the evidence of their value in clean, prosthetic surgery is not contested. In vascular graft surgery and orthopaedic joint surgery, infection rates should be less than 5% and 1%, respectively; antibiotic prophylaxis is extended for 24 hours in such surgery. However, there is no substitute for aseptic technique (together with ultraclean air in orthopaedics) as infection in these fields of surgery can be disastrous with high rates of mortality and morbidity and re-do surgery.

In dirty surgery, the rate of wound infection is so high with its attendant risks of superficial and deep wound disruption that a case for leaving the wound open can be made. Infection is thereby minimized and once there is a clean granulating wound it can be closed by delayed primary (within 5 days) or secondary closure. Antibiotic prophylaxis in such cases should be extended as treatment for 5 days. There are many other risk factors than contamination (see Table: *Risk factors for wound contamination*).

Risk factors for wound infection

Local	Operative technique (haematoma or roughly handled tissues)
	Thin devascularized skin flaps (local hypoxia)
	Inflammatory disease (without infection being present)
	Previous surgery (breast biopsy)
Systemic	Malnutrition
	Blood transfusion
	Age
	Immunosuppression of any cause
	Chemotherapy or radiotherapy
	Medical complications (diabetes, renal or liver failure, vascular disease)
	Shock of any cause (haemorrhagic, septic, myocardial)
	Cancer
	Remote infections
General factors	Long preoperative hospital stay
	Long operations
	Shaving (which ought to be immediately preop., if undertaken at all)
	Use of preoperative antiseptic showers
	Operating theatre and ward rituals

Management of wound abscess/infection

* Release pus, remove any retaining sutures, and ensure adequate drainage.
* Debride necrotic non-viable tissue; this may need several sessions, including general anaesthetic in the operating theatre.
* Antibiotic empirical therapy (or based on microbiological analyses) for associated cellulitis, lymphangitis, or systemic complications of sepsis or bacteraemia.
* Topical antimicrobials (such as povidone iodine—which is useful against methicillin-resistant *Staph. aureus* (MRSA)—or chlorhexidine).
* Keep wound moist with appropriate surgical dressings.
* In the presence of clean granulations consider grafting or secondary suture.

When taking pus from an infected wound, fresh specimens (large volumes of pus preferably in a sterile pot rather than on a swab) need to be sent for microbiological identification and sensitivities. Communication with a microbiologist gives the best results and the best choice of an antibiotic if needed.

Other wound infections that may need surgical intervention

Synergistic gangrene

This is caused by a mixed pattern of organisms and often a 'soup' is responsible—coliforms, staphylococci, *Bacteroides* spp, anaerobic strepto-cocci, and peptostreptococci have been implicated. It is more commonly seen in patients who are immunocompromised and even more unusual bacteria may be seen.

Risk factors for immunocompromisation and synergistic wound infection:

* malnutrition
* cancer
* diabetes
* anti-cancer therapies—chemo- and radiotherapy
* steroids and other drugs
* immunosuppressing diseases, e.g. acquired immunodeficiency deficiency syndrome (AIDS).

These infections can, in susceptible patients, follow even clean wound operations such as herniorrhaphy with several related eponyms—Meleney synergistic hospital gangrene (abdominal wall); Fourniér's gangrene (scrotum). This may be overlooked in the early stages as the infection is sub-dermal, but it is soon clear that the patient is profoundly unwell with SIRS and the risk of a multiple-organ dysfunction syndrome (MODS). There soon may be obvious non-viable changes in dermal tissues with severe pain; and crepitus may be felt or gas seen on imaging (X-ray or ultra-sound). Gas is not confined to *Clostridium perfringens* infection.

Therapy includes:

* IV fluids
* aggressive systemic organ support
* antibiotics
* early widespread debridement of non-viable tissue with laying open of wound
* hyperbaric oxygen (controversial)
* skin grafting once debrided areas are clean.

Clostridial gas gangrene

The spores of *Clostridium perfringens* are widely distributed, being present in soil and normal human faeces. Again, immunocompromised patients are more at risk and gas gangrene can follow surgery or a needlestick injury. Patients most susceptible are those with contaminated anaerobic tissues, particularly muscle, and those in whom foreign bodies are present. These are the typical conditions after military injuries, particularly high-velocity missile injuries where the kinetic energy ($0.5 \ mv^2$) is high and dissipates into widespread soft-tissue injury and cavitation. There is also a 'sucking' action at the entry wound which promotes the entry of foreign bodies such as clothing and soil. The exotoxins and proteases released by *Clostridia* spp. cause widely spreading gangrene with crepitus (and gas seen on X-ray) and severe septicaemia. Wide debridement is necessary with organ support, antibiotics, and hyperbaric oxygen.

Tetanus

This is a very rare complication of surgery. After implantation of spores there is a long prodromal period (a shorter period of a few days indicates a poor prognosis) while the neurotoxin is taken up by the anterior horn cells of the spinal cord. The local inflammation reaction at the implantation site or wound may be trivial or often resolved before the patient presents with painful spasms, respiratory failure, and aspiration pneumonia in the most severe form. Tracheostomy and prolonged paralysis and ventilation may be needed. The rarity of this infection may relate to the widely accepted programme of immunization with tetanus toxoid and, of course, the excellence of operating theatre environments.

'Superbugs'

The β-haemolytic organisms can cause rapidly spreading cellulitis and lymphangitis after surgery. Some carry superantigens and may relate to high mortality (referred to in 'outbreaks' a few years ago as the 'Gloucester flesh-eating virus'). They may be associated with the similar organism 'soups' seen in synergistic gangrene and need to be treated with the same aggression and urgency. Animal and human bites may result in these infections but they are rare after elective surgery.

MRSA was reported as being an important pathogen in 1961 and has since been implicated in several surgical ward epidemics. There are now epidemic strains (EMRSA). This epidemic potential is clearly a concern in surgery, particularly when a prosthesis has been implanted. MRSA is an opportunistic pathogen which colonizes theatre and ward environments as well as open wounds (such as chronic ulcers, pressure sores, and incised wounds which have broken down). It can be difficult to eradicate, and controversy over the need to attempt this escalates. In some hospitals, colonization may reach >40% of surgical patients and infection control can be a costly business. Containment involves ward and theatre closure, isolation of patients with full barrier nursing, identification of carriers, and the use of mupirocin and povidone iodine in all those so infected.

Multiply resistant, coagulase-negative staphylococcus (MRCNS) is another colonizing pathogen and the principal cause of infected intravascular devices, vascular grafts, and orthopaedic prostheses. Short preoperative stays reduce the risk of colonization before surgery. If antibiotic use is not controlled then the incidence of MRSA and MRCNS will increase with a corresponding decrease in the numbers of effective antibiotics. Vancomycin is still effective in treatment, although resistance is known, and there are new effective agents such as linezolid.

Clostridium difficile enteritis

Antibiotic-related colitis is common, but *Clostridium difficile* enteritis can be profound with blood loss and dehydration shock. Although the organism can be cultured from normal stools, the diagnosis is made by assay of toxin. The disease can be of epidemic proportions and is spread by poor ward hygiene. Older patients are particularly susceptible, and they may suffer relapses.

The antibiotics most commonly associated with the syndrome are broad-spectrum penicillins or cephalosporins, particularly when they are prolonged in use or changed over. Clindamycin had a particularly bad reputation but most antibiotics have been implicated. Treatment is usually effective using metronidazole or vancomycin with removal of existing antibiotic therapy.

Recognition follows suspicion and assay of the toxin. Sigmoidoscopy shows the classical pseudomembrane of fibrin and sloughed mucosa (hence its alternative name). There is a risk of perforation but colectomy is life-saving; however, aggressive IV replacement therapy is usually successful, although often needing high-dependency unit (HDU) monitoring and isolation barrier nursing.

Fungal infections

These can occur as complications of prolonged broad-spectrum antibiotic therapy, again particularly in immunosuppressed patients. Candida is a yeast that may result in infection of the gastrointestinal tract, mostly mouth and oesophagus, and respiratory tract. Rarely, there may be systemic candidiasis often related to intravascular catheter infection, which may require therapy with fluconazole or ketoconazole. Nystatin is only useful in managing oral thrush. The filamentous organisms of the *Aspergillus* genus, may be seen in patients who have prolonged stays on ITU; amphotericin is the antibiotic of choice.

Fungal infections are often missed or the diagnosis is delayed. The usual help can be gained by communication with a microbiologist when there is suspicion of a fungal infection, and appropriate recognition methods can be used.

Urinary tract infection

This, like wound infection, is a common and costly nosocomial complication. The risk factors for postoperative urinary infections are:

* presence of neoplasm
* urinary obstruction/urinary stasis
* presence of urinary catheter
* presence of urinary stent
* urinary calculi and other underlying disease.

The definition of a lower urinary tract infection (UTI) depends on symptoms (not present with a urethral catheter in place) of 'cystitis'—i.e. frequency, dysuria, haematuria. An MSU may show sterile pyuria but it needs a bacteriuria of 10^5 organisms/ml to be diagnostic. Lower numbers of bacteria may represent commensals. In the presence of significant UTI, bacteraemia may follow instrumentation and antibiotics should be given prophylactically and as treatment. Upper urinary tract infection can follow ascending infection or bacteraemia. It is more likely to present with high pyrexia (>30 °C) and rigors.

The organisms causing UTIs are mostly aerobic Gram-negative bacilli: principally *E. coli*, but also *Proteus* and *Pseudomonas* spp. (the latter can be an unwanted colonizing organism on urology wards and ITUs). Staphylococci may colonize the lower urinary tract when there is a catheter and *Candida* spp. may appear after prolonged catheterization, particularly after prolonged antibiotic use. Urinary tract infections are a common cause of postoperative pyrexia.

Treatment involves the use of large-volume fluid therapy to ensure an adequate diuresis and appropriate antibiotics, preferably chosen from the results of culture and sensitivities. Underlying obstructive and other disease should be attended to, with early removal of catheters and stents when possible (see also Chapter 19).

Respiratory tract infection

The alveolar–capillary interface, and ventilation–perfusion balance, is a delicate one. Postoperative respiratory tract infections can be anticipated in patients with restricted airways: where lung volumes are reduced but with a reasonable FEV_1 (fibrosing alveolitis, chest wall disease, after pneumonectomy and pneumoconiosis) (FEV_1, forced expiratory volume in 1 second); and in obstructive airways disease with a reduced FEV_1 of <70% (those with chronic bronchitis, smokers, and asthmatics). These patients can be accurately identified using spirometry—an FEV_1 of <1 litre is particularly poor. Arterial blood gases identify the 'pink puffer' with a low $PaCO_2$ and the 'blue bloater' with a high $PaCO_2$ (cor pulmonale and right ventricular failure). Preoperative physiotherapy and choice of the time for surgery when respiratory function is optimized may reduce postoperative respiratory tract infection. Cessation of smoking at least 4–6 weeks prior to surgery results in an improvement in respiratory function and less viscid bronchial secretions.

Atelectasis during the first 24–48 hours is recognized as poor basal air entry, dullness to percussion, and extra sounds. It is a common cause of early postoperative pyrexia and responds to good pain relief and physiotherapy. Chronic obstructive pulmonary disease may become acute, with an increase of pathogens such as *Haemophilus* spp. and pneumococci. Progression to bronchopneumonia can be prevented with physiotherapy and appropriate antibiotics. Aspiration leads to profound pneumonitis, which may progress to lobar pneumonia or lung abscess without bronchial lavage and respiratory support. Pneumonias involving aerobic Gram-negative bacilli are common after prolonged ventilation on ITU and are related to sepsis and MODS, including ARDS. Ventilation may be required if physiotherapy, antibiotics, and aids to breathing fail.

Postoperative peritonitis

Postoperative peritonitis may follow an anastomotic leak after oesophageal, rectal, colonic, pancreatic, or biliary surgery; or it may persist or follow inadequate source control at operation for community-acquired peritonitis (perforated peptic ulcer, pancreatitis, perforated appendix, gallbladder, or colonic pathology).

Postoperative ileus associated with peritonitis may be difficult to differentiate from obstruction during the early postoperative days. There is now evidence that not giving early enteral feeding leads to intestinal mucosal atrophy with colonization and translocation to mesenteric lymph nodes—thereby, through macrophage activation, acting as a 'motor' of sepsis. Certainly, attention should be given to nutrition whilst determining the cause of an ileus/obstruction and assessing whether re-laparotomy is necessary. Gastric ileus is treated with decompression. Enteral nutrition is provided by nasojejunal feeding or direct jejunal feeding by a jejunostomy, created at the primary operation.

Enteral feeding is always preferable to total intravenous parenteral nutrition which carries the risk of complications of insertion as well as a major risk of infection and further sepsis. Water, electrolyte, and acid–base balance can be usually managed using a peripheral IV line.

Signs of SIRS and MODS need to be monitored and early appropriate organ support instituted if necessary; in particular, signs of acute tubular necrosis associated with hypovolaemia, ARDS, and the need for cardiovascular support with fluids and inotropic support. (See below SIRS and MODS; complications of sepsis.)

Antibiotics need to be considered, but complications of resistance (MRSA, VRE (vancomycin-resistant enterococci), etc.), emergence (fungal infection, *Clostridium difficile* enteritis), toxicity, and allergy need to be taken into account. A second line of antibiotics, agreed by protocol, should be used to empirically cover the spectrum of likely organisms. This may either be monotherapy (using, for example, a carbapenem such as imipenem or meropenem) or combination therapy (such as tazobactam and metronidazole), but not with the same antibiotics used to treat the peritonitis that led to the first operation.

Second operations to exclude an abdominal cause of sepsis, such as a pelvic abscess or anastomotic leak, should be made on demand rather than on a routine 'second-look' basis. Although percutaneous drainage using imaging control may be appropriate, it cannot substitute for the need for peritoneal lavage or exteriorization of bowel ends after an anastomotic leak.

SIRS and MODS (complications of sepsis)

Many meanings have been ascribed to the term 'sepsis'. Now, it should not be used as an expression of infection, but should specifically relate to a systemic response (which may be triggered by infection). Similarly, terms such as 'Gram-negative sepsis', 'septic shock', and 'multiple organ failure' can be confusing. In 1992 the American College of Chest Physicians and the Society of Critical Care Medicine defined 'systemic inflammatory response syndrome (SIRS)', 'sepsis', and 'sepsis syndrome' (or severe sepsis). These definitions are surviving the test of time and need to be learnt (see the table below).

Systemic inflammatory response syndrome (SIRS)

Pyrexia (>38 °C) or hypothermia (<36 °C)
Tachycardia (>90 beats/min in absence of β-adrenergic blockade)
Tachypnoea (>20 breaths/min)
Raised WBC count (>12×10⁹/l) or low WBC (<4×10⁹/l)
Any two of the above 4 criteria confirms SIRS
Sepsis
SIRS with a documented focus of infection (can be of chest, wound, peritoneal, urinary, etc. origin)
Sepsis syndrome (or severe sepsis)
Sepsis with evidence of organ failure

SIRS may be regarded as an excessive systemic or hyperinflammatory response associated with vasodilatation and capillary leakage. It is a complex response to injury or infection and there are compensatory regulatory mechanisms which if interfered with may worsen SIRS. This feedback mechanism has been termed 'compensatory anti-inflammatory response syndrome' (CARS). Unchecked systemic inflammation may progress to multiple organ dysfunction syndrome (MODS) and multiple organ failure.

Initiation of SIRS and MODS

Several sources which can lead to these syndromes are initiated and promoted by a complex pattern of mediators (see the following table).

A simple mnemonic is to consider the 'Is', with some examples:

* **injury**—multiple trauma or extensive burns;
* **inflammation**—severe acute pancreatitis;

Initiating 'Is' of SIRS and MODS

INJURY
INFLAMMATION
INFECTION
ISCHAEMIA
Iatrogenic
Intoxication
Immune
Idiopathic

* **infection**—faecal peritonitis; and
* **ischaemia**—following shock of any cause or tissue ischaemia–reperfusion.

Less important (in surgery) are iatrogenic, intoxication, immune, and idio-pathic causes.

Infection is the most important cause in general surgical practice and may involve Gram-negative organisms (principally *E. coli* and its lipopolysaccharide endotoxin which stimulates macrophages to release mediators); but superantigens related to *Staph. aureus*, and the fungi are also important organisms (see figure below).

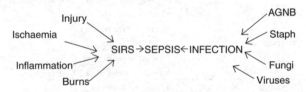

Initiating factors in sepsis.

Although non-infectious causes exist (e.g. multiple trauma or acute pancreatitis), blood cultures should always be at least considered in the investigation of patients with SIRS and MODS; specific antibody therapy may then be started if cultures are positive.

The mediators involved in SIRS (see following table) lead to the activation of complement with stimulation of macrophages and polymorphonuclear neutrophils (PMNs). Activated PMNs are involved in systemic inflammation and their interaction with endothelium leads to changes in coagulation with the release of platelet activating factor (PAF). Increased margination and white cell diapedesis can be measured as the expression of adherence molecules (selectins and integrins). PMNs release oxygen free radicals (superoxide O_2^-, hydrogen peroxide H_2O_2, and hydroxyl radicals OH^-) with proteases, and together with other molecules (when in excess) go beyond physiological protective mechanisms and lead to tissue damage.

With macrophages there is release of proinflammatory cytokines (principally interleukin-6 (IL-6), tumour necrosis factor (TNF), and IL-1), prostaglandins from the arachidonic acid cascade, leukotrienes through eicosopentanoic acid, the potent vasodilator nitric oxide, kinins, and histamine. Lymphocytes are also involved and there may be anergy. In untreated SIRS, CARS and other compensatory feedback mechanisms may be overwhelmed leading to organ failure.

Mediators involved in SIRS and MODS

Cytokines	Complement
Nitric oxide	Proteases
Prostaglandins	Kinins
Leukotrienes	Histamine
Platelet activating factor (PAF)	Oxygen free radicals

Definition of MODS (see table below)

Definitions of multiple organ dysfunction

Pulmonary	ARDS	PaO_2 <9.3 kPa
		PaO_2/FiO_2 <30
		(↓compliance, ↑PEEP, CXR appearance)
Renal	ATN	<120 ml urine/4 h
		(↑urea, creatinine, K^+)
Cardiovascular		lactate >1.2 mmol/l
		SVR <800 dynes/s/cm³
		(cardiac depression, ↓CO, arrhythmias)
Coagulation	DIC	↓platelets↑D-dimers
		(bleeding tendency)
Central nervous system		GCS <15 (in absence of head injury)
Hepatic		(↑bilirubin, AST, ↓albumin)
Intestinal		(stress ulceration, ileus)

NB (brackets indicate associated but non-definitive variables).
ARDS, acute respiratory distress syndrome; PEEP, positive end-expiratory pressure; CXR, chest X-ray; ATN, acute tubular necrosis; SVR, systemic vascular resistance; DIC, disseminated intravascular coagulation; GCS, Glasgow Coma Score; AST, aspartate aminotransferase.

Organ failure follows SIRS and several organs are involved. Various scoring systems have been devised to recognize early organ dysfunction; some are based on trauma (TRISS, Trauma and Injury Severity Score), others on physiological variables (APACHE, Acute Physiology and Chronic Health

Evaluation (severity of illness score)) or the extent of organ failure (Goris). They may be an adjuvant to therapy, and sequential scoring may anticipate the need for surgery or higher planes of monitoring or therapy (HDU and ITU).

Management of SIRS and MODS

Anticipate/predict complications
Resuscitate (fluids and oxygen)
Investigate
Remove precipitating cause
Treat with antibiotics (based on empirical therapy)
Give nutritional support

Management of SIRS and MODS (see following table)

SIRS and MODS are more likely in some presenting surgical illnesses and after specific types of surgery; they can be anticipated and avoided or, at the earliest sign, recognized and prevented quickly. Resuscitation is based on ABCDE (airway, breathing, circulation, disability, exposure (in trauma patients)), but a rapid response to high-flow oxygen (the rebreathing Hudson mask can give an FiO_2 of 60%) and a colloid or crystalloid (not 5% dextrose) fluid challenge should be given. Systems' scoring may be helpful and encouraging. Once organ failure is established (APACHE >20, Goris 2+ systems failure) mortality can reach 80–100%. Inotropes may be considered once the fluid deficit is corrected (based on pulse, BP, CVP, urine output, and markers of cardiopulmonary performance such as blood gases, oximetry, and Swan–Ganz or transoesophageal-measured cardiac variables). Fluid and oxygen therapy is as important in early hyperdynamic circulatory states, when oxygen consumption (VO_2) is high and oxygen delivery (DO_2) falls behind. The development of late 'cold' hypotensive shock is an ominous sign of myocardial and peripheral circulatory failure.

Investigation needs to identify the cause, particularly a focus of infection. Interventional radiology now has an important role; not only can collections of pus be accurately imaged (using ultrasound, CT, radionuclide scans, and MRI), but guided drainage is successful and may avoid the need for surgery. Occasionally, surgery is necessary for the evacuation of pus and has a place in excluding ischaemia, particularly in second-look operations or when there is an abdominal compartment syndrome (which may need bowel exteriorization—resection, or laparostomy). Catheter-related sepsis (central venous catheters (CVCs) and urinary catheters) usually require removal of the catheter before sepsis can be controlled.

Antibiotics are given on an empirical basis. This can involve combination chemotherapy or monotherapy to cover the likely organisms. Most hospital trusts and ITUs have strict protocols for antibiotic use. As an example, first-line combination antibiotic therapy for faecal peritonitis following a perforated sigmoid diverticulum should cover aerobes and anaerobes (a wide-spectrum penicillin or second- or third-generation cephalosporin together with an imidazole, such as metronidazole, would suffice); whereas for a nosocomial infection, for example a postoperative pneumonia, a second-line monotherapy drug might be used (such as a carbapenem, like meropenem or imipenem, or a quinolone, like ciprofloxacin). Samples should always be sent for microbiological culture whenever possible (blood, sputum, urine, pus) and sensitivities may justify a change in antibiotic therapy if the clinical response is unsatisfactory.

Specific treatments involving monoclonal antibodies to endotoxin or cytokines such as TNF have been disappointing. The cause of sepsis may initially be unclear, and interference with the complex septic process may upset the feedback mechanisms of SIRS and CARS. Nevertheless, the search to modulate mediators continues.

Respiratory compromise in sepsis

The most common cause of poor conscious levels in postoperative surgical patients relates to cardiopulmonary performance. Respiratory failure may be of type I (when there is failure of oxygen uptake) or type II (when, in addition, there is failure of carbon dioxide removal). Blood gas levels in failure include a PaO_2 of <8 kPa and a $PaCO_2$ >7 kPa; oxygen levels in this low range relate to the steep part of the dissociation curve when saturation can rapidly fall under 90%. There may be pre-existing COPD in a surgical patient with airflow obstruction, but in septic conditions there may be an acute fall in functional residual capacity (FRC) (e.g. in pneumonia) or increased pulmonary vascular dysfunction (e.g. in ARDS).

ARDS is recognized when the PaO_2/FiO_2 ratio is <30 and the PaO_2 falls under 9.3 kPa. The high FiO_2 (0.6) of a rebreathing mask may be inadequate and as compliance falls there is a need for CPAP or ventilation with increasing PEEP.

Cardiovascular compromise in sepsis

In sepsis there is a need for oxygen supplementation and assurance of adequate fluid intake before inotropes are considered. The fluid loss to the 'third space' may be large in septic states. Myocardial depression may occur with arrhythmias; but when cardiac preload and myocardial performance have been corrected, a fall in systemic vascular resistance (SVR <800 dynes/s per cm³) may need inotrope support. Dobutamine can improve myocardial contractility and heart rate by stimulating β_1-adrenergic receptors, but if there is hypotension this may be worsened (through β_2-adrenergic receptor stimulation, although there is some α-adrenergic receptor effect). Dopamine is similar, but is not as effective. The use of small 'renal' doses of dopamine is controversial. Noradrenaline (norepinephrine) is an effective α-adrenoreceptor stimulant and raises SVR but with some degree of renal vessel constriction. The titration of optimal fluid input, myocardial support, and inotropes may be complex. Pulmonary artery catheter measurements are used to measure cardiac pressures and aid in the measurement of preload and afterload and myocardial performance—particularly in sepsis and MODS, ARDS, and monitoring of inotropes (see the following table). Transoesophageal Duplex Doppler ultrasound scanning can less invasively measure many of these variables.

Measurements that are possible with pulmonary artery catheters

---

Determination of cardiac output (stroke volume, stroke index)

Systemic and pulmonary vascular resistance (SVR and PVR)

Oxygen delivery and uptake (DO_2 and VO_2)

Left ventricular stroke mark index

Renal compromise in sepsis

Loss of fluid to third-space compartments must also be corrected for optimal renal function. If, despite this and with the appropriate cardiopulmonary support, there is evidence of renal failure (oliguria, rising potassium concentration, rising urea and creatinine levels with sodium and water overload) renal replacement therapy may be required. Peritoneal dialysis is rarely appropriate and haemofiltration or dialysis is required.

The acid-base balance will also need to be addressed. In sepsis, there may be a renal failure to excrete hydrogen ions, and a respiratory compromise (e.g. ARDS) when there is a failure to remove CO_2. In sepsis, there is also an added metabolic acidosis.

Gastrointestinal compromise in sepsis

In sepsis, many gastrointestinal protective mechanisms are lost. With starvation and increased metabolic rate there is a rapid atrophy of enterocyte function with falls in IgG in gastric mucus and gut-associated lymphoid tissue function. This may be severe in shock states, particularly after ischaemia–perfusion injury. In jaundice, there is also a loss of protective enteral bile salts.

The normally sterile upper gastrointestinal tract becomes colonized, principally with aerobic Gram-negative bacilli in sepsis, and in conditions where there is a risk of sepsis development, such as multiply injured patients being ventilated on ITU. There is translocation of bacteria to the mesenteric lymph nodes, and following macrophage stimulation the release of proinflammatory cytokines and other mediators which cause sepsis add to the development of ileus. The colonization of the gut has been termed the 'motor' of sepsis and multiple organ failure. Translocation and sepsis has been convincingly proven in animal models but is clinically controversial. Nevertheless, efforts to selectively decontaminate the digestive tract (SDD) have been made using topical, poorly absorbed, antimicrobials (amphotericin B, tobramycin, polymyxin E) with parenteral cephalosporins to reduce nosocomial infections on ITU, particularly pneumonia. The effect on mortality is less clear. Other methods to decontaminate the GI tract, including the use of probiotic bacteria and early enteral nutrition with novel diets (containing nucleic acids, arginine, and polyunsaturated fatty acids), are promising.

The stomach is at risk of acute stress gastritis in sepsis. The use of antacids (proton-pump inhibitors or H_2-receptor antagonists) reduces gastric acidity and further increases the risks of gastrointestinal colonization. Cytoprotective agents such as sucralfate are an alternative.

Chapter 2
Venous thromboembolism (deep vein thrombosis and pulmonary embolus)

Deep vein thrombosis

Thrombus formation in the deep venous system involves endothelial damage with the exposure of collagen and activation of the intrinsic and extrinsic clotting cascades. The resulting layering of the platelets and fibrin forms a mesh that traps more platelets and both red and white blood cells. Possible outcomes include:

* resolution with a complete return to normal;
* organization (healing by granulation tissue and scarring) and loss of valves leading to venous hypertension and loss of calf muscle pump;
* major vein obstruction, e.g. of the ileofemoral segment with phlegmasia alba dolens (painful white leg) or phlegmasia caerulia dolens (dusky red leg);
* postphlebitic syndrome with oedema, secondary varicose veins, haemosiderosis, venous eczema, venous ulceration.

Of the possible outcomes, pulmonary embolism (PE) is the most serious. It may be multiple in the postoperative period and a massive fatal pulmonary embolus is often preceded by smaller emboli that may go unrecognized. It is the tragedy of unexpected death—particularly in young, fitter patients—and the recognition of the frequency of the problem that has led to doctors appreciating the importance of identifying risk factors, implementing effective prophylaxis according to careful protocols, and identifying effective mechanisms for diagnosis and treatment when deep vein thrombosis, and particularly pulmonary embolism, occurs. Repeated small pulmonary emboli may lead to pulmonary complications such as pulmonary hypertension.

Aetiology

With regard to the aetiology of venous thrombus it is essential to remember the time-honoured Virchow's triad:

* endothelial damage;
* reduced venous flow rate through the deep veins; and
* increased coagulability of the blood.

Risk factors

These are many, and may be grouped according to those that are relatively frequent and widely applicable and those that are often specific but less common.

* *Frequent and widely applicable risk factors:*
  (1) elderly patients;

(2) type and duration of surgery, e.g. major pelvic surgery;
(3) immobility, particularly preoperative;
(4) malignancy, particularly involving the abdomen and pelvis;
(5) previous deep vein thrombosis (DVT);
(6) obesity.

+ *Significant specific factors which are sometimes less applicable:*
    (1) disorders of coagulability: thrombocytopenia, altered coagulation cascade affecting antithrombin-3, lupus anticoagulant factor, heparin cofactor, protein C, α_2-macroglobulin, protein S, α_1-antitrypsin, and activated protein C—abnormalities and defects in fibrinolysis are also significant;
    (2) sedentary occupation, pregnancy and the puerperium, general or local injury, bed rest, varicose veins, cardiac failure, arterial ischaemia, medications, including the oral contraceptive.

Note: smoking is not a risk factor.

Risk factors may be classified into:

+ **High risk**—elderly patients undergoing major pelvic surgery for malignancy or hip surgery. Immobility and obesity are cofactors which may enhance the risk. Previous DVT or PE is a particularly high risk factor.
+ **Medium risk**—involves major operations, particularly of long duration.
+ **Low risk**—young patients undergoing a short operation, e.g. herniorrhaphy.

Site of thrombus

A thrombus may frequently affect the sinusoids and deep veins of the calf, and if confined has a low risk for breaking off proximally. The ileofemoral segment and tributaries of the internal iliac vein may also be affected, with a higher risk of pulmonary embolus.

Diagnosis

Diagnosis is unfortunately imprecise. When there is inflammation around the thrombus then the patient may complain of tenderness in the calf, particularly on walking, and examination may reveal oedema of the dorsum of the foot and ankle, together with local tenderness in the calf and a positive Homans' sign (pain on extension of the ankle following stretching of the soleus muscle, the sinusoids of which are affected by the thrombotic process). The dramatic appearance of phlegmasia caerulia dolens is rarely forgotten. This is an intensively painful, congested lower limb associated with an extensive ileofemoral DVT, where the periphery is not only oedematous but dusky (phlegmasia alba dolens is where there is impairment of the arterial supply in addition to the venous thrombosis). A grumbling temperature of 37.5–38 °C, classically around the 6th to 8th day, may be the only sign of a DVT.

Diagnostic tests

These include:

* **Bipedal ascending contrast venography**. This is accurate but invasive and uncomfortable for the patient, and time-consuming with regard to radiological time.

* **Duplex Doppler venous imaging with B-mode ultrasound**. This has the advantage of being non-invasive, widely applicable, but is slightly less accurate in the diagnosis of calf deep vein thrombosis compared to ascending contrast venography. It is almost 100% accurate above the knee. The criteria for diagnosis being when a vein is not compressible it is considered to contain thrombus. If there is doubt, duplex Doppler imaging should be repeated in 2–3 days or ascending contrast venography should be carried out.

* **Isotope venography**. This is a simple test, but is less accurate than the above.

* **[125I]fibrinogen-uptake test**. This is a very sensitive test but has largely been abandoned because of the risk of human immunodeficiency virus (HIV) contamination of pooled blood products.

* **Plethysmography**. This has low accuracy for non-occlusive thrombus and is cumbersome and not widely applicable.

* **Thermography**. This is too insensitive and non-specific.

Prevention

First, and foremost, the operating surgeon should be aware of the risk factors so that any of them can be minimized whenever possible before elective surgery, although this is obviously not applicable in the emergency situation. Prophylaxis involves either mechanical methods or anticoagulant therapy, or a combination of both.

Mechanical methods

* Graduated, TED (thromboembolic deterrent) compression stockings are widely used; these are usually worn below the knee, unless there are obvious long saphenous varicose veins. It is important to be wary of the use of these stockings in patients with peripheral vascular disease (PVD) and they are contraindicated when PVD is severe as it may risk peripheral ischaemia or infarction.

* Intermittent pneumatic compression using single or multichamber devices is effective and is used intraoperatively. It is more cumbersome, but may be used in combination with the graduated stockings.

* Simple elevation of the heel on a foam sponge prevents sustained pressure on the calf and is a common-sense precaution. It should not be excessive; otherwise this leads to hyperextension of the knee joint and if a muscle relaxant is given this can cause postoperative discomfort.

* Electrical stimulation is now rarely, if ever, used.

The combination of all these methods, except electrical stimulation, is quite frequently used and there is evidence that the use of pneumatic devices, combined with graduated elastic compression stockings, is synergistic.

Anticoagulant methods

Anticoagulation used for prophylaxis is partial, since full anticoagulation, using warfarin or full-dose heparin, may be effective but the incidence of bleeding complications is unacceptably high. Low-dose unfractionated subcutaneous heparin, either the calcium or sodium salts of heparin, may be given preoperatively and then twice daily subcutaneously in a dose 5000 units.

Low molecular-weight fractionated heparin (LMWH) is becoming an increasingly favoured method since it can be given once daily, thus reducing the number of injections, discomfort for the patient, and nursing time, and has been shown to be at least, if not more, effective than unfractionated heparin. The initial dose should be given 2 hours before surgery, at a dose of 2500–5000 units daily depending on risk (and type of LMWH preparation). This regimen is of proven value in the prophylaxis of pulmonary embolism after hip surgery (LMWH administration may be prolonged in such cases) and it can be combined with the mechanical methods described above. Heparin is usually stopped when the patient is mobile enough to go home.

Other methods

• Dextran 70—now rarely used.
• Antiplatelet agents—these are unproven for DVT prophylaxis.

Outcome of effective prevention

Unfortunately, even with effective, correctly administered prophylaxis, up to 20% of all patients still develop deep vein thrombosis and up to 0.2% may have a fatal pulmonary embolus. The great benefit of effective prophylaxis is the reduction in mortality from pulmonary embolus.

It should not be forgotten that patients remain at risk, often after discharge from hospital, and therefore prophylactic measures can be continued at home for several weeks—easily achieved with graduated stockings. With the advent of low molecular weight heparin a once-daily dose for those patients who are at high risk should certainly be considered, particularly after total hip replacement.

Treatment of a deep vein thrombosis

Although confirmatory evidence of a diagnosis of deep vein thrombosis can often be achieved by duplex Doppler or venography, it may on occasions be necessary to treat on the basis of suspicion.

1. **Heparin treatment**—until recently sodium heparin was administered intravenously at a dose of 70 U/kg (this is usually between 5000 and 10 000 units), followed by an infusion of 20–30 U/kg per hour (1000–2000 units/hour). The dosage is monitored by measuring the

activated partial thromboplastin time (APTT), but this should only serve as a guideline since its accuracy and relevance has been questioned. Heparin levels can be accurately measured if necessary.

2. **Subcutaneous low molecular-weight heparin**—usually given subcutaneously once daily for a week at a dose of approximately 170 U/kg rounded to the nearest 1000 units, e.g. for a 70-kg subject, 12 000 units would be administered (a volume of 0.6 ml). Check with local protocols and which LMWH is being used.

3. **Warfarin therapy**—is usually started after 24–48 hours of heparin therapy, providing there is no surgical contraindication. The loading dose is usually 10 mg, followed by 5 mg on the second and third day; thereafter, the dose is adjusted accordingly to the international normalized ratio (INR), which is kept at 2.0–2.5. It is important to remember that a large number of other medications, particularly antibiotics, interfere with vitamin K and hence may affect the INR. The duration of warfarin treatment is usually between 3 and 6 months according to the risk factors.

Management of acute extensive venous thrombosis

* Fibrinolytic agents, including streptokinase, urokinase, and tissue plasminogen activator have been used selectively in patients with recent venous thrombosis to good effect.

* Surgical thrombectomy for distal thrombus is not recommended. However, in the rarer case of phlegmasia caerulia dolens the ileofemoral thrombus may be removed using a Fogarty catheter passed in an antegrade fashion via the femoral vein. Thrombus can be squeezed from the leg by compression of the calf with an Esmark elastic bandage. Re-thrombosis is prevented by full anticoagulation postoperatively, although arterial shunting has been used to prevent thrombosis.

* The risk of embolism is considerable and prophylactic measures for this are presented later.

* The risk of valve damage and the development of the postphlebitic syndrome has to be considered.

Pulmonary embolus

An embolus is an abnormal mass of undissolved material in the circulatory system which is transported through the system until it enters a vessel where it causes obstruction. In the case of pulmonary embolus this is usually a thrombus from the ileofemoral segment or deep veins of the calf which travels towards the heart, passing through the chambers of the heart and entering the pulmonary circulation where it causes obstruction of the pulmonary vasculature, depending on its size (with appropriate clinical consequences from no signs or symptoms to sudden death).

Pulmonary embolus is both over- and underdiagnosed and is easily missed in patients with cardiorespiratory disease, the elderly, and patients presenting with unexpected dyspnoea.

- 10% of all hospital deaths are due to pulmonary embolism.
- 33% of patients with a clinically suspected pulmonary embolus have diagnostic pulmonary angiography, the remaining two-thirds have no evidence of pulmonary embolism.
- The natural history of pulmonary embolus is imprecise, but it is estimated that approximately 30% of untreated patients with a PE will die.

Risk factors

Include:

- surgery, particularly orthopaedic lower limb joint-replacement surgery or pelvic surgery
- trauma or burns
- malignancy
- immobility
- paralysis of the legs
- pregnancy or the puerperium
- old age
- cardiac failure
- inflammatory bowel disease
- nephrotic syndrome.

Diagnosis

The clinical symptoms and signs are non-specific. The patient may complain of tenderness in the calf with swelling, associated with episodes of breathlessness, pleuritic pain, and occasionally a small haemoptysis.

- The absence of the key features of dyspnoea, tachypnoea, and pleuritic chest pain render the diagnosis highly unlikely (less than 3%).

- 98% of emboli originate from thrombi in the leg and pelvic veins.
- In patients with a proven diagnosis, a major predisposing risk factor may be found in 80–90%.
- Diagnosis is often made at postmortem.

Investigations

The useful tests following clinical examination include an ECG and a chest X-ray, both of which may show features to strengthen the diagnosis. The latter is often portable but may be of help particularly in excluding other pathologies. Measurement of blood gases should also be done, but it is important to recognize that a normal PaO_2 does not exclude pulmonary embolus. The investigation plan depends on whether the patient is stable or unstable.

The stable patient

In the stable patient, the ventilation–perfusion (VQ) scan is a pivotal test and must be performed urgently, preferably within 4–6 hours. The perfusion phase being the most important (with regard to the ventilation phase, ^{81}Kr-/$^{99}Tc^m$-labelled DTPA (diethylenetriaminepentaacetic acid) aerosols are better than ^{133}Xe-labelled ones). Results of the VQ scan are often (70%) reported as intermediate, representing a 16–60% risk of pulmonary embolus; therefore one must also take into account the clinical findings.

Duplex Doppler ultrasound of the leg veins is increasingly valuable since 90% of emboli actually arise from the leg veins.

Contrast venography is both invasive and uncomfortable, and 30% of patients with angiographically proven pulmonary emboli have a normal venogram.

Plethysmography is accurate for proximal deep vein thrombosis when causing obstruction, but tests miss 40% of thrombi in asymptomatic patients with proven pulmonary emboli, particularly where the deep vein thrombosis is distal. This poses a clinical question—is the patient likely to have another embolus? The answer if the above tests are positive is in the affirmative, but if both the VQ scan and the Doppler ultrasound of the leg veins are negative, and the clinical suspicion is high, then the question cannot be answered without performing a pulmonary angiogram.

Haemodynamically unstable patient

The key test here is the echocardiogram for the patient who collapses with hypotension. It shows well-defined abnormalities with a large central pulmonary embolus and also excludes, in the differential diagnosis, aortic dissection, ventricular septal rupture, and cardiac tamponade.

Where there is doubt either a pulmonary angiogram or spiral CT should be performed as an emergency, particularly if the facility and possibility for embolectomy is to be considered. The latter is very sensitive for proximal emboli down to the size of segmental arteries.

The likelihood of pulmonary emboli

This should be estimated by the clinician before the VQ scan is undertaken.

1. Group A—high clinical probability (80–100%):
   - more than one predisposing factor;
   - appropriate symptoms and signs without other cardiorespiratory diseases (the symptoms and signs including dyspnoea, tachypnoea, pleuritic pain, haemoptysis, shock, and syncope).

2. Group B—low probability (0–19%):
   - the absence of risk factors and the presence of other disease that accounts for symptoms and signs.

3. Group C—intermediate probability (20–79%):
   - the patient does not fall into either of the above two categories;
   - a lung VQ scan in this group enables classification on the basis of the presence or absence of segmental perfusion defects.

VQ scan findings

- *High probability of pulmonary embolism shown by:*
   (i) two or more large (>75%) segmental perfusion defects without corresponding ventilation abnormalities;
   (ii) one large and two moderate (25%) segmental perfusion defects;
   (iii) four or more moderate segmental perfusion defects.

- *Intermediate probability of pulmonary embolism, shown by:*
   (i) one moderate or less than two large segmental perfusion defects without corresponding abnormalities in ventilation or on chest radiograph;
   (ii) corresponding ventilation–perfusion defects and radiographic parenchymal monoplasty in the lower lung zone;
   (iii) single, moderate-match, ventilation–perfusion defects with normal findings on chest radiography;
   (iv) corresponding ventilation–perfusion defects and small pleural effusion.

- *Low probability of pulmonary embolism, shown by:*
   (i) multiple-match, ventilation–perfusion defects regardless of size with normal findings on chest radiograph;
   (ii) corresponding ventilation–perfusion defects with radiographic parenchymal opacity in upper or middle lung zone;
   (iii) corresponding ventilation–perfusion defects and a large pleural effusion;
   (iv) any perfusion defects with a substantially larger abnormality on chest radiograph;
   (v) more than three (<25%) segmental perfusion defects with normal results on chest radiograph.

Management options for suspected pulmonary embolism

- Patients with normal or very low probability scans should not be treated.
- Patients with high probability lung scan must be treated.
- Patients with non-diagnostic scans should be treated according to whether or not they have cardiorespiratory disease.

Patients without cardiorespiratory disease

If the patients are not treated 14% will be at risk of a further thromboembolic event. Mortality in this group in unknown. Assess the odds. Balance the risk of treatment against the risk of recurrent embolism. Patients with a high or intermediate clinical suspicion have a 16–66% probability of an underlying embolus and a 14% risk of recurrence. Anticoagulant treatment is associated with a mortality rate of 0.1%. (The use of duplex Doppler ultrasound can refine this and treatment should be instituted if the ultrasound is positive.)

Patients with cardiorespiratory disease

Attach equal importance to low and intermediate scan reports. The mortality of untreated patients will be in excess of 8.5%, therefore these scan reports should be a low threshold for initiating anticoagulation in this group.

Treatment

The standard treatment has been anticoagulation with heparin followed by warfarin. Intravenous sodium salts of unfractionated heparin was the standard method of treatment, which has the disadvantage of limiting the patient's mobility because of the infusion pump. Probably more appropriate to those patients with a minor embolism, and for reducing the risk of major haemorrhage, is the use of subcutaneous LMWH. Additionally, patients can be taught to administer LMWH at home, with clear economic advantages in terms of reducing the nursing time in hospital and also the stay in hospital while waiting for the INR to reach satisfactory levels.

Acute massive embolism may be associated with significant pulmonary artery occlusion. Emergency embolectomy can save the patient's life in these circumstances, whereas with small emboli, anticoagulation or fibrinolytic treatment alone may be as effective.

The concern that early ambulation may dislodge thrombi in the lower extremities has often led physicians to restrict patients to bed, but progressive ambulation is desirable in those with less extensive embolism.

The place of follow-up VQ scans

It must be remembered that 16% of patients fail to achieve 90% resolution of the perfusion scan and 28% of patients with existing cardiopulmonary disease fail to show complete resolution. These points are important in the interpretation of follow-up VQ scans. Resolution can occur up to 3 months. There is a considerable body of opinion that suggests that follow-up VQ scans are not cost-effective. Similarly, follow-up, non-invasive leg tests, such as duplex Doppler ultrasound or impedance plethysmography are not considered cost-effective.

Inferior vena cava filters

These have a role when:

* anticoagulants are contraindicated in a patient with a massive or multiple pulmonary emboli;
* pulmonary emboli have recurred whilst a patient is receiving adequate effective anticoagulant therapy;
* the pulmonary embolus is severe in a patient with right ventricular failure and hypertension and the occurrence of a pulmonary embolus might be fatal.

The insertion of an inferior vena cava filter may be life-saving. However, their value is debatable in patients who have multiple emboli and where there is a continuing predisposition, since the filters themselves, although now much improved, are not without complications.

The role of thrombolysis

Open pulmonary embolectomy and catheter-tip embolectomy or catheter-tip fragmentation may be considered in two groups of patients:

* patients with proven pulmonary emboli who present with or develop systemic arterial hypertension; and
* patients with proven pulmonary emboli who have persistent hypoxaemia while receiving high concentrations of inspired oxygen.

The precise approach is still debated and will depend on local expertise, but intravenous thrombolytic therapy is by far the most extensively used modality. The selection of intravenous thrombolytic therapy, reduced-dose thrombolytic therapy, delivered by pulse spray directly into the embolus, open embolectomy, and catheter-tip embolectomy or catheter-tip fragmentation, all depend upon the experience of the clinician and local facilities, including monitoring facilities. Most clinicians reserve thrombolytic therapy for haemodynamically unstable patients with refractory shock.

Chapter 3
Cardiovascular complications after surgery in general

Introduction

Cardiovascular complications after anaesthesia and surgery are a major cause of morbidity and mortality. Identifying patients most at risk preoperatively, and the use of invasive monitoring in the perioperative period have increased the safety of surgery. Nevertheless, myocardial infarction, dysrhythmias, congestive cardiac failure and cerebrovascular accidents occur relatively frequently, reflecting the need for better understanding of the basic pathophysiology, diagnosis and management of the cardiovascular complications.

Essential physiology

Cardiac output is the amount of blood pumped out of each ventricle per minute:

$$\text{Cardiac output} = \text{stroke volume} \times \text{heart rate.}$$

Determinants of cardiac output

* **Preload**—the degree to which the myocardium is stretched before it contracts. Mainly determined by circulating blood volume. Also affected by: atrial contraction, venous tone, intrathoracic pressure, intrapericardial pressure, and posture.
* **Afterload**—the resistance against which the heart has to eject. It is determined mainly by peripheral vascular resistance and arterial vaso-constriction/dilatation. Also affected by viscosity of blood, compliance and inertia of large arteries, and the radius of the ventricular cavity.
* **Myocardial contractility**—the intrinsic inotropic state of the heart muscle is affected by the autonomic impulses, circulating cate-cholamines, hypoxia, acidosis, hypercapnia, ischaemia, and drugs.
* **Heart rate.**

The Frank Starling principle describes the length–tension relationship in the cardiac muscle where the more the muscle is stretched, the greater the tension developed in the muscle, and hence the greater the force of contraction. As the stretch becomes more extreme, no further tension is developed, and eventually the force of contraction declines. The curve is moved up and to the left with increased contractility, but shifts downward and to the right in heart failure (see Fig. below).

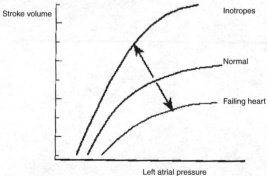

The Frank Starling curve.

The Frank Starling curve illustrates the relationship between the end-diastolic volume and the stroke volume, or, put in a clinical context, the relationship between atrial pressure and cardiac output.

Coronary blood flow (CBF)

* Is normally about 225 ml/min at rest.
* The heart has a very high (70–80%) oxygen extraction ratio, even at rest.
* Increased delivery of oxygen to the myocardium at times of increased need can therefore only be achieved by increasing the blood flow.
* The major determinants of myocardial oxygen consumption are myocardial contractility, heart rate, and intramyocardial tension.
* CBF to the left ventricle mainly occurs during diastole.
* Increasing heart rates lead to a shortening of diastole, and a reduction in CBF.

Aids to assessment of cardiovascular complications

History

This should include the past and present history of cardiovascular disease, the patient's symptomatic status (NYHA (New York Heart Association) classification I–IV), and current medication.

Clinical examination

- General examination
- Cardiovascular examination: blood pressure (BP), pulse rate and rhythm, jugular venous pressure (JVP), apex beat
- Heart sounds 1 and 2 (3rd and 4th sounds indicative of heart failure)
- Murmurs—location, timing, nature, intensity, radiation, other features
- Signs of congestive heart failure; basal crepitations, peripheral oedema, hepatomegaly
- Carotid and peripheral pulses

Investigations

Include these in general:

- Blood: biochemistry, haematology, cardiac enzymes
- Blood gases
- ECG
- Chest X-ray

Other specific tests are used as indicated:

- Echocardiography: transthoracic or transoesophageal
- Radionuclide scan/stress test
- CT scan, MRI, carotid Doppler in cases of stroke
- Cardiac catheterization

Identification of higher risk patients

- Myocardial infarction (MI) within 6 months
- Unstable angina
- Signs of CCF
- Aortic stenosis
- Premature ventricular beats >5/min.

* Untreated hypertension
* Arrhythmias

Monitoring cardiovascular status

(1) Simple monitoring (e.g. on surgical ward) includes:
    * ECG: heart rate, rhythm
    * non-invasive blood pressure
    * urine output
    * peripheral temperature
    * pulse oximetry

(2) More intermediate monitoring (e.g. on high-dependency unit) includes:
    * central venous pressure
    * arterial line: blood pressure, blood gases

(3) Advanced monitoring (e.g. on intensive care unit) involves:
    * pulmonary artery catheterization with direct measurements of pulmonary artery wedge pressure and cardiac output; derived haemodynamic variables such as vascular resistance, left ventricular stroke work index, etc. may also be determined
    * mixed venous oxygen saturation, and oxygen delivery/consumption
    * transoesophageal Doppler cardiac output

Management of cardiovascular complications

Checklist for patients who have cardiac complications

This entails:

- resuscitation (ABCDEs);
- history and examination;
- review of notes and charts;
- management plan;
- appropriate investigations;
- specific treatment;
- consider transfer to higher level of care and senior consultation.

Optimization of cardiac output

- This involves giving oxygen with spontaneous or assisted ventilation.
- Cardiac preload can be optimized by giving fluids (crystalloid, colloid, blood, or diuretics or nitrates).
- Cardiac afterload may be adjusted with vasodilators and adequate pain control.
- Contractility can be improved by giving inotropes, restore coronary blood flow.
- Heart rate and rhythm can be optimized using antiarrhythmic agents, chronotropic drugs, and transvenous pacing.

Myocardial infarction

The risk of perioperative MI in the general surgical population is 0.07%. If surgery is performed within 3 months of MI, the risk of reinfarction may be as high as 25% and it is important to identify the high-risk group and take precautions to reduce the incidence of MI and subsequent mortality.

Risk factors

* Previous MI
* Unstable angina
* Disabling angina
* Silent ischaemia
* Hypertension

Pathophysiology

Ischaemic necrosis results from an imbalance in the supply and demand of oxygen in the myocardium. Haemodynamic alterations occurring perioperatively influence the development of MI. Tachycardia results in increased oxygen demand and reduced supply because of shortened diastole. Hypotension results in reduced coronary perfusion pressure thereby reducing oxygen supply, and hypertension results in increased oxygen demand. Left ventricular overfilling results in increased oxygen demand and reduced supply secondary to augmented tissue pressure.

Clinical features

Chest pain, crushing or constricting in nature, retrosternal, radiating to the jaws or both arms and wrists. There may be an atypical presentation (painless, heart failure, or gastrointestinal symptoms), which is common in the elderly, diabetics, or perioperatively.

Nausea, vomiting, dyspnoea, and autonomic disturbances occur.

The physical examination is often negative.

Investigations

Electrocardiography

Typical changes accompanying acute MI are:

* ST segment elevation >1 mm in precordial leads or 2 mm in limb leads which persists for more than 24 h;
* reciprocal ST depression in the opposite leads;
* development of new Q waves if they are wide (above 0.04 s) or deep (more than one-third of the height of the following R wave);

* T-wave inversion (not diagnostic by itself);
* location of these changes on the ECG identify the region of the infarction.

Enzyme changes

Enzyme	Peak (hours)	Duration (days)
CK-MB	12–24	1.5–3
CK-18	18–30	2–5
ALT/AST	20–30	2–6
LDH	30–48	5–14

CK-MB, creatine kinase, membrane-bound; ALT, alanine aminotransferase; AST, aspartate aminotransferase; LDH, lactate degydrogenase.

Enzyme changes

Membrane-bound creatine kinase (CK-MB) estimation is the most useful diagnostic test. If the ratio of CK-MB to CK is >6–8% then MI is highly likely. Troponin T assay is now a useful adjunct to the diagnosis of myocardial injury.

Echocardiography

Is helpful in equivocal cases and may reveal immobility of discrete area of ventricular wall and help to titrate the dose of angiotensin-converting enzyme (ACE) inhibitors

Treatment of myocardial infarction

Immediate

* Transfer to coronary care unit (CCU).
* Monitor and treat complications.
* Prescribe pain relief with nitrates and opiates.
* Give oxygen.
* Give aspirin.
* Give atropine to reduce reflex vagal activity.
* Thrombolysis is usually contraindicated, consider reperfusion strategy with percutaneous transluminal coronary recanalization (PTCA).

Subsequent treatment

Aspirin reduces the short-term mortality by 23% and there may be some modest patency advantage for heparin added to tissue plasminogen activator (TPA). Their use, however, may be contraindicated in the perioperative period. IV β-blockers reduce mortality by preventing cardiac rupture, oral β-blockade after MI is proven to reduce sudden death and reinfarction.

ACE inhibitors and nitrates for continuing pain and patients in heart failure may be considered.

Complications

- Cardiac arrest (ventricular fibrillation, VF)
- Pump failure
- Arrhythmias
- Ventricular septal defect (VSD)
- Cardiac rupture
- Pericardial tamponade
- Ventricular aneurysm
- Mitral regurgitation

Prevention

To be forewarned is to be forearmed and a delay of elective surgery for 3–6 months after MI is obvious sense. Extended monitoring in the intensive care unit of the high-risk patients may be planned after assessment with echocardiography, radionuclide cardiac imaging, or angiography. The treatment of ischaemic heart disease (IHD) can be optimized preoperatively, including coronary revascularization strategies.

Cardiac failure

Definition

Inability of the heart to meet the body's oxygen requirement.

Aetiology

* Pressure overload—caused by hypertension or aortic stenosis.
* Volume overload—caused by fluid overload, aortic or mitral regurgitation.
* Cardiac muscle dysfunction—related to coronary artery disease or cardiomyopathy.
* High-output failure—following sepsis or hyperthyroidism.

Pathophysiology

Both systolic and diastolic function are impaired, although a systolic component often predominates. Impaired systolic function with ventricular dysfunction leads to a decrease in ejection fraction. The ventricle lies on the flat part of the left ventricular function curve (see figure of the Frank Starling curves above) thereby impairing its ability to increase the stroke volume by increasing the preload, the ventricle is very sensitive to increase in afterload.

Impaired diastolic function with reduction in ventricular compliance leads to marked increase in filling pressures at relatively normal end-diastolic volume, thereby limiting the ability of the ventricle to respond positively to fluid challenge.

Compensatory mechanisms

* Acute—increase in heart rate, vasoconstriction (sympathetic and renin–angiotensin mediated), venoconstriction
* Chronic—increase in chamber size and muscle mass, salt and water retention

Clinical features

* Impaired systolic function leading to fatigue, confusion, agitation, cold clammy extremities, oliguria, and tachypnoea
* Impaired diastolic function of left ventricle (LV) with pulmonary oedema and hypoxaemia
* Impaired diastolic function of right ventricle (RV) causing peripheral oedema, hepatic congestion, and splanchnic congestion

Investigations

* ECG—evidence of ischaemia, infarction, or arrhythmias
* Chest X-ray—bat's wing shadowing, upper lobe blood diversion, kerley B lines, pleural effusion, and cardiomegaly
* Echocardiography—myocardial contractility, pericardial effusion, valvular pathology, and septal defects
* Enzyme estimation—CK, CK-MB, LDH, and AST
* Blood gases—low PO_2, rising base deficit, variable PCO_2.
* Swan–Ganz—low cardiac output (CO) and cardiac index (CI), high pulmonary arterial wedge pressure (PAWP), high central venous pressure (CVP), low mixed venous saturation

Management

Aims to achieve adequate oxygen supply/demand balance by appropriate manipulation of preload, afterload, and myocardial contractility.

Monitoring involves ECG, BP, skin temperature, urine output, CVP, arterial pressure, and pulmonary artery (PA) catheterization.

Treatment

* Sedation, pain relief, and oxygen.
* Diuretics.
* Vasodilators: glyceryl trinitrate (GTN), sodium nitroprusside (SNP), or hydralazine reduce the preload and the afterload.
* Inotropes: adrenaline (epinephrine) and dopamine improve myocardial contractility, whereas dobutamine, dopexamine, enoximone, and milrinone improve myocardial contractility and reduce the afterload.
* Positive-pressure ventilation with or without positive end-expiratory pressure (PEEP) reduce the preload and afterload
* Intra-aortic balloon pump (IABP) or ventricular-assist devices improve forward flow, augment coronary perfusion, and reduce afterload.
* Specific treatment involves antiarrhythmics or cardioversion for arrhythmias, valve replacement for organic valve pathology.

Arrhythmia

Arrhythmias occurring during the perioperative period are an important cause of cardiovascular morbidity.

Predisposing factors

* Age >70 years
* Pain and anxiety
* Increased catecholamine concentration
* Hypoxia
* Hypercarbia
* Electrolyte disturbances (hypokalaemia, hyperkalaemia, hypomagnesaemia)
* Hypovolaemia
* Pyrexia, sepsis
* Drugs

Clinical features

The patients may be asymptomatic or present with palpitations, dizziness, or sweating. There may be features of cardiac failure, an MI, or of underlying cardiac disease.

Investigations

These include ECG, measurement of serum electrolytes and cardiac enzymes, and blood gas/oximetry.

General principles of management

* Monitoring involves ECG and oximetry; invasive monitoring may be indicated in haemodynamically unstable patients.
* The severity of haemodynamic instability determines the urgency with which the arrhythmia needs to be treated.
* Urgent DC cardioversion may be needed in patients with severe instability.
* Need to correct hypoxia, electrolyte disturbances, and hypovolaemia before resorting to treatment with antiarrhythmic agents.
* Ventricular arrhythmias produce greater haemodynamic disturbance than supraventricular rhythm.
* Arrhythmia in the absence of haemodynamic instability can be managed by oral antiarrhythmic agents or elective cardioversion.

Management of narrow-complex tachycardia

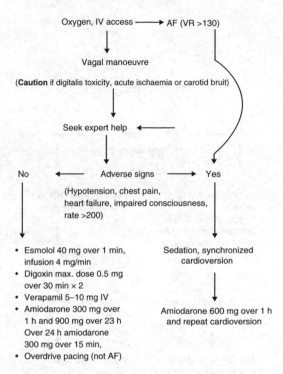

Management of narrow-complex tachycardia.

Management of broad-complex tachycardia (QRS >0.12 s)

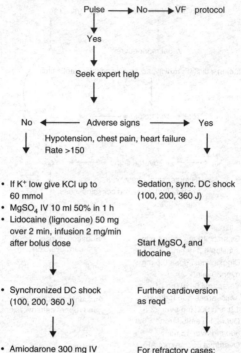

Management of broad-complex tachycardia (QRS >0.12 s).

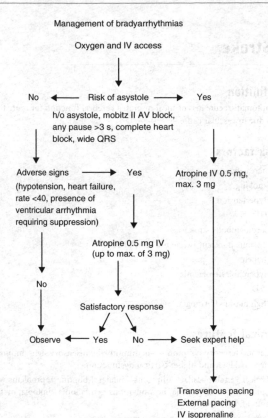

Management of bradyarrhythmias

Stroke

Definition
Symptomatic acute loss of focal or global cerebral function for more than 24 h due to vascular cause.

Risk factors
* Increasing age
* Smoking
* Hypertension
* IHD
* Cardioembolic stroke
* Previous transient ischaemic attack (TIA)
* Diabetes
* Hypercholesterolaemia
* PVD
* High plasma fibrinogen

Clinical features
* Carotid territory symptoms—hemimotor/hemisensory signs, monocular visual loss, and higher cortical dysfunction.
* Typical vertebrobasilar symptoms—bilateral blindness, problems with gait or stance, dysarthria, homonymous hemianopia, diplopia, nystagmus, and vertigo.
* Non-hemispheric symptoms—syncope, dizziness

Investigations
* Biochemical: electrolytes, glucose, coagulation screen
* CT scan: to exclude haemorrhage, ischaemia, and localization
* Extracranial Doppler sonography: internal carotid artery (ICA) stenosis/occlusion, vertebral artery occlusion, distal flow reduction
* Transcranial Doppler sonography
* CT angiography
* MRI
* ECG
* Echocardiography in suspected cases of cardioembolism

Complications

* Cerebral oedema
* Hydrocephalus
* Raised intracranial pressure
* Secondary haemorrhage
* Seizures
* Aspiration
* Cardiac arrhythmias

General principles of management

Complete neurological assessment with early involvement of the neurophysician.

The aetiology of stroke should be taken into account when choosing therapy. The most common causes of mortality after stroke are transtentorial herniation and cardiopulmonary complications. Monitor blood pressure, oxygenation, temperature, and blood glucose.

Risk reduction and monitoring are critical elements of therapy. Degree of disability and independence influence prognosis and therefore therapy. Specialized stroke rehabilitation units for convalescence.

Prevention

Reducing risk factors and instituting prophylactic medical or surgical therapy can help prevent stroke with optimal treatment of hypertension, diabetes, hypercholesterolaemia, cardiac failure, and arrhythmias in the preoperative period.

Antiplatelet therapy can be given in cases of mild to moderate carotid artery disease. However, for symptomatic patients with carotid artery disease (70–99%), carotid endarterectomy with medical therapy significantly reduces the incidence of stroke.

Anticoagulation should be given to patients with cardiac dysrhythmias.

Patients with a recent stroke should have their surgery delayed (3–6 months) and extremes of hypotension or hypertension in the elderly should be avoided in the perioperative period.

Output reduces progressively and the right atrial pressure rises. Tamponade can be difficult to distinguish from myocardial failure but diagnosis is usually clinical: chest X-ray and transthoracic echocardiography often fail to confirm the diagnosis, but transoesophageal echocardiography is extremely useful in difficult situations.

Treatment requires transfer to the operating room for re-exploration, relief of tamponade, and haemostasis.

Complications involving other organ systems

Renal insufficiency

Up to 15% of patients develop some evidence of renal dysfunction following cardiac surgery. The causes are preoperative problems (renal impairment, nephrotoxins, etc.) or hypoperfusion associated with cardiopulmonary bypass, low cardiac output syndrome, or hypotension.

Diagnosis is made on oliguria (urine output <0.5 ml/kg per h) and elevated serum urea and creatinine.

Management

* Ensure adequate position of the urine catheter.
* Optimize preload.
* Optimize cardiac output.
* Start 'renal' dose of dopamine (3 µg/kg per min), which is conventional but is increasingly questioned.
* Use a diuretic once the cardiac output is adequate (furosemide (frusemide) or bumetanide as a bolus or continuous infusion).
* Haemodialysis or ultrafiltration is required in established renal failure, volume overload, hyperkalaemia, acidosis, or uraemia.

Gastrointestinal tract complications

May occur independently or as part of a multisystem failure following cardiopulmonary bypass. The mechanism is either reduced perfusion due to low cardiac output or abnormal perfusion on cardiopulmonary bypass.

The main complications are:

* Gastrointestinal bleeding, which is often preceded by a history of gastritis or previous ulcer disease, and H_2-antagonists generally used for prophylaxis. Endoscopy is required for diagnosis and treatment, and coagulopathy needs correction.
* Mesenteric ischaemia and infarction, which presents with a severely ill patient with any combination of ileus, sepsis, acidosis, diarrhoea, bleeding, renal failure, low or even high cardiac output. The treatment is laparotomy and bowel resection (and occasionally successful embolectomy) but it has a poor prognosis.
* Biliary complications.
* Pancreatitis.
* Liver dysfunction, which is commonly in relation to multisystem organ failure and sepsis.

Haematological complications

Some 3–5% of patients require re-exploration for bleeding after heart surgery. The causes being 'surgical' bleeding (in two-thirds of the cases) and a coagulopathy (in the rest), usually caused by the extracorporeal circuit (related to heparin, platelet damage and dysfunction, fibrinolysis and depletion of coagulation factors.

Management requires control of hypertension and the giving of blood products according to the results of coagulation studies (protamine, platelets, fresh-frozen plasma, cryoprecipitate).

Re-exploration is indicated if bleeding is:

* >500 ml in the first hour;
* 400 ml/h during each of the next 2 h;
* 300 ml/h in the first 3 h;
* 1000 ml in total during the first 4 h.

Infectious complications

Prophylactic antibiotics are given for the first 24 h postoperatively.

The most common infections are sternal wound infections which are superficial or deep (mediastinitis), leg wound infections, and pneumonia.

Sternal wound infections

Risk factors include diabetes, obesity, chronic obstructive pulmonary disease (COPD), and low cardiac output. They present with fever, purulent drainage, leucocytosis, and there may be sternal dehiscence when mediastinitis is present.

Management requires antibiotics and local drainage. Sternal dehiscence and mediastinitis require re-operation, debridement, and irrigation. Sternal reconstruction may be required with muscle or omental flaps.

Leg wound infections

The risk factors include poor peripheral perfusion, tissue oedema, obesity, diabetes, and poor surgical technique. They are a very common cause of prolonged postoperative morbidity.

Suction drains may help to reduce the incidence, but management involves antibiotics and leg elevation. Debridement and reconstruction may occasionally be necessary.

Pneumonia

Some degree of lung collapse is common after cardiac surgery and analgesia, respiratory exercises, and physiotherapy are crucial.

Diagnosis is based on purulent sputum, cough, fever, and leucocytosis. The sputum culture may reveal a positive growth of a microorganism.

There is infiltrate or lobar shadowing on the chest X-ray and management is based on antibiotics and physiotherapy.

Neurological complications

The incidence of major neurological complications is less than 1%, but less severe neuropsychological problems may occur in up to 25% of patients.

Neurological complications include:

* focal neurological deficit or stroke;
* neuropsychological disturbance: confusion, agitation, disorientation, depression, personality changes;
* peripheral nerve injury: caused by sternal retraction;
* phrenic nerve palsy: left internal thoracic artery dissection, cold injury to the phrenic nerve.

Major neurological deficits have risk factors in the history of a past stroke, in older age, and if there is calcification of the aorta.

Causes include:

* cerebral hypoperfusion with low perioperative perfusion pressure, and significant carotid stenosis;
* emboli to the brain from an intracardiac thrombus, atherosclerotic aorta, or air embolism;
* intracerebral bleeding due to vascular malformation or hypertension and anticoagulation.

Assessment requires a neurological examination, CT scan, and carotid Doppler ultrasound.

Management involves the use of heparin, providing there is no evidence of intracerebral bleeding, as well as management of intracranial pressure and early physiotherapy and rehabilitation.

Pulmonary complications

Risk factors include smoking, COPD, obesity, and older age.

The causes of acute respiratory failure include:

* atelectasis, pneumothorax, pleural effusion;
* pulmonary oedema;
* pneumonia, bronchospasm;
* prolonged mechanical ventilation.

Assessment requires a physical examination, with attention to the presence of air entry or wheeze. Position of the endotracheal (ET) tube is checked on a chest X-ray. Arterial blood gases should be measured and checked with ventilator settings.

Management requires identifiable problems (sedation, analgesia, pleural drainage) to be treated with optimization of cardiac output and ventilator settings (PEEP, FiO_2). Bronchodilators and diuretics may be necessary.

Other respiratory complications include:

* pneumothorax;
* pneumonia;

* atelectasis;
* bronchospasm;
* adult respiratory distress syndrome;
* chronic respiratory failure.

Complications after pulmonary surgery

Persistent air leak

This may develop from the lung parenchyma or a major airways stump. Air leak through the chest drains is the obvious sign.

Management includes:

* checking drainage unit for leaks;
* chest X-ray to visualize lung expansion and position of chest drains;
* addition of suction.

If the lung is fully expanded the majority of air leaks will seal spontaneously. Obstruction of the major airways with sputum will prevent full expansion, so physiotherapy and bronchial suction may be required. If an air leak persists for more than 2 weeks, consider pleurodesis. Massive air leaks require bronchoscopy and possible re-exploration.

Atelectasis

This follows retained secretions or hypoventilation due to pain.

Management includes:

* physiotherapy;
* adequate analgesia;
* adequate pleural drainage;
* bronchoscopy;
* minitracheotomy.

Arrhythmias

The most common are supraventricular tachycardias, mainly atrial fibrillation, and are treated with digoxin or amiodarone, and correction of hypokalaemia and hypoxia.

Respiratory failure

Risk factors include patients with borderline lung function, infection of the remaining lung parenchyma, atelectasis, and fluid overload.

Failure is managed by:

* treating the specific cause (fluid restriction, antibiotics, etc.);
* controlling bronchial secretions;
* applying mechanical ventilation if necessary.

Bronchopleural fistula

This is more common after pneumonectomy and can be acute or chronic (>2 weeks after surgery). It presents with fever and cough with fluid or blood or respiratory failure. An alteration in fluid level in the pneumonectomy space may be seen on chest X-ray.

The cause is a residual tumour in a bronchial stump, or a poor surgical technique with failure to close a bronchial stump adequately, or ischaemia or infection of a bronchial stump.

Management requires:

• pleural drainage
• bronchoscopy
• antibiotics
• consideration of re-operation.

Empyema

Occurs in a persistent intrapleural space after pulmonary resection and presents with fever, pleural effusion, and an air fluid level seen on a chest X-ray. Purulent pleural fluid with positive cultures are obtained on aspiration.

Management requires:

• chest tube insertion;
• antibiotics according to sensitivity;
• decortication.

Chapter 4
Complications of fluid and electrolyte balance in surgical patients

Water

Water is lost from the body in urine, as sweat and insensitive loss, in respiration, and in faeces. Normally the kidney balances water intake and loss. Water balance is controlled by the release of antidiuretic hormone (ADH), also called arginine vasopressin, by the posterior pituitary. Increased secretion of ADH results in increased reabsorption of water by the kidney, thereby producing a smaller volume of more concentrated urine.

Water deficit

The commonest cause of water deficit in surgical patients is reduced intake, which can be due to many causes. Water deficit leads to confusion, particularly in the elderly patient. Oesophageal and bowel obstruction are the other commonest presenting causes, together with the perioperative use of sedatives and analgesics. Patients may also suffer from iatrogenic water deficit if they are given too much sodium in intravenous fluids or continue to receive diuretics with a reduced fluid intake. Increased loss of water in vomit, diarrhoea, fistula and drain fluid, and diabetes insipidus in head injury can result in water deficit in the presence of a normal intake.

Diagnosis

Patients with water deficit usually complain of thirst. Study of the patient's fluid-balance charts may show a negative fluid balance or a relative water deficiency, i.e. an excess intake of electrolytes relative to water. Oliguria, high urine osmolarity, and increased serum sodium concentrations results and there may be associated tachycardia, hypotension, and decreased elasticity of the skin.

Avoiding the complication

The patient's carers (doctors and nurses) need to monitor fluid intake accurately and encourage the confused to drink regularly. Patients who cannot drink should be given early adequate replacement using the enteral route via a percutaneous endoscopic gastrostomy (PEG) or jejunostomy, or intravenously. Causes of increased water loss should be considered and addressed (such as prolonged pyrexia or large drain fluid loss).

Treating the complication

Whenever possible water should be given orally. Failing this, water can be given enterally via a nasogastric or a fine-bore feeding tube, provided the enteral route is accessible and functioning. When the intravenous route is the only one available a solution such as 5% glucose should be used: which also furnishes 200 kCal/l. Glucose solutions are not appropriate for treating causes of shock such as haemorrhage or sepsis. The normal requirement for water is 3 litres/day so this has to be given as well as the extra water to correct the deficit of total body water volume. To avoid overcompensation regular monitoring of the patient is required. Increased urine output is a good indicator of hydration and serum electrolytes should be measured daily. It is best to correct the deficit gradually, rather than rapidly, to avoid water intoxication.

Water excess

The normal response to surgery is an increased release of ADH, which leads to water retention in the first 24 h after surgery. This reduction in urine output may be misinterpreted as a fluid deficit, which wrongly prompts additional but consequently excessive intravenous fluid replacement. The water retention corrects itself with a spontaneous diuresis, usually on the second or third postoperative day, and does not need to be treated. Other causes of water excess in surgical patients are the overzealous administration of intravenous fluids containing a high proportion of free water (5% glucose, 4% glucose/0.18% sodium chloride), and inappropriate ADH secretion by tumours. Urological patients undergoing transurethral resection of the prostate (TURP) may suffer from the TURP syndrome. During TURP 1.5% glycine solution is used to irrigate the bladder, but this may lead to the excessive absorption of water into the circulation at a rapid rate.

Diagnosis

There is a reduction in the serum sodium, serum osmolality, and haemoglobin levels. Examination of the fluid-balance charts may show an excessive administration of intravenous fluids containing free water. It should be remembered that increased ADH secretion after surgery causes a drop in serum sodium levels on the first day postoperatively and that this is normal and corrects itself spontaneously. Water excess due to TURP syndrome usually presents in the theatre recovery room and presents as confusion, hypoxia, and irritability. In extreme cases of TURP syndrome patients may suffer fits and coma. The syndrome may occur on the ward postoperatively and is more likely if the patient is given postoperative intravenous fluids that contain free water.

Avoiding the complication

Patients rarely require more than 3 litres of water/day in temperate climates. Attention to fluid balance should avoid an excessive administration of intravenous fluid containing free water. Appreciation of the increased secretion of ADH following surgery should avoid the interpretation of postoperative reduced urine output and decreased serum sodium as an indication for more intravenous fluid. TURP syndrome is more likely following prolonged prostatic resection and becomes more likely when more than 9 litres of glycine irrigation is used. In these cases a prophylactic dose of diuretic during surgery may be used to increase water excretion. Postoperatively, TURP patients should receive 0.9% sodium chloride for the first 12 h.

Treating the complication

Water retention due to increased ADH secretion following surgery requires no treatment, and is corrected spontaneously. Established water retention due to ADH secretion by tumours and iatrogenic intravenous free water is treated by restricting water intake with careful electrolyte infusion. Water excess due to TURP syndrome is normally corrected with restriction of water intake, but in severe forms it may require the use of diuretics. The use of hypertonic sodium solutions in patients with the TURP syndrome is best avoided as the additional sodium load may cause fluid retention, which can lead to circulatory overload in the elderly.

Sodium

Sodium is mainly an extracellular ion and the normal serum sodium concentration is in the range 135–145 mmol/l. The control of sodium is achieved through renal mechanisms acting under the influence of renin/angiotensin and aldosterone. Aldosterone release results in sodium retention, angiotensin II secretion leads to sodium and water retention. It is important to realize that the serum sodium level may not rise since sodium retention is accompanied by renal retention of water. There may be sodium overload in the presence of a normal serum sodium level. Sodium must always be considered in conjunction with water, as the two are interrelated. The normal sodium requirement is 1 mmol/kg per day, i.e. 70 mmol for a 70-kg man.

Sodium deficit

A low serum sodium level (hyponatraemia) may be due to a sodium deficiency or, more frequently in surgical practice, sodium dilution due to excess water. Sodium deficit may exist with a normal serum sodium value as the kidney excretes additional water when sodium is lost to keep the serum sodium level nearer to normal. In surgical patients, sodium may be lost in vomit, diarrhoea, sequestration in the bowel and fistula, and drain fluid. Excess water intake in IV fluids containing free water, or water retention in renal failure, may result in a low serum sodium level due to dilution. A low serum sodium value on the first day postoperatively commonly occurs following water retention in response to ADH secretion as part of the stress response.

Diagnosis

Diagnosis can be difficult. It is easy to confuse a low sodium level due to dilution with a true sodium deficiency, thereby resulting in incorrect treatment. Diagnosis depends on a careful history, study of fluid-balance charts, and consideration of serial electrolyte results. A history of sodium loss, e.g. vomiting, is more suggestive of sodium deficit; the administration of IV fluids containing free water may point to a water excess. A normal serum sodium level in the presence of an elevated serum urea and haemoglobin are suggestive of a true sodium deficit. In true sodium deficit there may be low blood pressure, reduced skin turgor, and a low central venous pressure (CVP), but there is no single definitive diagnostic sign and careful consideration of the whole picture is important.

Avoiding the complication

Patients should be given adequate sodium to replace losses. Following major surgery there may be major losses of sodium into the bowel and this needs to be taken into account when prescribing IV fluids. Careful attention to fluid balance and regular measurement of electrolytes should be made. Causes of sodium loss should be treated, such as with the use of antiemetics to prevent vomiting.

Treating the complication

Treatment should only be undertaken when an accurate diagnosis has been made. Rapid correction of electrolyte imbalance should be avoided if possible as this can cause rapid fluid shifts between the internal fluid compartments. Hyponatraemia due to water excess should be treated by water restriction or with diuretics in urgent situations. True sodium deficit should be treated by the administration of a sodium-containing feed or with intravenous fluids containing a high proportion of sodium relative to water (e.g. 0.9% sodium chloride or Hartmann's solution). When treating sodium deficiency with intravenous fluids it is wise to measure electrolytes at least twice a day.

Sodium excess

There may be sodium excess with a normal serum sodium level as the kidney retains water when sodium is retained. Hypernatraemia is usually due to excessive water loss rather than sodium retention. In the surgical patient the common causes of hypernatraemia are dehydration, diabetes insipidus in head injury/pituitary tumour, and the administration of diuretics in the absence of adequate water intake. The commonest cause of sodium excess in surgical patients is overadministration of IV fluids containing sodium. Just 1 litre of either 0.9% sodium chloride or Hartmann's solution contains more than the normal daily requirement of sodium. If patients are given excessive quantities of sodium in intravenous fluids the kidney cannot excrete the excess and water is retained in response to the hypernatraemia. Retention of water and sodium results in fluid overload, leading eventually to oedema, raised blood pressure, breathlessness, and congestive heart failure. The elderly patient with pre-existing heart disease is particularly vulnerable to complications from excessive sodium administration.

Diagnosis

The cause of hypernatraemia can be diagnosed by attention to the history, fluid-balance charts, and electrolyte results. A history of restricted water intake or excessive urine output point to a problem with water balance. A history of positive fluid balance and the application of excessive sodium in intravenous fluid suggest sodium excess. Symptoms and signs of congestive heart failure in the absence of other causes indicate a serious overloading of the circulation with sodium.

Avoiding the complication

Causes of excessive water loss should be treated to prevent hypernatraemia developing. To avoid sodium excess, patients should not be given more sodium in replacement fluids than they require. As a general rule, no patient requires more than 1 litre of 0.9% sodium chloride/day in an intravenous fluid maintenance regime. Remember, 1 litre of 0.9% sodium chloride contains 154 mmol of sodium.

Treating the complication

In hypernatraemia, the treatment is directed to correcting the cause of the excess water loss, for example ADH should be given in diabetes insipidus with appropriate water replacement. In sodium excess, the intake of sodium should be restricted and a replacement fluid given that contains free water. The kidney normally corrects this abnormality, when presented with the correct fluid balance, by producing a diuresis. In this situation there is often fluid overload and the kidney excretes the excess retained water with the excess sodium. Care must be taken to avoid correcting the situation too rapidly, and it is best to allow a negative fluid balance to occur as the kidney produces a diuresis. When there is a serious sodium excess leading to congestive heart failure, the patient should optimally be transferred to a high-dependency or intensive care unit with central venous monitoring. The use of diuretics in this situation may improve the hypernatraemia more rapidly.

Potassium

Potassium is the main intracellular ion. The serum concentration of potassium is 3.5–4.5 mmol/l and the intracellular concentration is 140 mmol/l. There is approximately 100 times more potassium in the intracellular space than in the extracellular space. Serum potassium levels are not a good indicator of overall potassium balance as losses from the extracellular space are corrected by the migration of potassium from the intracellular space. The serum potassium concentration only shows a significant fall when there is a substantial loss from the intracellular space. Potassium concentration is controlled by the kidney in response to mineralocorticoids, particularly aldosterone.

Potassium is the most dangerous ion to give intravenously, as potassium has effects on the heart and rapid administration may lead to cardiac dysrhythmias and cardiac arrest. The normal daily requirement of potassium is 1 mmol/kg, i.e. 70 mmol for a 70-kg man.

Potassium deficit

Hypokalaemia is a serum potassium concentration below 3.5 mmol/l, but the total potassium loss is often larger than expected as the migration of intracellular potassium to the extracellular space delays the drop in the serum concentration. The causes of hypokalaemia in surgical patients include reduced intake in bowel obstruction and patients who are unable to eat. Increased losses occur in conditions where sequestration of body fluid occurs, such as prolonged postoperative ileus, and when additional loss occurs in the urine as in Addison's disease. A low potassium level occurs in patients who are given replacement fluid that does not include potassium for more than a few days. The surgical patient with bowel obstruction nearly always has a potassium deficit which needs correction prior to surgery. Diabetic patients who receive insulin/glucose infusions may develop hypokalaemia if the infusion is given too rapidly.

Diagnosis

A serum potassium concentration below 3.5 mmol/l indicates hypokalaemia, but it does not give a good indication of the total potassium deficit, which is usually substantial. The ECG changes of hypokalaemia are flattening of the T wave and depression of the ST segment. There should be a clinical cause that is consistent with the diagnosis.

Avoiding the complication

Potassium should be given early to patients who have conditions known to be associated with potassium loss, such as intestinal obstruction. Maintenance fluid should contain potassium after 24 hours of fasting,

20 mmol of potassium chloride can be added to each litre of replacement fluid. Causes of potassium loss should be addressed, e.g. the supplementation of steroids in Addison's disease. Patients receiving intravenous fluids should have daily electrolyte measurements to monitor their potassium levels.

Treating the complication

Where appropriate, hypokalaemia can be treated by oral supplementation or by the addition of extra potassium into enteral feeds. Intravenous replacement is potentially dangerous and advice should be sought if there is any doubt of the correct way to proceed. Potassium is given peripherally as a potassium chloride solution diluted in large volumes of intravenous fluids. No more than 40 mmol of potassium should be added to 1 litre of intravenous fluid, concentrations above this are damaging to veins and may cause thrombophlebitis. It is usual to give fluids containing potassium at a slow rate, no more than 1 litre in 4 h, to avoid cardiac effects. In severe hypokalaemia, the patient should be admitted to a high-dependency or intensive care ward. For rapid correction of severe hypokalaemia in the preoperative situation, 80 mmol of potassium chloride can be diluted in 100 ml of 0.9% sodium chloride and infused over 4 h. It is essential that this is done in an intensive care unit, the solution is given through a central line via a controlled infusion device, the ECG is monitored continuously, and measurements of electrolytes are repeated at the end of the infusion before any more potassium is given. In severe cases of hypokalaemia the patient may need to be given 200–300 mmol of potassium to achieve satisfactory serum levels.

Potassium excess

A potassium level above 5.0 mmol/l is abnormal, and above 6.0 mmol/l is usually an indication for urgent treatment. A rapid increase in potassium is more dangerous than a slow rise, as some adaptation occurs as in chronic renal failure. The commonest cause of hyperkalaemia in the surgical patient is sepsis leading to renal impairment. Patients with pre-existing renal failure are more likely to develop hyperkalaemia perioperatively as the initial response to the tissue damage of surgery is a release of potassium from damaged cells. Stored blood contains high levels of potassium and rapid blood transfusion may elevate the serum potassium. Diabetic patients with hyperglycaemia may also have a raised potassium concentration. Elevated serum potassium also occurs after burns due to potassium release from damaged tissues.

Diagnosis

Diagnosis is made when the serum potassium exceeds 5.0 mmol/l. Hyperkalaemia may produce the following ECG changes: tall-peaked T waves; widening of the QRS complex; prolongation of the PR interval; and loss of the P wave.

Avoiding the complication

Potassium intake should be restricted in high-risk patients. Patients with established renal failure are at particular risk and regular measurements of serum potassium should be made. Hyperkalaemic patients receiving enteral and total parenteral feeding should be given feed that contains reduced amounts of potassium.

Treating the complication

Patients with hyperkalaemia should have a restricted potassium intake. When active treatment is required the treatment selected depends on the urgency of the clinical situation. For less urgent cases, cation exchange resins can be used. Calcium Resonium 15 g orally every 6 h or 30 g rectally can be administered. Calcium Resonium starts to reduce serum potassium within 4 hours and lasts for 12 hours. For more urgent cases a glucose/insulin infusion can be used—50 ml of 50% glucose containing 10 units of soluble insulin is infused intravenously over 20 minutes and can reduce the serum potassium level within 15 minutes and lasts for 3 hours. In extreme cases, 10 ml of 10% calcium chloride injected intravenously over 1 min reduces the serum potassium level for 1 h. A persistent hyperkalaemia associated with renal failure may require treatment with renal dialysis.

Other electrolytes

Other electrolytes

The other electrolytes—calcium, magnesium, and phosphate—can usually be ignored in the short term as the body contains large pools of these electrolytes. Patients who are unable to eat normally for long periods should have these electrolytes measured twice a week and deficits corrected by the administration of supplements. Hypocalcaemia can occur acutely after parathyroidectomy and needs treatment by infusion of calcium chloride 10%. Acute pancreatitis is associated with disturbances of calcium and phosphate balance and daily electrolyte measurements should be made.

Colloids

Colloids are solutions containing substances of large molecular weight that are mainly retained in the intravascular compartment after infusion. Colloids expand the intravascular volume three times faster than crystalloid solutions and are sometimes referred to as 'plasma expanders'. There are four main colloids: albumin; dextrans; gelatins; and starches. Rapid infusion of colloids can lead to circulatory overload and heart failure; this is a particular risk in the elderly and patients with pre-existing heart disease.

Albumin

Albumin is a natural protein in the circulation and plays an important role in oncotic balance. Human albumin solution (HAS) is derived from pooled human serum. The use of HAS is controversial and there is probably no place for its routine use on surgical wards. However, there may be a place for its use in septic patients in intensive care units on the advice of an intensivist. Albumin should not be used as a replacement for acute blood loss as it has no advantage in this role over synthetic colloid solutions.

Dextrans

Dextrans are solutions containing glucose polymers. There are two solutions; Dextran 70, molecular weight 70 kDa and Dextran 40, molecular weight 40 kDa. Dextrans interfere with blood clotting. These solutions are little used since the introduction of the gelatins and starches and they will not be discussed in detail. There is no difficulty in blood grouping after a patient has received a dextran solution as long as the haematologist is aware of the fact.

Gelatins

Gelatins are short-acting colloid solutions derived from animal collagen. The molecular weight of these solutions is around 35 kDa. There are two types of gelatin solutions: succinylated gelatins (e.g. Gelofusine) and polygelines (e.g. Haemaccel). Gelatins are used for the short-term expansion of fluid volume (1–4 hours) after blood loss, in sepsis, and during anaesthesia. Both types of gelatin are provided in solutions of sodium chloride, approximately 150 mmol/l, and this has to be taken into account when considering sodium balance. There are differences between the two types of gelatins and this may influence the choice of gelatin used in particular patients. Succinylated gelatin contains low calcium (<0.4 mmol/l) and potassium (<0.4 mmol/l) levels compared to polygelines (calcium 6.25 mmol/l, potassium 5.1 mmol/l). Polygeline solutions may cause transfused blood to clot in infusion lines and is probably best avoided in patients with hyperkalaemia. Anaphylaxis is a rare complication of the use of gelatins.

Starches

A range of starch-based colloids are produced based on hydroxyethyl starch (HES). The molecular weight, concentration, and substitution (number of hydroxyethyl groups per 10 glucose molecules) determines the duration of persistence in the plasma. Starches with a molecular weight below 70 kDa are excreted by the kidney. Starches with a molecular weight above 70 kDa are metabolized by α-amylase, and the chains broken down and then excreted by the kidney. The short-acting starches are used for the same indications as the gelatins. The longer acting starches are mainly used in the treatment of patients with sepsis in intensive care units. Long-acting starches should be used with caution as they remain in the circulation up to 24 hours and it is easy to overload the circulation if they are given in excess. Starch solutions may affect clotting.

It is important to understand the characteristics of the starch solutions used as they vary greatly in their properties. Before using these solutions it is wise to read the manufacturer's data sheet to avoid inappropriate use. A rough guide is that the long-acting starches are the hexastarches (eloHAES 6%), the shorter acting starches are the pentastarches (e.g. HAES-steril 6%, HAES-steril 10%).

Volume overload

It is possible to overload the circulation with all the intravenous fluids discussed above. The clinical manifestation of the overload depends upon the type of fluid used and the speed of its administration. The elderly and patients with pre-existing heart disease are at particular risk.

Overload occurs when the volume of input exceeds the volume of elimination. Overload of the circulation with water occurs when patients are infused with excessive amounts of intravenous fluid containing free water, e.g. 5% glucose, 0.18% sodium chloride/4% glucose. Glucose solutions are rapidly lost to the extravascular space and are of little use in the resuscitation of shocked patients. Overload of the circulation with electrolyte fluids and gelatin colloids presents as sodium overload.

Diagnosis

The clinical picture in water overload is one of confusion, restlessness, and eventually fits. Haemodilution is present and measurement of electrolytes shows a reduced serum sodium level. A serum sodium concentration below 130 mmol/l is an indication for urgent treatment. Examination of the fluid-balance chart shows a positive fluid balance and an excess administration of intravenous fluid containing free water.

Sodium overload presents as oedema and increasing breathlessness. The oedema is dependent and will manifest as ankle oedema in ambulatory patients and as sacral oedema in supine patients. In more serious cases the patient shows signs of heart failure: raised jugular venous pressure; severe breathlessness; and pulmonary oedema. If the CVP is measured it will be found to be raised. Examination of the fluid-balance chart shows a positive fluid balance and an excessive administration of electrolyte solution (0.9% sodium chloride, Hartmann's solution, gelatin colloids). The serum sodium is often normal or slightly raised as the kidney retains water to dilute the excess sodium.

Avoiding the complication

It is important to administer the correct volume and combination of fluid to avoid fluid overload. Attention to fluid balance by studying the daily fluid charts and serial electrolyte measurements is important. When a patient starts to take oral or enterally administered fluids the volume of intravenous fluid administered needs to be reduced.

Treatment of the complication

The treatment of fluid overload is described earlier under the sections on water excess and sodium excess. In more serious cases it is wise to seek advice and consider transfer of the patient to the high-dependency or intensive care unit. The use of central venous pressure monitoring is useful in severe or clinically complicated cases.

Chapter 5
Complications of nutrition

Complications of nutrition

Many patients (perhaps as many as 30–50%) show evidence of protein-energy malnutrition (PEM) at the time of admission for surgery. It was clearly shown over 60 years ago that malnutrition significantly increases the morbidity and mortality of surgery, especially with regard to wound healing and resistance to infection. Awareness of the importance of nutrition is therefore important when planning surgical treatment. Postoperative complications have a significant effect on nutritional requirements. Nutritional support is of even greater importance in patients who may already have had a prolonged period of fasting and may be under considerable stress. Finally, poorly planned or executed nutritional support may itself give rise to potentially life-threatening complications.

Causes and risk factors for PEM

- Decreased food intake—dysphagia, subacute intestinal obstruction, chronic abdominal pain, psychosocial or cultural factors, iatrogenic;
- Decreased absorption—enteropathies, fistulas, short-bowel syndrome, chronic pancreatitis, mesenteric vascular insufficiency;
- Impaired utilization—sepsis, cancer;
- Increased requirements—catabolic states (sepsis).

Assessment of nutritional status

An assessment of nutritional status is a key element in taking a history and performing a physical examination. Simple clinical tests have not been shown to be inferior to more sophisticated ones. It has been shown that many patients are admitted to hospital without being weighed and that even when patients are known to be underweight, referral to a dietician is frequently overlooked. Nutritional assessment can be performed using the following techniques.

Clinical

Look at the patient's general appearance, and ask about evidence of recent weight loss and loss of muscle bulk (from temporalis, forearm, and dorsal interosseous muscles). Enquire about usual weight, recent weight loss, and dietary habits.

Anthropometric

Measure weight (absolute, as a percentage of 'usual', and of 'standard' from life insurance tables), body mass index (BMI) (weight in kg/height in m^2—a BMI of usually <20 denotes serious nutritional depletion), thickness of the skin fold over the triceps muscle (denotes amount of body fat stores), and muscle circumference in the mid-arm area (denotes body protein stores). Anthropometric measurements, with the exception of weight, are best performed by trained dieticians.

Laboratory

Check serum levels of albumin, prealbumin, transferrin, retinol-binding protein and total lymphocyte count, although many of these are only used in nutritional research. In general, abnormal laboratory results are less indicative of nutritional impairment and more of an underlying illness. Hypoalbuminaemia, for example, is rarely, if ever, a consequence of simple malnutrition, but more likely related to sepsis.

Functional

These tests are often overlooked and seldom performed—measurement of hand grip strength and respiratory muscle function (FEV_1, maximum inspiratory pressure, if normal pulmonary function can be assumed). These tests may indicate the effects of nutritional impairment on muscle function.

Scoring systems

Many of the tests described above have been used to produce weighted scoring systems that quantify nutritional risk, e.g. Subjective Global Assessment, Prognostic Nutritional Index.

Nutritional requirements and the metabolic responses to stress and starvation

The principal sources of dietary energy are carbohydrates (which provide 4 kCal (16.7 J)/g) and lipids (which provide 9 kCal (37.7 J)/g). Nitrogen is needed from protein (6.25 g of protein = 1 gN) to maintain structural and functional proteins in the body. The body has stores of both carbohydrate (liver and muscle glycogen) and lipid (adipose tissue) energy. Protein is stored chiefly in muscle.

When determining the amount and type of nutritional support required, it is important to take into account the normal requirements of the patient and then the effect of disease or its treatment upon them. During simple starvation, the metabolic rate falls to enable the body stores to last as long as possible, so protecting the patient. Eventually, when the carbohydrate and lipid stores start to become depleted, the body's protein reserves are broken down to provide energy. Even small amounts of carbohydrate can prevent this.

Metabolic effects of stress	Nutritional consequences
Increased metabolic rate	Increased calorie requirements
Increased protein catabolism	Muscle wasting despite feeding
Insulin resistance	Impaired glucose tolerance
Increased lipid oxidation	Energy requirements best met by feeding lipids

In contrast, injury (including surgery) and infection lead not only to the breakdown of energy stores but also to the rapid loss of protein stores.

In patients with sepsis, improvements in nutritional status will not occur in response to nutrition alone—treating the cause of sepsis is essential to achieve effective nutritional support.

When designing nutritional prescriptions, these factors should be taken into account. The following table serves as a simple guide:

Typical nutritional requirements for adults

	Normal	Stressed
Energy	25 kCal[a]/kg per day	35 kCal[b]/kg per day
% Energy as carbohydrate:lipid	75:25	50:50 or even 25:75
Nitrogen	1 gN/200 kCal[c]	1 gN/120 kCal[d]

[a]104 J; [b] 145 J; [c]837 J; [d]502 J

Very few patients require more than 35 kCal (~147 J)/kg per day, even if they are critically ill.

Methods of nutritional support

Nutritional support should be considered in all patients who have evidence of impaired nutritional status, or in those who are unlikely to achieve a nutritional intake appropriate to their requirements within 5 days. Nutritional support can be provided by enteral or intravenous routes. In general, the gut should be used if it is working. Enteral feeding is less expensive and, in units without special expertise in intravenous nutrition, may be safer. It may also reduce morbidity in critically ill patients by preserving gut epithelial integrity, although this is controversial.

Enteral nutritional support—when nutritional support is indicated and the gut is working

Oral feeding

This is the method of choice in the conscious patient with an intact gut and a normal swallowing mechanism. Hospital food is unfortunately often unpalatable and intake is frequently suboptimal.

Dietary supplements

A variety of sip feeds are available. All come in a selection of flavours and usually provide 200 kCal (832 J) in a 200 ml carton, with approximately 1.5 g of N. Many patients find them unpalatable and they may reduce their food intake, so that total energy intake remains the same.

Tube feeding

The gut can be intubated and feeding given in several ways:

* nasoenteric (nasogastric and nasoduodenal/nasojejunal);
* percutaneous endoscopic gastrostomy (PEG);
* percutaneous endoscopic (transgastric) jejunostomy (PEJ);
* surgical enterostomy (gastrostomy or jejunostomy)—may be placed at the time of surgery to provide for postoperative nutritional support (e.g. after oesophagectomy).

If enteral feeding for longer than 6 weeks is contemplated then a PEG or jejunostomy should be considered rather than a nasoenteric tube, because the risks of aspiration and oesophageal stricture are less. In general, jejunal feeding is preferred to gastric feeding as the incidence of reflux and diarrhoea is smaller. Most commercially available feeds provide 1 kCal (4.18 J)/ml and approximately 5 g of N/l. Feeding should start at approximately 30 ml/h and then increase progressively over the next 24 hours until the desired rate is reached (approx. 100 ml/h). It is customary to provide a 4-h rest period in a feeding regimen and deliver the required feed in the remaining 20 hours.

Parenteral feeding—when nutritional support is indicated and the gut is unavailable

Parenteral feeding may be required when the gut cannot be used. This can arise in the following circumstances:

(1) When the gastrointestinal tract is 'blocked' due to:
   • mechanical obstruction
   • paralytic ileus
   • intestinal pseudo-obstruction

(2) When the intestinal tract is inflamed because of:
   • inflammatory bowel disease
   • severe infective enteritis
   • radiotherapy
   • chemotherapy

(3) When the gastrointestinal tract fails to function adequately for other reasons
   • intra-abdominal sepsis
   • multiple organ failure
   • acute pancreatitis

Intravenous feeding

This can be delivered via:

• **Peripheral veins**—insertion takes little or no special skill and is safe. Nutrition is limited by the osmolality and pH of the feed, which tend to cause thrombophlebitis. Use of ultrafine polyurethane catheters, low-osmolality feed (based upon lipid) and heparin can allow effective 'peripheral parenteral nutrition –PPN' for up to 14 days in many cases.

• **Central veins**—catheter insertion carries a small but significant complication rate. The risk of thrombosis is much smaller than with PPN, but the consequences of line infection are significantly greater.

To minimize the risks of line infection, all intravenous feeding catheters should be inserted under sterile conditions in the operating theatre and thereafter used only for parenteral nutrition. They should be maintained by dedicated and trained nursing staff and handled according to strict aseptic techniques.

Complications of nutritional support

Nutritional support is frequently associated with complications. In the case of parenteral nutrition these may be life-threatening. They can generally be avoided by the creation of nutrition teams in whom experience and skill can be developed and maintained.

Complications can be divided into mechanical, infective, and metabolic causes.

Mechanical

Enteral

* Dislodgement, fracture or migration of feeding tubes (peritonitis, fistula formation, intestinal obstruction, aspiration)
* Tube occlusion

Parenteral

* Pneumothorax, arterial or cardiac injury, pericardial tamponade (usually at percutaneous insertion)
* Dislodgement or fracture of intravenous lines (air embolus, foreign-body embolus)
* Line occlusion (thrombotic, with lipid or calcium deposits)
* Thrombophlebitis
* Central vein thrombosis
* Atrial thrombosis
* Pulmonary embolus

Infective

Enteral

* Enteric infection associated with contaminated feed

Parenteral

* Exit-site infection
* Tunnel infection
* Catheter-related sepsis
* Infective endocarditis
* Sepsis associated with contaminated feed

Metabolic

Enteral

* Diarrhoea and dehydration (often related to overfeeding or use of hyperosmolar feeds)
* Nutritional deficiencies

Parenteral

* Hyperglycaemia
* Fatty liver
* Reactive hypoglycaemia (too abrupt a cessation of feed)
* Cholestasis (gallstones, intrahepatic cholestasis, leading to progressive liver failure)
* Hyperlipidaemia (with excessive lipid infusion)
* Metabolic acidosis (associated with excessive chloride administration)
* Nutritional deficiencies (folate, vitamins A and K, fatty acids, zinc, and selenium deficiency not uncommon, biotin and molybdenum deficiency have been described)

Chapter 6
Complications of blood transfusion and coagulation

Acute (immediate) transfusion reactions

These occur during or within 1–2 hours of completion of a transfusion. The most important causes are:

1. **Acute immune haemolysis**—which is life-threatening, is usually caused by ABO incompatibility, but less commonly, there may be other red cell antibodies. Clinically there is fever and hypotension, and there may be loin pain or pain at the infusion site. In an anaesthetized patient, hypotension and bleeding due to disseminated intravascular coagulopathy (DIC) may be the only finding. Immediate action is to stop the drip, but keep the intravenous line open. Treatment for shock is instituted and there may be a need to treat DIC. Check full blood count (FBC), perform a direct Coombs test and a coagulation screen with blood cultures and tests of renal and liver function. Save urine (test for haemoglobulinuria) and the transfusion pack must be kept for repeat serological testing.

2. **Acute non-immune haemolysis**—the most serious cause is bacterial contamination of blood causing marked fever and shock. Blood in the pack may be discoloured. Action should be taken as in acute immune haemolysis but Gram stains of blood and blood cultures are also necessary on both patient and donor blood. Broad-spectrum antibiotics must be instituted whilst waiting for the results of tests.

Other acute immune-mediated reactions include:

1. **Hypersensitivity to donor plasma proteins**—which usually presents as urticaria and is quite common, occurring in up to 1% of transfusions. It may require antihistamines (e.g. chlorphenamine (chlorpheniramine) 10 mg IV). A record must be made in the notes, as prophylactic antihistamine may be needed with or without hydrocortisone (100 mg IV) before subsequent transfusions. Anaphylaxis from anti-IgA antibody in IgA-deficient subjects is rare, although IgA deficiency occurs in about 1:500 people. Adrenaline (epinephrine) (0.4 ml 1:1000 SC or IM), hydrocortisone (100 mg IV), fluid volume (saline), and oxygen support may be required. Inform the haematologist.

2. **Transfusion-related acute lung injury (TRALI)**—is increasingly recognized as a severe acute complication, with 14 cases (2 deaths) reported to the Serious Hazards of Transfusion Scheme (SHOT) in 1997–98. It is caused by donor leucoagglutinins. Clinically fever, hypotension, non-productive cough, dyspnoea, and hypoxia are seen. Early respiratory support with intubation, oxygen, and possibly ventilation are required.

3. **Febrile, non-haemolytic reactions**—are usually caused by antibodies to donor leucocytes (all UK blood/blood products are now leucodepleted).

Other acute non-immune-mediated reactions include:

1. Congestive cardiac failure from volume overload.
2. Hypothermia, hyperkalaemia, and hypocalcaemia need to be considered after massive transfusions.

Delayed transfusion complications

These may occur days or weeks after a transfusion. There is fever with haemolysis in association with red cell alloantibodies. Transfusion-transmitted malaria is a much less common, but very important, consideration. Graft versus host disease (GvHD) is increasingly recognized as a serious delayed complication of transfusion in susceptible subjects, most commonly patients with lymphomas and certain other immunocompromised groups. Mediation is through viable, transfused donor T lymphocytes. GvDH presents with fever, skin rash, diarrhoea, and abnormal liver function tests, usually within 4 weeks of blood transfusion. This group of patients should receive only irradiated blood.

Post-transfusion purpura (PTP) is an important delayed immune reaction mediated by antiplatelet antibodies, usually anti-PIA (platelet impedance aggregation) in the recipient. A profound thrombocytopenia develops 1–2 weeks' post-transfusion. Patients are almost always multiparous females. Administration of high-dose intravenous immunoglobulin and transfusion of PIA[1]-negative platelets may be necessary.

Massive transfusions, where volumes equal to or more than the patients blood volume are administered within 24 h, carry additional complications. Early volume replacement with crystalloids and colloids is essential to counter shock. Depletion of coagulation factors and platelets may occur and regular FBCs and coagulation screens are required to recognize this and anticipate replacement requirements. Hypothermia should be avoided and warmed solutions and blood may be used. A proper blood warmer is necessary. Biochemical and ECG monitoring is required for the early recognition of hyperkalaemia, hypocalcaemia, and renal problems.

Infectious agents transmitted by blood-product transfusion

The statistical risk is not high in comparison with the identification/documentation errors described earlier, but it assumes a high public profile. Careful donor selection and improved testing procedures have further reduced transmission rates.

Approximate estimated risk of infectious donation per million donations (USA, 1991–93)

Human immunodeficiency virus (HIV)	2.03
Hepatitis B virus (HBV)	15.83
Hepatitis C virus (HCV)	9.7

The possibility of cytomegalovirus (CMV) transmission is important in the newborn and in immunodeficiency states. CMV-negative blood is available for these situations. New variant Creutzfeldt–Jakob disease (nvCJD) transmission is a theoretical possibility at present, and the universal leucodepletion programme is designed to prevent this possible risk.

Complications of coagulation

Surgery with anticoagulation

Minor surgery

Warfarin does not need to be reversed; the aim is for a target International normalized ratio (INR) of 2.0. If the INR is less than 2.5, surgery can proceed, but if greater than 2.5 the surgery should wait until help from a haematologist is given.

Major surgery

Standard practice

Stop warfarin 3 days before surgery. Start standard perioperative heparin prophylaxis when INR is less than 2.0. This will normally be with low molecular-weight heparin (LMWH). Monitoring with activated partial thromboplastin time (APTT) is not required with LMWH. Warfarin can be restarted as soon as the patient has an oral intake.

Major surgery in patients with mechanical heart valves

The short-term risk of thromboembolism in these patients when they are not fully anticoagulated is very small. Management, therefore, can follow standard practice as above, but this should be discussed with a cardiologist first. If a patient is considered at high risk, manage as below.

High-risk patients

For patients at high risk of venous thromboembolism (VTE) management should involve the giving of unfractionated heparin (UFH) by continuous infusion when the INR is less than 2.0, aiming for an APTT ratio of 1.5. Switch to LMWH postoperatively when the patient is stable. Warfarin can be restarted as soon as the patient has an oral intake. Heparin can be stopped when the INR is within the therapeutic range for 2 consecutive days. If heparin is continued, the platelet count should be checked at 5 and 10 days.

Assessment and prophylaxis for VTE

Risk assessment for VTE

This depends on the patient's features and diseases, and the surgical procedure. Age, obesity, varicose veins, immobility, pregnancy and the puerperium, previous VTE, and thrombophilia all pose an increased risk. Diseases and procedures giving increased risk include: malignancy, heart failure, trauma or surgery, polycythaemia, inflammatory bowel disease, lower limb paralysis, recent myocardial infarction, and nephrotic syndrome. Anticardiolipin syndrome is a less commonly acquired thrombophilic state which should be suspected if there is recurrent fetal loss, unexplained prolonged APTT, thrombocytopenia, or arterial/venous thrombosis at an early age.

Consideration of these factors gives low-, moderate-, and high-risk groups:

(1) Low risk (deep vein thrombosis (DVT) <10%):
  - minor surgery (<30 min) no risk factor other than age
  - major surgery (>30 min) age <40 years, no other risk factor

(2) Moderate risk (DVT 10–40%):
  - major surgery, age >40 years, no other risk factor
  - major medical illness, trauma, or burns
  - minor surgery, previous VTE or thrombophilia with no previous thrombosis

(3) High risk (DVT 40–80%):
  - major orthopaedic surgery, fracture, hip, pelvis, lower limb
  - major pelvic/abdominal surgery for malignancy
  - major surgery, previous VTE

Inherited thrombophilia

This is much less common than the above acquired risk factors, but has assumed a high profile recently, mainly in relation to thrombosis associated with oral contraceptive usage. Thrombosis at an early age (arterial <35 years, venous <40 years), in unusual sites (e.g. mesenteric, retinal), a strong family history (two or more first-degree relatives) all warrant further testing. Test for antithrombin III (ATIII), protein S, protein C, and activated protein C resistance, which is usually associated with the factor V Leiden defect.

Prophylaxis

Low-dose heparin is widely used and effective. LMWH is more effective in elective orthopaedic surgery, does not show definite clinical advantage in other situations, but is more convenient (once-daily administration) and has better bioavailability. A typical management regime using, for example, tinzaparin, would be:

Moderate risk   3500 IU daily SC

High risk   70 IU/kg daily SC

Prophylaxis should begin preoperatively and continue until the patient is reasonably mobile. The platelet count should be checked at 5 days, 10 days if heparin is continued. Check with anaesthetists about the use of an epidural. A dose of heparin less than 12 h before an epidural may cause complications.

Preoperative assessment of bleeding problems

The patient history is most important. The factors to enquire about are previous bleeding or bruising, the site, the duration, whether lifelong or recent, or if a transfusion was required. Response to previous surgery needs to be recorded together with a drug, alcohol, and family history. Examination should look for petechiae, bruising, capillary abnormalities, hepatomegaly, and haemorrhage into joints or muscle compartments.

Investigations should include: FBC, prothrombin time (PT), and APTT. These should be done if there is a suspicion from the history or examination and always if proposed investigative or surgical procedures involve the liver or biliary tract. Further assays may be required depending on the situation, e.g. fibrinogen, D-dimers in suspected DIC, or bleeding time (BT), when screening tests are all normal, but where there is clear clinical evidence of abnormal bleeding/bruising.

Prolongation of the PT by more than 5 s, APTT by more than 10 s, or a significantly reduced platelet count ($<70 \times 10^9$/l) should always be discussed with the haematologist before surgery is undertaken. Replacement with fresh-frozen plasma (10–15 ml/kg), cryoprecipitate (1 bag/10 kg), platelet concentrates, or specific factor concentrates may be required.

Chapter 7
Pressure sores: causes and potential complications

Risk factors

Although all patients are at risk of developing pressure ulcers, some are more at risk than others. For example, tissue oxygenation may be compromised in smokers and during anaesthesia. Low haemoglobin levels, because of a reduction in oxygen delivery, also increase risk. Patients with peripheral vascular disease, diabetes, or cardiac disease are also at greater risk. Age is another important factor, perhaps because of changes in elastin and collagen networks in ageing tissue. Gender may have an effect on the viscoelastic properties of tissues relating to female hormonal changes.

Poor nutritional status, mostly related to reduced serum albumin levels, has also been associated with an increased risk of pressure damage. Poor nutrition may, however, be more appropriately associated with the presence of pressure ulcers (see below) rather than an increased risk of developing them. Patients with a low body mass index (BMI = wt(kg)/ht (m)^2) are at greater risk because bony prominences are not protected by a thick layer of subcutaneous tissue. Conversely, obese patients are also at increased risk, perhaps because of reduced blood supply (and therefore oxygen) to their excess fatty tissue and because of poor mobility.

Intraoperative episode

Intraoperative episode

During surgery each patient is subjected to complex metabolic and circulatory changes following anaesthesia and surgical trauma. The cardiovascular system is in a state of flux, oxygen demand is increased, and changes can be rapid and wide ranging, particularly during induction of anaesthesia. An episode of haemorrhagic shock can reduce arterial blood pressure, cause vasoconstriction, and thereby affect the microcirculation, particularly in skin, and so increase the risk of pressure damage. Anaesthetic agents can cause episodes of hypotension which also decrease capillary critical-closing pressures and increase the risk of skin ischaemia. Pressure damage acquired in the operating theatre has a more complex aetiology than other hospital-acquired ulcers.

Risk assessment

A major problem for healthcare professionals is the timely, and accurate, identification of vulnerability so that effective prevention strategies may be implemented. This identification process is carried out on a day-to-day basis through formal risk-assessment scores, the most well known being the Norton Score, Braden Scale, Douglas Score, and the Waterlow Score. There are several inaccuracies related to these scoring systems: they have not been the subject of rigorous clinical testing and their scientific value is questionable. These criticisms may have arisen because risk-assessment scores have tended to become a substitute for, rather than an aid to, clinical judgement.

The damage process

The damage process

For a pressure sore to develop, two conditions must apply. First, the localized external pressure must be of a greater intensity than the capillary pressure so that the microcirculation is occluded. Second, this occlusion, which in effect stops the oxygen supply to the cells, must last long enough for tissue damage to occur. Therefore, although the two extrinsic factors—intensity and time—are important, occlusion of the blood supply, and therefore the potential for ischaemia and tissue necrosis, depends on the intrinsic factors of capillary blood flow and the tension of the capillary walls. The equilibrium of each vessel is dependent on three variables: (1) the radius of the cylindrical vessel; (2) the total tension of the wall; and (3) the difference in pressure across the wall (blood pressure minus tissue pressure). Low pressures exerted over a long duration, or high pressures of short duration, result in experimentally induced pressure ulcers. It is also thought that repeated, intermittent external pressures are more likely to cause pressure ulcers than the first pressure loading and that the actual damage caused by repeated pressure insults may be more severe. This may relate to reperfusion injury with the production of oxygen free radicals, which trigger a chain of bio-chemical responses. If the circulation is occluded and the venous and lymph flow is inhibited, the waste products of metabolism accumulate within both the cells and the interstitial spaces, and cellular processes begin to fail as energy is depleted. Metabolites continue to be produced resulting in tissue acidosis, which in turn leads to capillary permeability, oedema, and cell death.

The trauma caused by the disruptive pressure forces also initiates haemostatic mechanisms. There is a subsequent increase in platelet activation with thrombosis which causes occlusion of the microcirculation and dislocation of endothelial cell-junction complexes. Visible manifestation of early damage is the skin pallor that characterizes the ischaemic episode. When the pressure is removed, the reddened skin characteristic of reactive hyperaemia may be visible. This reaction may not be immediate and can be delayed for 5–10 minutes, depending on the rate of capillary refill, following the release of pressure. Reactive hyperaemia is a normal response after a period of external pressure, and therefore may have a beneficial effect. The response, sometimes called the 'blood flow debt', is prompted by tissue oxygen deprivation and the accumulation of metabolites and is independent of the nervous system. It may be that a delayed recovery time (slower capillary refill) is indicative of a susceptibility to tissue damage and ulcer formation. Reactive hyperaemia may be impaired in acute illness, may diminish with age, and may be reduced by immobilization and bedrest, or in spinal cord injury.

Classification and grading of pressure damage

Classification and grading of pressure damage

Pressure ulcers can be classified according to the depth of the initial damage. Type 1 ulcers are characterized by superficial skin damage and caused by exclusion of the blood supply to the skin. Type 2 ulcers, sometimes called 'closed' pressure ulcers, are severe ulcers resulting from damage within the deeper layers of muscle adjacent to the bone. As it is thought that resting muscle tissue is less able to tolerate ischaemia than skin, this may explain the more extensive damage associated with type 2 ulcers. The superficial layers of intact skin conceal damage to endothelial cells and the possible activation of haemostatic mechanisms, platelet thrombosis, and occlusion of major blood vessels. These 'closed' ulcers may also provide an indicator of the presence of generalized endothelial damage that may be related to disseminated intravascular coagulation (DIC). Pressure ulcers can also be graded according to the degree of damage. Although several systems have been developed, that of the European Pressure Ulcer Advisory Panel is recommended for clinical use (see table below).

Grading of pressure ulcers

Grade 1	Non-blanchable erythema of intact skin. Discolouration of the skin, warmth, oedema, induration, or hardness may also be used as indicators, particularly on individuals with darker skins.
Grade 2	Partial-thickness skin loss involving epidermis, dermis, or both. The ulcer is superficial and presents clinically as an abrasion or blister.
Grade 3	Full-thickness skin loss involving damage to, or necrosis of, subcutaneous tissue that may extend down to, but not through, underlying fascia.
Grade 4	Extensive destruction, tissue necrosis, or damage to muscle, bone, or supporting structures with or without full-thickness skin loss.

Source: European Pressure Ulcer Advisory Panel.

Prevention

Research has shown that the damage caused by pressure may not always be immediately apparent. This delayed manifestation may be of hours but it could be of days, which makes it difficult to identify when the damage took place and also its exact cause. Because of this, it is essential that there is continuity of preventive care, especially when patients are moved through different clinical areas within the hospital. This is particularly important for surgical patients who are cared for by different groups of nursing staff in the ward, operating theatre, recovery room, and during transport. Pressure-relieving care should not be neglected in accident and emergency departments, intensive care units, and rehabilitation wards.

Traditionally, the prevention of pressure ulcers has focused on altering the duration of pressure by changing a patient's position. Technological innovations in mattress production have concentrated on preventing long periods of pressure intensity. As a first-line approach, static mattresses and overlays are available (for both ward and intraoperative use) that reduce interface pressures. For patients at higher risk, there are several dynamic mattresses and overlays that are based on alternating pressure or on low-air-loss systems. These are mainly for ward use and it is only recently that any dynamic systems (alternating pressure overlays) have become available for intraoperative use.

Complications of pressure ulcers

Pressure ulcers can result in longer hospital stays and they are expensive to manage in terms of special beds, dressings, and nursing time. There is also the potential for complications. The worst, although relatively rare, are septicaemia and osteomyelitis and the potential for these life- and/or limb-threatening conditions must always be considered. Systemic antibiotics may be required together with repeated, extensive debridement of necrotic tissue and the release of pus. Any exudating ulcer involves protein loss and the potential for causing, or exacerbating, malnutrition and anaemia. Dietary supplements of protein and calories, as well as fluid electrolytes and vitamins, may therefore be necessary. Effective pain control is also an essential aspect of the treatment of a patient with a pressure ulcer. Care should be taken with spinal or epidural anaesthesia as they may add to immobility.

Treatment should involve the use of an adequate pressure-relieving/reducing mattress or overlay, which is an expensive resource. Some ulcers are difficult to heal and there is always the possibility of further damage occurring if immobility persists. Debridement of necrotic tissue should be undertaken early. Methods of debridement include surgical, enzymatic, autolytic, larva therapy, or a combination of these. In some circumstances this may involve surgical debridement under anaesthesia. This is not only traumatic for the patient but also involves the additional risk of anaesthesia, but it usually ensures excision of all dead tissue with adequate drainage of infection. Ignoring dead or infected material physically prevents wound contraction and epithelialization, and is a constant source of white-cell and macrophage-activation proinflammatory cytokine and other mediator release which leads to sepsis and impairment of healing.

Pressure ulcers are a painful and distressing complication of hospitalization. They are also an increasing cause of litigation—every patient with a pressure ulcer is a potential claimant against the NHS. Pressure ulcers are also used as a performance indicator of quality care and are an important element of risk management frameworks. All the evidence suggests they can be prevented through comprehensive strategies that should be in place in all clinical environments. Continuity of pressure-relieving care is essential.

Chapter 8
Complications after drugs used perioperatively or in surgical intervention

General advice on the use of medicines

Medicines bring undoubted benefits to healthcare, but there is always the potential for risk. Strategies to avoid this risk include being aware of the possible risks and reducing the unnecessary exposure of patients to medicines. The maxim that 'more is rarely better—it is usually less safe and always more expensive' is invariably true.

The *British National Formulary* (BNF) is an excellent, comprehensive, and very readable pocket-size textbook on most aspects of medicine use. It is also provided free of charge to all hospital doctors and pharmacists and is regularly updated. It is important that all practising doctors are familiar with it.

When writing a prescription, never use abbreviations, be clear about your intentions, and be specific about the dose, the route of administration, and the duration of treatment. Always check your doses, especially for new or unfamiliar medicines, and for patient groups with whom you are not familiar, e.g. paediatrics. Be aware of interactions and the common adverse side-effects.

Advice is always available from pharmacists and experienced colleagues. Most hospitals have a medicines information centre in the pharmacy. This is staffed by an experienced pharmacist, with access to a range of specialist drug and therapeutics textbooks, journals, and databases. This is a free service, and well worth getting to know, as is your local medical library service.

Use a framework for dealing with prescribing, such as the mnemonic NESCAFE, i.e.:

Necessary

Effective

Safe

Cost

Appropriateness

Follow-up

Evaluation

Be aware that medicines prescribed for a patient for a particular purpose will only be required as long as that purpose still exists. Discontinue all medicines that are no longer required. Ensure that *pro re nata* (PRN; when required) medicines, which were used in hospital, are not automatically prescribed on discharge. This is how patients could start using benzodiazepines for night-time sedation at home.

Medicines used in theatres

Theatres are areas that are not subject to the usual prescription surveillance, when large amounts of medication are used sometimes rapidly, and as such are also an environment where errors can occur.

The following points should be noted.

• When a particular medicine is routinely used, it is tempting for practitioners to rely on what an ampoule or box looks like (e.g. colour, style, manufacturer's livery) to identify it. This is no substitute for reading the label, noting the drug concentration and its expiry date. Manufacturers will often specialize in drugs for a therapeutic area and will market drugs with opposing effects in similar packages.

• Colour coding is often suggested as a way to differentiate between different types of medicines. This approach has difficulties due to the large number of products used, and the number of manufacturers used to source them. Packaging and manufacturers both change very regularly. Colour blindness amongst staff could also be a problem. There is no substitute for reading the label.

• Get all calculations independently checked by another healthcare professional familiar with the calculation. Never tell them the answer, but get them to recalculate and confirm that you both have the same answer.

• All parenteral solutions should be made up freshly when required. Microbiological considerations generally mean that once made up solutions should have a maximum shelf-life of less than 24 hours. Often chemical instability will dictate a shorter shelf-life.

• Unlabelled syringes are obviously dangerous and subject to potential confusion.

• Obtain and use blank labels specifically designed for parenteral drugs.

• All administration of medicines legally requires that a prescription be written. You should ensure that all such details of prescribing and administration are recorded on either the patient's main drug chart or the theatre drug chart.

Adverse drug reactions (ADRs)

ADRs can be divided into two types:

(1) *Predicted:*
   - dose-related
   - logical, from a knowledge of their pharmacology

(2) *Idiosyncratic:*
   - allergic reactions
   - autoimmune
   - illogical

ADRs account for significant morbidity and mortality. They are responsible for 5% of hospital admissions. In hospital, 7% of patients will suffer a serious ADR, of which 0.1–0.3% are fatal. There is a national formal scheme whereby doctors and hospital pharmacists can report ADRs to the Committee on the Safety of Medicines (see BNF for details). Many hospitals run their own scheme. In a new initiative hospital pharmacists can now report ADRs directly. Be aware that no matter how good a prescriber you are, your patients will suffer from ADRs. However, a good medication history and knowledge of therapeutics will minimize this risk. Certain patient populations and disease states will pose additional problems for prescribing and such patients are at an increased risk of suffering from ADRs:

- paediatrics
- elderly
- those with renal and hepatic impairment
- multi-organ failure
- multiple drug therapy

Always consider medicines as a cause of toxicity, and beware of treating one medicine's toxic side-effects with another medicine, e.g. the short-term use of opiates causing constipation leading to long-term laxative use, or antinauseants causing parkinsonism, with the result that the patient is given a diagnosis of Parkinson's disease and treated for such.

Drug interactions

Detailed information on drug interactions is beyond the scope of this text. First refer to the BNF, and then to specialist texts or a drug information centre.

Drug interactions occur because one medicine interferes with the pharmacokinetics (the effect of the body on the drug, i.e. absorption, distribution, metabolism, and excretion) or pharmacodynamics (the effects of the drug on the body) of another medicine.

Medicines that interfere (inhibit or induce) with the enzymatic (usually hepatic via cytochrome P450) degradation pathways for chemicals cause changes in the pharmacokinetics of other medicines.

+ Enzyme inducers include rifampicin, most antiepileptics, and cigarette smoke.
+ Enzyme inhibitors include quinolones, chloramphenicol, omeprazole, and cimetidine.

The result of the interaction is that the effects of one medicine are enhanced or reduced.

For those drugs that are toxic at low doses, a drug interaction, which further enhances their effect, will be very dangerous. (These drugs with a low ratio of therapeutic dose to toxic dose are known as drugs with a low therapeutic ratio.)

Medicines with a low therapeutic ratio include:

+ warfarin and other anticoagulants
+ digoxin
+ antiarrhythmics, e.g. lidocaine (lignocaine) and disopyramide
+ methylxanthines, e.g. theophylline and aminophylline
+ some antibiotics, e.g. gentamicin and vancomycin
+ antiepileptics, e.g. phenytoin and carbamazepine

Medicines in surgery

Perioperative maintenance medication for chronic conditions

It is vital that a preoperative medicines assessment is carried out to record the patient's medication history. This should include the recent history of:

* medication obtained via the patient's doctor;
* medication purchased over the counter—'self medication';
* medication borrowed from relatives or friends;
* possible illicit substance use;
* herbal or 'natural' remedies;
* compliance;
* allergic reactions/ADRs;
* medication stopped within the last 3 months, e.g. corticosteroids.

The anaesthetist needs to be aware of any medicines being taken by patients prior to surgery. One of the aims of a preoperative medicines assessment is to ensure that during surgery anaesthetists are aware of potential problems. They can then ensure that patients have a stable and controlled regulation of vital body systems. This is especially so with regard to the cardiovascular, respiratory, metabolic, endocrine, central nervous, and coagulation systems.

Abrupt, temporary discontinuation of medicines due to overzealous 'nil by mouth' (NBM) policies can lead to:

* withdrawal reactions (e.g. benzodiazepines and fitting, and withdrawal symptoms if opiate-dependent);
* rebound effects (hypertensive crisis with withdrawal of antihypertensives);
* impaired reactions to surgery (impaired stress reaction with corticosteroids);
* unmasking of clinical disease (e.g. antiepileptics).

All of which can lead to a stormy and hazardous postoperative phase.

NBM policies must enable the continuation of vital medicines wherever possible. If the oral route is definitely compromised, then alternative formulations of medicines for other routes of administration are usually available. If they are not, then other suitable therapeutic options could be used by the anaesthetist. (Refer to the table below.)

Oral drug therapy guidelines for surgical patients

BNF class	Drug group (examples)	Risk	Use preoperatively when nil by mouth	Alternative postop. if unable to take oral medication	Management
Gastrointestinal	Antispasmodics, motility stimulants (mebeverine)	Increased risk of ileus	Omit preoperative dose		Monitor U+E
	H₂-receptor antagonists (ranitidine)	Reduce risk of acid aspiration	Give 2 h preoperatively	IV ranitidine	
	Proton-pump inhibitors (omeprazole)	Reduce risk of acid aspiration	Give 2 h preoperatively	IV ranitidine	
Cardiovascular	ACE inhibitors (ACEI) (lisinopril, enalapril)	Hypotension Renal failure Reduced cerebral blood flow	Minimum withholding time depends on ACEI (>12 h captopril, >24 h lisinopril). Can be continued with caution. Discuss with anaesthetist	Alt. IV antihypertensive agent/IV diuretic. Some ACE inhibitors absorbed sublingually, e.g. captopril	Monitor BP and U + E Avoid NSAIDs
	Angiotensin II antagonists (losartan)	Hypotension Renal failure	Can be continued with caution. Discuss with anaesthetist	Alt. IV antihypertensive agent/IV diuretic	Monitor BP and U + E Avoid NSAIDs
	Alpha-blockers (doxazosin)	Hypotension	Continue—improves c/v stability	Alt. IV antihypertensive	Monitor BP

(continued)

Oral drug therapy guidelines for surgical patients (*continued*)

BNF class	Drug group (examples)	Risk	Use preoperatively when nil by mouth	Alternative postop. if unable to take oral medication	Management
	Antiarrhythmics	Prolong n/m block Bradycardia Reduce cardiac output	Continue	Use IV alternative within same class	ECG monitoring Monitor U + E
	Anticoagulants (warfarin)	Haemorrhagic risk	*Minor*: INR 2.0 on day of op. *Major*: stop 3 days before. Aim or INR <2. High-risk patients start on continuous heparin infusion or treatment dose of LMWH. (See local haematology guidelines)	Heparin (UFH or LMWH) prophylaxis until oral intake resumed and INR within therapeutic range for 2 consecutive days	INR, APTT (if on UFH), platelet counts (>5 days UFH) Check BNF for interacting drugs
	Antiplatelets (aspirin, clopidogrel, dipyridamole)	Haemorrhagic risk	Usually stop 7 days prior to surgery. Seek advice in patients with severe IHD or history CVA/TIA. Can restart immediately postop.		
	Beta-blockers (atenolol, propranolol)	Hypotension Bradycardia Bronchospasm	Continue—improves c/v stability. Rebound if withdrawn	Give alt. IV β-blocker or GTN patch if patient symptomatic	Monitor BP and pulse

				Monitor BP and pulse
Calcium antagonists	Hypotension Bradycardia (verapamil)	Continue	IV antihypertensive	Monitor BP and pulse
– diltiazem, verapamil	Additive effect with enflurane, halothane			
– dihydropyridines	Additive effect with isoflurane			
Central-acting hypertensives (clonidine, methyldopa)	Hypotension	Rebound if withdrawn—hypertensive crisis with one missed dose. Continue		Monitor BP
Digoxin	Increased toxicity with suxamethonium Arrhythmias	Continue	IV digoxin. Convert PO to IV dose using conversion factor (0.65 tablets, 0.80 elixir)	Monitor digoxin level and K^+
Diuretics—thiazide and loop (bendroflumethiazide, furosemide)	Arrhythmias Prolonged n/m block	Continue	IV diuretics	Monitor BP, fluids, U + E
Diuretics—potassium-sparing (amiloride, spironolactone)	Tissue damage Reduced kidney perfusion Hyperkalaemia	Omit on morning of surgery	Add potassium to fluids where needed	Monitor U + E
Nitrates	Hypotension	Continue	Topical, buccal, sublingual, and IV forms available	Monitor BP

(continued)

Oral drug therapy guidelines for surgical patients (*continued*)

BNF class	Drug group (examples)	Risk	Use preoperatively when nil by mouth	Alternative postop. if unable to take oral medication	Management
	K$^+$ channel activators (nicorandil)	Hypotension	Continue	Alternative antianginals (see nitrates)	Monitor BP
	Vasodilators (hydralazine)	Reflex tachycardia Hypotension	Continue	IV alternatives available	Monitor BP and pulse
CNS	Anticonvulsants	Induce hepatic enzymes (phenytoin, barbiturates, carbamazepine) Anaesthetics may depress hepatic drug elimination Resistance to non-depolarizing muscle relaxants	Continue	Phenytoin—IV at 90% of current dose Phenobarbital—IV Carbamazepine—rectal (125 mg PR = 100 mg PO) Sodium valproate—IV	May need increased doses of induction agents and opiates. Phenytoin levels pre- and postop.
	Antipsychotics (haloperidol, thioridazine)	Sedation Arrhythmias	Continue (antiemetic effect useful)	IV alternatives available	
	Benzodiazepines (diazepam, temazepam)	Tolerance Additive effects Withdrawal syndrome	Continue	IV and rectal forms if necessary	May need lower/higher doses for sedation

Lithium	Prolongs n/m blockade Toxicity	Discontinue 24–48h before major operations. Restart postop.	Haloperidol ± lorazepam in some cases	Check levels, monitor fluids and U + E. Avoid NSAIDs
Monoamine oxidase inhibitors (MAOIs)	Hypertension, hyperthermia, convulsions, coma with opioids, esp. pethidine and sympathomimetics. Can be fatal	Stop 2 weeks before surgery. Newer reversible MAOIs are reversible after 24–48h. Psychiatric advice needed. Alternatively, use 'safe' anaesthesia. Discuss with anaesthetist	Withhold whilst on opioids	
Tricyclic antidepressants (TCAs)	Increase effect of exogenous catecholamines, e.g. adrenaline resulting in arrhythmias	Omit preoperative dose. Avoid proarrhythmic anaesthetic agents. Use reduced doses of sympathomimetic agents	Extended half-lives so can be omitted for few days	
Selective serotonin-reuptake inhibitors (SSRIs)	Serotonin syndrome, e.g. pethidine, pentazocine	Omit preoperative dose. Avoid interacting agents	Extended half-lives so can be omitted for few days	
Anti-Parkinsonian drugs	Arrhythmias Hypertension (L-dopa) Symptoms exacerbated by some antiemetics	Continue	No IV but ng L-dopa possible	Avoid metoclopramide and prochlorperazine

(continued)

Oral drug therapy guidelines for surgical patients (*continued*)

BNF class	Drug group (examples)	Risk	Use preoperatively when nil by mouth	Alternative postop. if unable to take oral medication	Management
Endocrine	Insulin	Increased risk of postop. infection Altered requirements	Glucose, potassium, insulin (GKI)	GKI (see local protocol)	Monitor blood glucose and K⁺
	Oral hypoglycaemics (tolbutamide, gliclazide)	Perioperative hypoglycaemia Lactic acidosis (metformin)	*Minor* surgery—omit on day of op. *Major* surgery—stop once patient NBM either on day of op. or day before if long-acting agent or metformin used	GKI for major surgery (see local protocol)	Monitor blood glucose and K⁺
	Corticosteroids (long-term/last 3 months)	Hypotension Impaired stress reaction Delayed wound healing Altered immune function Risk of bleeding with NSAIDs	Continue at increased dose	Increase dose to cover surgery. Dose depends on usual steroid dose, duration, indication, e.g. 25–50 mg IV hydrocortisone every 8 h	Monitor glucose and K⁺

Combined oral contraceptive (COC) (oestrogen-containing)	Increased risk of DVT/PE in major surgery	Discontinue 4 weeks prior to major surgery. Progestogen-only pill is suitable alternative	Restart with first merses that occur at least 2 weeks after discharge	Thromboprophylaxis
Progestogen-only contraceptives (includes injectables)	No added risk of thrombo-embolic risk	Continue		
Hormone replacement therapy	Slight increased risk of DVT/PE	Can be continued if patient wishes. If to discontinue then need to stop 4 weeks prior to surgery	Restart after discharge as for COC	Thromboprophylaxis
Thyroxine and anti-thyroid drugs (carbimazole)	Impaired stress reaction if hypothyroid	Continue	May discontinue therapy for several days due to long half-life	TFTs to ensure dose adequate
Musculoskeletal/joint disease NSAIDs (diclofenac, piroxicam)	GI haemorrhage Impaired wound healing Renal impairment	Stop to allow platelet recovery. 1 day prior to surgery for short-acting drugs, 3 days for long-acting	PR preps available	U + E
Methotrexate	Impaired wound healing Renal impairment	Stop 1–2 weeks prior to surgery	Restart once wound healed	U + E. Caution with NSAIDs

(continued)

Oral drug therapy guidelines for surgical patients (continued)

BNF class	Drug group (examples)	Risk	Use preoperatively when nil by mouth	Alternative postop. if unable to take oral medication	Management
	Azathioprine	Major wound complications	Stop 3 weeks before surgery	Restart once wound healed	
Topical eye preps	Steroids, pilocarpine, β-blockers (timolol)	Bradycardia due to systemic absorption (β-blockers)	Continue		

The above table is not exhaustive, although most drug groups not included in the above table can be omitted pre/perioperatively. If in doubt contact an anaesthetist or the ward pharmacist for further advice.

Abbrev.: NBM, nil by mouth; preop., preoperatively; postop., postoperatively; U + E, urea and electrolytes; IV, intravenous; PO, orally; PR, rectally; ACE, angiotensin-converting enzyme; BP, blood pressure; NSAIDs, non-steroidal anti-inflammatory drugs; c/v, cardiovascular; n/m, neuromuscular; ECG, electrocardiograph; INR, International normalized ratio; LMWH, low molecular-weight heparin; UFH, unfractionated heparin; APTT, activated partial thromboplastin time; BNF, *British National Formulary*; IHD, ischaemic heart disease; CVA, cerebrovascular accident; TIA, transient ischaemic attack; GTN, glyceryl trinitrate; DVT, deep vein thrombosis; PE, pulmonary embolus; TFTs, thyroid function tests; GI, gastrointestinal.

Hypertension

Antihypertensives (some not all) can cause a rebound hypertension if abruptly discontinued. These include α-blockers such as prazosin and doxazosin and β-blockers such as propranolol and atenolol.

Diabetes

Altered insulin and carbohydrate requirements due to fasting and surgery mean that patients need individual assessment. Oral hypoglycaemics (e.g. gliclazide, chlorpropamide, glibenclamide) should be stopped once the patient is NBM (or the day before if they are long-acting drugs) and a sliding-scale insulin regimen used. A sliding scale will also be used for diabetics generally using insulin.

Corticosteroids

Patients who have been taking systemic glucocorticosteroids (prednisolone, dexamethasone, and hydrocortisone) for at least 3 months (or have completed a long course in the last 3 months) will be at risk of an impaired reaction to stress, cardiovascular instability, delayed wound healing, and depressed immune function. An increased dose will be necessary to cover surgery to prevent an Addisonian-like collapse. Appropriate prophylactic antibiotic therapy is necessary due to this depressed immune function.

Oral contraceptives and hormone replacement therapy (HRT)

The action to be taken depends on the type of oral contraceptive being used, and the type of surgery. For minor surgery (e.g. laparoscopic sterilization or tooth extraction) or for contraceptives that do not contain oestrogen then no action is required.

Oral contraceptives containing oestrogen should be discontinued 4 weeks before major elective surgery, or surgery to the legs. Alternative contraceptive methods should also be used. For emergency surgery when this is not possible, prophylactic low-dose heparin should be considered.

HRT does increase the risk of thromboembolism. In women with other risk factors for thromboembolism it may be worth temporarily stopping HRT.

Anticoagulants

There is an obvious risk of haemorrhage in patients using warfarin. Options available include switching to heparin therapy, or for minor operations reducing the INR to 2.0 for the day of the operation. For major operations the INR may need to be less than 2.0, with continuous heparin to keep the activated partial thromboplastin time (APTT) at 1.5. Specialist haematological advice is usually necessary.

Antidepressants

Monoamine oxidase inhibitors (MAOIs) (e.g. tranylcypromine, phenelzine) should be stopped 2 weeks before surgery due to the potential for serious interactions with sympathomimetic drugs (e.g. adrenaline (epinephrine) and pethidine). The newer reversible inhibitors of monoamine type A (RIMA) such as moclobemide, are reversible after 24–48 hours.

Tricyclic antidepressants (e.g. amitriptyline, lofepramine) can be continued, but patients are at an increased risk of arrhythmias and hypotension. The effects of exogenous catecholamines (e.g. adrenaline) can be potentiated. Any withdrawal should be planned and gradual in order to prevent a relapse.

Lithium therapy can be continued for minor surgery and stopped 2 days before major surgery. Fluid and electrolytes should be monitored.

Anticonvulsants

These should be continued to enable seizure control. However, usually these drugs will have induced hepatic enzyme function so that increased doses of induction agents and opiates may be needed. Some anaesthetic drugs may depress hepatic drug excretion. Close monitoring of anticonvulsants, which have a low ratio of therapeutic to toxic effects, will be needed, e.g. phenytoin.

Anxiolytics

There is a definite risk, especially for short-acting benzodiazepines like lorazepam, of a withdrawal reaction. In addition, there may be a possible additive effect with other sedative agents used in anaesthesia, or conversely tolerance may be a problem.

Respiratory therapy

Patients with asthma or chronic obstructive pulmonary disease (COPD) will require bronchodilators or corticosteroids to maintain good pulmonary function. This therapy should be continued perioperatively.

Glaucoma therapy

Ocular therapy for glaucoma can be continued without compromising a NBM policy. You should be aware that systemic absorption of some eye drops can occur, especially with β-blockers, e.g. timolol.

Medicines affecting thyroid function

Thyroxine or antithyroid drugs should be continued if possible to avoid metabolic changes. However, thyroxine has a long half-life and may be omitted for a single day or two.

Immunosuppressants

Immunosuppressants, e.g. methotrexate and azathioprine, will impair tissue healing. There is obviously a balance between risk and benefit about temporarily discontinuing these medicines perioperatively.

Commonly used perioperative drugs

Opiates

+ Most patients who have never before had opiates suffer from nausea and vomiting. Prescribe an antinauseant like metoclopramide or prochlorperazine at the same time as morphine.

+ All opiates cause respiratory depression, which is dependent on their potency, and the dose used. Beware of patients with a decreased respiratory reserve.

+ All opiates cause constipation, if this is a long-term problem a stimulant laxative such as senna can be used. Beware of patients with an acute abdomen as the purgative effect may result in perforation.

+ All opiates can cause behavioural toxicity, particularly dysphorias. This may be a problem especially in older patients.

Doses of opiates should be appropriate to the patient, their body weight, and any concomitant disease:

+ use low doses in the elderly and debilitated patient;

+ use low doses or avoid in patients with renal or hepatic impairment;

+ avoid the use of opiates in patients with a head injury or raised intracranial pressure (can interfere with pupilliary responses).

Antinauseants

Antinauseants, which block central dopamine receptors (e.g. metoclopramide and prochlorperazine), can cause significant behavioural toxicity, sedation, and acute dystonic reactions. These facial and skeletal muscle spasms are more common in the young, in females, and in elderly and debilitated patients. They tend to occur soon after therapy has started. The dystonias, such as oculogyric crisis or torticollis, can be treated if severe by parenteral antimuscarinics, e.g. procyclidine or benzatropine.

Other extrapyramidal side-effects can occur on prolonged therapy, e.g. Parkinsonian symptoms with tremor and akathisia.

Antihistamines such as cyclizine are suitable alternatives to prochlorperazine and metoclopramide, although not as efficacious. They can cause drowsiness and often show anticholinergic side-effects such as dry mouth and blurred vision.

5-HT$_3$ antagonists, such as ondansetron, are useful as second- or third-line therapy in patients who cannot tolerate standard antinauseants, and they also have a specific use in cytotoxic chemotherapy. They should be considered as prophylaxis in patients known to be at risk of a decreased level of consciousness (oral surgery), or who have a history of uncontrolled postoperative nausea and vomiting

Non-steroidal anti-inflammatories (NSAIDs)

Although these medicines are devoid of the respiratory depression and drowsiness caused by opiates, and are very effective analgesics, there are specific safety concerns especially with their long-term use.

NSAIDs cause gastric irritation and should be avoided in patients with active peptic ulceration who are at an increased risk of haemorrhage or perforation. NSAIDs are contraindicated in patients with a history of hypersensitivity (asthma, urticaria, angiodema, and rhinitis) to aspirin or other NSAIDs and in patients with inflammatory bowel disease.

Caution is required with the use of NSAIDs in patients with renal, hepatic, or cardiac impairment as NSAIDs may cause a decrease in renal function. Patients also taking angiotensin-converting enzyme (ACE) inhibitors (e.g. captopril, enalapril, lisinopril) maybe at a higher risk of renal impairment due to a drug interaction.

When used intravenously, additional contraindications include bleeding diathesis, operations with a high risk of haemorrhage, history of confirmed or suspected cerebrovascular bleeding, history of asthma, hypovolaemia, and dehydration.

NSAIDs are more effective when used regularly rather than on a PRN basis. They have a useful opiate-sparing effect and have additive effects in combination with simple analgesics such as paracetamol.

Paracetamol/opiate combinations

Combinations of paracetamol with a low-dose opiate (dihydrocodeine, codeine, dextropropoxyphene) are popular as minor to moderate analgesics. Evidence for the efficacy of adding low-dose opiates to paracetamol is limited and controversial. However, they are popular with clinicians and patients.

Increasing the dose of opiates will of course improve efficacy but will produce the same problems listed above with opiates in general.

The benefits of therapy with paracetamol are optimized by using a regular dose, rather than a PRN regimen, if patients have constant pain. The efficacy of regular paracetamol should not be underestimated.

Thromboprophylaxis (see Chapter 2—Venous thromboembolization)

Consider appropriate therapeutic and mechanical measures to prevent deep vein thromboses (DVTs) and pulmonary embolisms (PEs). The use of either unfractionated heparin or low molecular-weight heparin (LMWH) should be encouraged. Costs of both are approximately equal, LMWH may be slightly more effective especially in orthopaedic surgery and is easier to administer once a day.

IV therapy (see Chapter 4— Complications of fluid and electrolyte therapy)

Correct fluid replacement is vital if a patient is NBM. However, the volume and type of fluid should be appropriate. Total volume, tonicity, and electrolyte content are important.

Requirements

For an 80-kg adult this equates to 2–3 litres a day, incorporating 150 mmol of sodium and 40–60 mmol of potassium. This maintenance therapy can be achieved by prescribing 1 litre of sodium chloride 0.9% infused over 8 hours followed by 1–2 litres of dextrose 5% each infused over 8 hours. Both dextrose 5% and sodium chloride 0.9% are available with 20 mmol/l or 40 mmol/l of potassium chloride.

For the elderly, the volume and amount of sodium and potassium should be reduced.

Prescribing

It is good practice to prescribe each individual bag of IV fluid separately on the fluid prescription chart. This forces a daily review of IV fluid therapy. IV fluids should be prescribed on the current day's chart: 'flicking' back over previous charts to find the next solution can result in adverse events. Systems that allow a prescription to cover an unlimited period of administration are inherently dangerous, and can lead to unintentional fluid overload. Fluid overload in the elderly with concomitant congestive heart failure can be fatal.

Intravenous additives

IV therapy, which involves a sealed sterilized system (i.e. a bag of infusion fluid) is generally safe and free from contamination. It is, however, worth inspecting all containers for the presence of particles.

Once sealed systems are breached, e.g. by adding medicines to a bag of fluid for infusion, then microbial contamination becomes a potential problem. The physical and chemical stability of adding medicines and nutrients to infusion fluid is problematic. Such decisions are best referred to the pharmacy.

The guidelines are:

• Only add a medicine to an infusion if it is really necessary (i.e.: constant plasma concentration required; avoidance of a high, potentially toxic, plasma concentration; dilute concentration required to avoid local tissue damage).

• Always use a commercially available preparation if suitable (e.g. dopamine and potassium infusions are available premixed and sterilized).

• Use a strict aseptic technique, wash your hands and use gloves.

• All preparations should be freshly made and used immediately.

• After adding additives shake the infusion very well. Some additives are denser than the infusion fluid and can settle unseen at the bottom of an infusion bag. This readily happens with potassium chloride solutions, and can result in a bolus of all the additive being infused—with potentially lethal consequences.

• In general, an expiry of up to 24 hours can be given once additives have been made.

• After adding additives check for signs of incompatibility immediately and then periodically after. Look for precipitates, colour changes, hazy or cloudy solutions. Look in the bag and the intravenous line. Some incompatibilities are often only seen after the fluid has mixed with other fluids being infused at the same time through Y sites, for example.

• Clearly label the infusion solution with the name of the medicine, the amount added, the date and time of addition, the patient's name, and the date and time of expiry. Labels designed for this are usually available from the pharmacy.

• Always seek expert advice from the pharmacy as some medicines are inherently unstable.

• Wherever possible use a centralized intravenous additive service. Contamination of parenteral fluids is a problem from which patients still suffer morbidity and mortality.

• Total parenteral nutrition (TPN) is expensive, is complicated to make, and is an ideal medium for the growth of microorganisms if contaminated. The compounding of TPN should be carried out within the pharmacy under strict aseptic conditions.

• Never add medicines to blood, albumin, colloids, mannitol solutions, sodium bicarbonate, and lipid solutions due to the risk of instability or haptan formation.

The BNF contains lots of useful information on this topic.

Using the oral route of administration

The IV route of administration is obviously mainly used perioperatively. However, consider switching to oral as soon as possible. The oral route reduces the risk of adverse events, decreases the administration workload, and reduces the cost, but is only to be used when the gut is effective.

Antibiotics (e.g. see Chapter 1—Infective complications)

Antibiotic regimens for prophylaxis and treatment should be:

* targeted at the likely pathogens, so choice is empirical—they can be changed based on the results of culture and sensitivity testing, but only if the patient is not responding;

* prescribed to ensure a high tissue concentration at the time of incision and postoperatively or during their use in treating infection;

* of short duration to minimize adverse drug reactions and reduce environmental exposure. It is unusual to need to give antibiotics in surgery for more than 5 days. Certainly this should be reviewed between 3–5 days and beyond. Exceptional cases would be acute prostatitis or epididymitis.

Surgery altering the pharmacokinetics of medicines

Pharmacokinetics is the effect of the body on the drug (absorption, distribution, metabolism, and excretion). Absorption of drugs from IM injections and the gastrointestinal tract will be affected by fluid-balance changes, changes in gastrointestinal motility, and shifts in vascular perfusion. Fluid-balance changes and shifts in vascular perfusion will affect the distribution of drugs. Metabolism and excretion of medicines are affected by changes in hepatic and renal function.

Chapter 9
Neurological complications after surgery in general

Postoperative confusion

Acute confusional states are a common postoperative complication, associated with increased mortality, increased frequency of other complications, prolonged hospitalization, and a higher rate of discharge to residential or nursing-home care. It can be defined as a syndrome characterized by widespread cerebral dysfunction caused by a wide spectrum of organic factors. The reported incidence is unknown, varying between 2 and 60%, which reflects the differences in data collection and definition of confusion within different study populations. The onset of symptoms is commonly seen between the second and fifth postoperative days.

Risk groups

Males are affected more than females, with the elderly at a higher risk than younger age groups. It has been shown that 9–15% of patients over 65 years will experience postoperative confusion. History and examination may be useful as known preoperative factors are:

* age >70 years;
* history of alcohol abuse;
* impaired preoperative cognitive function;
* poor preoperative functional status;
* deranged postoperative electrolyte balance;
* thoracic surgery;
* open cardiac surgery;
* aortic aneurysm surgery.

Perioperative factors

Hypotension

Hypotension and reduced cardiac output during surgery result in diminished cerebral perfusion. Depending on the duration of cerebral hypoperfusion, the resulting injury can range from mild to severe brain injury. Mild brain injuries can leave the patient obtunded for 72 hours before they regain a normal level of consciousness, normally without serious neurological consequences. More severe injuries are associated with a poorer prognosis.

Hypoxia

Intraoperative hypoxic insults are commonly associated with severe brain damage, secondary to cerebral oedema. This is the most devastating complication associated with general anaesthesia and, while the prognosis for a full functional recovery is usually poor, prompt management with hyperventilation, intravenous steroids, and intravenous mannitol may limit the damage.

Postoperative factors

Haemodynamic disturbance

Hypotension, hypovolaemia, postoperative anaemia, acute myocardial infarction, cardiac arrhythmias, and congestive cardiac failure due to fluid overload are all recognized factors for postoperative confusion. This is a preventable complication, and should be anticipated in the preoperative assessment.

Sepsis

Postoperative infections are a very common source of confusion, especially in the elderly. At the first signs of postoperative confusion a full sepsis screen should be considered. Common conditions to exclude are:

• chest—pneumonia, atelectasis;
• urinary tract infection—especially if the patient is, or has been, catheterized;
• cardiovascular—bacterial endocarditis in at-risk patients;
• wound—local infection;
• line infection—especially central venous or long lines;
• central nervous system—meningitis after open cranial surgery.

Drugs, drug interactions, and drug withdrawal

Drugs used during the procedure, interactions between concurrent medication, and the withdrawal of prescription (and sometimes nonprescription) drugs have a significant contribution to postoperative complications and confusion. The list of potential candidates is immense, but commonly implicated drugs are:

• anticholinergics
• opiate analgesics
• antidepressants, e.g. benzodiazepines
• anticonvulsants
• neuroleptics
• alcohol

The use of opiate analgesics, especially by the intravenous or patient-controlled analgesia system (PCAS) routes, has shown a higher incidence of confusion in the immediate postoperative period. The analgesic effect of opiates administered by the intramuscular or PCAS routes are similar. However, studies have shown the adjuvant use of non-steroidal anti-inflammatory drugs (NSAIDs) not only reduces opiate requirement but also the resultant adverse effects, and therefore the combination of NSAIDs and IM opiates is to be recommended.

Benzodiazepine use is common among the elderly and chronic use is known to cause habituation, tolerance, and dependence. Withdrawal from the longer acting agents (e.g. diazepam) is more likely to induce confusion than the shorter acting ones (e.g. temazepam)

Alcohol withdrawal is an important diagnosis that should be considered for all patients exhibiting abnormal behaviour (see delirium tremens below).

Inadequate pain relief

Uncontrolled and chronic pain are debilitating, with patients becoming withdrawn and uncommunicative. Commonly dismissed, careful attention to an individual's analgesic requirements can rapidly improve an acute confusional state.

Respiratory disorders

Infection and hypoxia have already been discussed. A late cause of confusion is pulmonary embolus. Commonly occurring 10–12 days after surgery, especially following abdominal, pelvic, or lower limb procedures, the clinical features include sudden dyspnoea, pleuritic chest pain, haemoptysis, and acute confusion. This is an important diagnosis to consider, occurring in 1.6% of the general surgical population, and fatal in 0.4% of cases.

Metabolic disturbances

Electrolyte imbalances, either iatrogenic or secondary to the surgical procedure, are common and preventable. Hyponatraemia, hypokalaemia, hypercalcaemia, and hypoglycaemia are commonly encountered. Impaired renal or liver function causes encephalopathy and confusion.

Neurological events

Postoperative stroke, transient ischaemic attacks, cerebral oedema, and fat emboli are common events in susceptible patients. Known risk factors, e.g. carotid artery disease, long bone fracture, postneurosurgery, help to identify the source of the problem.

Nutritional deficiencies

Confusional states are higher in the elderly who are thiamine-deficient.

Delirium tremens

Delirium tremens is an acute confusional state resulting from the abrupt withdrawal of alcohol in patients with a regular, heavy drinking habit. Prodromal features can present within 6 hours after the last drink (tremor, sweating, gastrointestinal discomfort, nausea, anorexia, and a mild confusional state with agitation), although it usually takes 2 or more days before the florid symptoms (confusion, agitation, disorientation, paranoia, tactile and visual hallucinations, e.g. formication) appear. There is a significant mortality rate (9%).

The true incidence is unknown, but studies suggest approximately 12% of known alcoholics will display features of acute confusion postoperatively, despite prophylaxis. A relationship between serum potassium levels and the progression of delirium tremens has been recorded. Careful monitoring of serum potassium levels is mandatory in the at-risk groups.

Optimal management requires a combination approach. Preoperative awareness and prophylactic sedative agents (chlordiazepoxide 10 mg, four times a day; clomethiazole capsules (192 mg clomethiazole base)—*day 1*: three capsules four times a day, *day 2*: two capsules four times a day, *day 3–7*: 1 capsule four times a day), followed by the controlled reintroduction of alcohol (oral, nasogastric, gastrostomy) in the postoperative period is the favoured treatment plan. This regime is cost-effective, reduces morbidity, and has improved mortality rates.

However, it should not be assumed that agitation in a patient with alcohol dependence is always due to withdrawal. These patients still remain susceptible to the other cause of postoperative confusion (see postoperative confusion below). It is vital that all possible causes are investigated, adequate hydration ensured, and normokalaemia maintained. Incidental hypoglycaemia requires careful management to avoid the physiological effect of intravenous glucose in reducing the serum potassium concentration.

Postoperative falls

Falls in the elderly are common, with a 10-fold increase in hospitalized patients over 65 years of age. Falls are associated with an increased risk of other injuries, particularly fractures of the femoral neck, which has significant morbidity and mortality. Falls have a multifactorial origin; but while many of the causes can be anticipated, the proportion preventable does vary depending on interrelated factors. The overall controlling factor appears to be the diminished functional and physiological reserve of elderly patients, which cannot be quantified. The principal causes seen in surgical patients are:

(1) **Postural hypotension**—diastolic blood pressure increases when a patient stands, the result of increased venous return due to venoconstriction to maintain cerebral perfusion. This is an autonomic reflex, but can be impaired in:

   • the elderly: a large fall in both systolic and diastolic pressure results in dizziness and falls;
   • hypovolaemia: since there is a reduced circulating volume to maintain cerebral perfusion;
   • autonomic failure: commonly seen in diabetic patients;
   • drug interactions: especially patients on antihypertensives, phenothiazines, tricyclic antidepressants, or levodopa;
   • prolonged bed rest: due to cardiovascular deconditioning;
   • epidural anaesthesia: transient, due to loss of vascular tone.

(2) **Cardiac arrhythmias**—disturbances in cardiac conduction reduce effective cardiac output. Atrial fibrillation, paroxysmal bradycardias (e.g. complete heart block), and tachyarrhythmias (e.g. ventricular tachycardias, ventricular fibrillation) are common causes, especially in the elderly. There may be a preceding warning (e.g. palpitations), or they may occur suddenly.

(3) **Vasovagal**—common after a general anaesthetic due to transient compromise of the autonomic reflex. Seen in all age groups.

(4) **Locomotor instability**—the elderly have restricted movement due to numerous, often interrelated, conditions. It accounts for over 50% of falls in the elderly postoperative patient. Osteoarthritis, Parkinson's disease, visual deterioration, balance disorders, and cervical spondylosis are common conditions in the older age groups. They have no relation to the surgical procedure performed, but are important to identify as they may be the first indication to the medical profession of an ongoing problem for which the patient is reluctant to seek help and advice.

(5) **Extracranial arterial disease**—transient ischaemic attacks are common in the older age groups. Either the anterior (carotid) or posterior (vertebral) cerebral circulation can be involved and present with an

abrupt onset of focal neurological features. Vertebrobasilar insufficiency is seen after manipulation of the neck during anaesthesia in patients with cervical spondylosis, due to compression of the vertebral artery.

(6) **Metabolic imbalances**—hypoglycaemia is common among patients who have been starved prior to general anaesthesia. The elderly fail to recognize the features of hypoglycaemia, which is only detected after a fall.

Postoperative cerebrovascular disorders (stroke)

Stroke is a clinical syndrome defined as an acute focal neurological deficit due to cerebrovascular disease, which lasts longer than 24 hours. It is the third commonest recorded cause of death in the Western world and its incidence within the general population (2:1000) indicates that there is a subgroup of susceptible surgical patients at increased risk of this disease. It is therefore to be expected that a surgical patient may experience a stroke, either related or unrelated to their treatment. The risk factors for peri- and postoperative stroke are numerous and interrelated, but result in: (1) cerebral infarction (85%); or (2) intracerebral haemorrhage; or (3) subarachnoid haemorrhage. Characterized by a sudden onset of hemiplegia, accompanied by dysarthria, dysphagia, visual disturbances, cognitive impairment, and emotional lability, recovery is dependent on the size of the infarct, the area of the cerebral cortex affected, and the presence of a suitable collateral circulation.

Causes

Early causes
Embolus

Atherosclerosis within the major vessels supplying the cerebral circulation is the main source of cerebral embolism. Symptomatic atherosclerosis is commonest at the carotid bifurcation, but may also arise from the aorta and the common carotid and vertebral arteries. Detachment of portions of thrombotic plaque from atherosclerotic internal carotid arteries is the most frequent cause of non-haemorrhagic stroke (90%). This risk is significant during carotid surgery (see Carotid endarterectomy below).

* **Air embolus**—infrequently seen. A known complication after air insufflation of the fallopian tubes for investigation of female infertility.
* **Traumatic**—subdural or extradural haemorrhages, either spontaneous or secondary to injury (post-traumatic, iatrogenic at time of surgery), compromise cerebral blood flow and cause watershed infarcts. Meticulous control of bleeding at the time of surgery should avoid this catastrophic complication.

Intermediate causes
Embolus

Embolic phenomena occur after open cardiac surgery (2–5% following valve replacement), or in patients with uncontrolled arrhythmias (commonly atrial fibrillation). The embolus is constructed from either air which enters through the atriotomy or aortotomy, debris detached when removing a heavily calcified valve, or due to turbulent flow within heart chambers. This is becoming less common due to the safety and efficiency of modern extracorporeal perfusion equipment.

Intracranial haemorrhage

Principally due to rupture of microaneurysms, which occur at well-defined sites (e.g. circle of Willis, basal ganglia, pons). Frequently seen in patients with known hypertension. Uncontrolled blood pressure during surgery can precipitate a bleed in the immediate recovery period.

Late causes

Embolus

Postoperative myocardial infarction can lead to the formation of a thrombus within the left ventricle. Separation of thrombi can cause an embolic stroke.

Complications of postoperative stroke

Cerebral oedema

Reactionary swelling of infarcted brain tissue can compress adjacent tissue, causing further ischaemia and brainstem distortion. This may lead to coma and death. Suspected if a patient has been lucid and then slowly loses consciousness; requires careful supportive management in a specialist unit.

Aspiration pneumonia

Most patients' experience swallowing difficulties and overspill aspiration. Assessment by a speech and language therapist determines if patients need to be nil by mouth.

Decubitus ulcers

Restricted movement predisposes to pressure sores. These can develop rapidly and are difficult to treat. They cause significant discomfort to the patient and exacerbate an already distressing condition. Secondary infection can occur if the patient is incontinent of urine and faeces.

Extension of stroke

Further vascular occlusion can extend the stoke by involving other vascular territories. This increases the disability.

Depression

Anxiety and depression are common reactions to stroke. May represent damage to the frontal or limbic systems.

Constipation

Retention of urine, faecal and urinary incontinence, disturbance of bowel and bladder function are all commonly encountered. Patients can either become faecally incontinent, or more commonly constipated. Disturbance in bladder function commonly manifests as urgency incontinence or dribbling incontinence. Urinary tract infection commonly supervenes.

Postoperative neuropsychiatric disturbances

Anxiety is intimately linked with surgery and can be considered a normal psychophysiological response. However, there is an increased incidence of psychiatric complications in a proportion of postsurgical patients, especially the elderly. Termed 'postoperative psychosis', this condition can not be considered a separate clinical entity as no single factor can be shown to be exclusively responsible. It is now believed that the physical illness and the operative procedure can simply reveal a latent, underlying, psychiatric tendency. One study diagnosed an acute confusional state in 20%, depression in 9%, dementia in 3%, and a functional psychosis in 2% of elderly postoperative patients. Depression is seen in 4.5% of all postoperative patients. Certain surgical procedures appear to increase the risk of a depressive illness (i.e. cancer surgery, open cardiac surgery, neurosurgery, breast surgery, transplantation, and craniofacial surgery), and this is affected by pre-existing psychiatric illness, complications of the surgery, and chronic illness.

Depression has a variety of clinical manifestations. Insomnia, anorexia, apathy, reversal of the night–day rhythm, and withdrawn behaviour are frequently seen. It commonly presents as a late complication of surgery.

Clinical manifestations

Depression in children

Approximately 20% of children show features of clinical depression after surgery. This presents as tantrums, disruptive behaviour, destructive tendencies, and increased maternal dependency (e.g. clinging). Presurgical ward visits, the input from a dedicated nurse practitioner, and play therapy can reduce this incidence. Interestingly, unlike the elderly, children do not show acute confusional states, believed to relate to a child's inability to rationalize death (which does not develop until 9 years of age).

Cardiac surgery

Depression is seen in 15% of patients after open cardiac surgery. This is unrelated to age, sex, severity of disease, or the complications after surgery. It seems to be related to the duration of extracorporeal bypass. It has been suggested that bypass may produce a form of organic brain disorder that sensitizes patients to neuropsychiatric disorders.

Neurosurgery

Extensive focal or generalized brain damage can lead to changes in personality, which presents as decreased intelligence, disinhibition, and a lower attention span.

Breast surgery

Some 20% of postmastectomy patients show depressive characteristics. This is associated with a perceived loss of self-esteem and concern over survival, but studies have shown this is reduced by counselling, dedicated breast-care nurses, and support groups. Interestingly, there is no significant difference in the incidence of depression in women undergoing breast conservation as compared to mastectomy.

ITU syndrome

This condition is seen in intensive therapy unit (ITU) patients, especially those mechanically ventilated for a protracted period. Restlessness, confusion, and disorientation occur in the initial stages, with longer term memory and social skill impairments. It is believed to be due to sleep deprivation, pain, drug interactions, anxiety, and fear. Recovery is slow but usually complete.

Chapter 10
Postoperative complications related to anaesthesia and intensive care

Anaesthesia

Intraoperative and postoperative anaesthetic complications occur in a minority of patients. With proper evaluation and preoperative investigation the patients at the highest risk of the following complications can be predicted and appropriate steps taken to avoid these problems.

However, unavoidable intraoperative complications do occur with no warning in low-risk patients and it is the responsibility of the anaesthetist to act decisively.

Patients at high risk of complications are those who:

* are elderly (>65 years);
* have significant comorbidity and intercurrent disease, especially of the cardiorespiratory system;
* are undergoing thoracic and major abdominal surgery;
* require prolonged surgery (>2 hours);
* need emergency surgery (within 6 hours).

Critical incidents

A critical incident is one where there is the potential of harm to the patient either in terms of increased morbidity and mortality or hospital stay. The majority of critical incidents are acted upon before serious harm occurs. The purpose of critical incident reporting is to promote safe practice as the majority of critical incidents are caused by human error. Factors that are liable to promote critical incidents include: failure to check; unfamiliarity with the environment, the equipment, or the procedure; inexperience and fatigue.

For these and other reasons numerous authorities have produced guidelines relating to the monitoring of patients under anaesthesia, the experience of anaesthetists doing certain procedures, and the timing of operations.

Intraoperative complications

Anaphylaxis

This is an exaggerated immune response to a substance to which the body has been sensitized. True anaphylaxis is triggered by IgE, whereas anaphylactoid reactions are not. Both types of reaction present and are treated similarly.

Implicated substances include: latex (which is present in a vast amount of theatre equipment); intravenous induction agents; muscle relaxants (especially suxamethonium); colloid solutions; and antibiotics. In a significant number of patients no cause is found.

Presenting features are:

* Cardiovascular:
  - tachycardia
  - hypotension
  - flushing
* Respiratory:
  - oral and laryngeal oedema
  - bronchospasm
* Cutaneous:
  - erythema
  - urticaria

Treatment

This involves:

* Immediate stopping of the implicated substance.
* Airway management with 100% oxygen.
* Adrenaline (epinephrine)—this is the most important drug in the acute management of anaphylaxis. In addition to supporting the circulation it stabilizes mast-cell membranes and reduces the release of the vasoactive substances responsible for anaphylaxis. An initial intramuscular injection of 0.3–1.0 mg is given and repeated according to response. Intravenous adrenaline should be reserved for severe anaphylaxis with incipient cardiac arrest in a monitored patient, and prior intravenous access must be established with the administration of fluids.

The second line of treatment involves the injection of intravenous hydro-cortisone 100–200 mg or chlorphenamine (chlorpheniramine) 10 mg.

Blood samples need to be taken to establish the exact nature of the reaction.

Cardiovascular complications

Arrhythmia

Bradycardia

This is the most common arrhythmia associated with anaesthesia. Many anaesthetic agents have vagolytic properties; in addition, many anaesthetic and surgical procedures are prone to causing vagal stimulation (laryngoscopy, peritoneal insufflation, perineal stimulation).

Treatment involves withdrawal of the offending stimulus and the administration of an anticholinergic drug such as atropine. Some anaesthetists routinely administer these drugs to patients who are prone to bradycardia.

Tachycardia

Tachycardia should be avoided because it reduces the diastolic time, which in turn reduces coronary perfusion. This is particularly a problem in patients with ischaemic heart disease in whom any reduction in coronary blood flow is poorly tolerated.

Tachycardia is treated by appropriate analgesia and fluids and withdrawal of drugs whenever possible, but β-blockers should continue up to the time of surgery, IV if necessary.

Many other arrhythmias can occur under anaesthesia, e.g. atrial fibrillation. Standard treatments should be used, with the proviso that electrical cardioversion can be used early in the anaesthetized patient.

Hypotension

Hypotension in the anaesthetized patient is a common occurrence. In the young and fit it is rarely a problem, but in the elderly and those with cerebrovascular and ischaemic heart disease it should be avoided. Recovery-unit staff must be aware of the possibility of reactive haemorrhage after the restoration of normal blood pressure.

Causes of hypotension under anaesthesia

* Reduced venous return to the heart:
    - preoperative fluid deprivation
    - preoperative fluid losses
    - haemorrhage, both pre- and intraoperatively
    - surgical pressure on the inferior vena cava (IVC)
* Reduced myocardial contractility:
    - pre-existing cardiac disease
    - cardiac depression by anaesthetic agents
    - sepsis (see below)
    - hypoxaemia
* Reduced afterload
    - anaesthetic agents
    - sepsis
    - epidural analgesia

Respiratory complications

Airway obstruction

The resting tone in the muscles of the tongue and pharynx hold the tongue and soft palate forward of the posterior pharyngeal wall. This protection is lost in the unconscious patient, whether this is due to anaesthesia or other causes.

Airway opening manoeuvres include:

* Chin lift
* Head tilt
* Jaw thrust forward
* Oropharyngeal airway
* Nasopharyngeal airway
* Laryngeal mask airway

* Endotracheal intubation
* Tracheostomy

Endotracheal intubation remains the 'gold standard'. In addition to opening the airway, it provides protection against tracheal soiling. There are many other causes of respiratory obstruction under anaesthesia:

* Kinked/blocked anaesthetic circuit
* Kinked/blocked endotracheal (ET) tube
* Oropharyngeal pathology:
  - tumour
  - anaphylaxis
  - haemorrhage and swelling
  - infection, e.g. epiglottitis
  - laryngospasm
* Tracheal pathology:
  - laryngomalacia
  - tumour intrinsic or extrinsic
  - tracheal stenosis
* Bronchial pathology
  - bronchospasm
  - retained secretions

Difficult intubation/failed intubation

The effective management of the difficult airway relies upon adequate preoperative assessment of the patient, and surgical factors involved in deciding the optimal method of managing the airway. The patient factors predisposing to difficult airway management or intubation include obesity, short stature, short and immobile neck, recessive jaw with restricted mouth opening, protruding teeth, or oropharyngeal pathology.

The surgical factors causing airway difficulty are:

* Need for airway protection—full stomach;
* Airway shared with the surgeon—ENT, maxillofacial, or thyroid surgery;
* Length of surgery—patients undergoing long operations should generally be intubated and ventilated;
* Patient positioning—patients whose airways are not easily accessible during surgery, e.g. prone patients should be intubated.

Management of a failed intubation—or worse, a failure to intubate or ventilate—revolves around the fact that failure to oxygenate rather than failure to intubate is the cause of morbidity and mortality. The onus is to keep the patient oxygenated until spontaneous respiration is adequate. The patient should then be woken up and a decision made about further airway management.

Hypoxaemia

The advent of pulse oximetry has allowed the early detection of hypoxaemia in the anaesthetized patient. The early detection of hypoxaemia should allow treatment before serious end-organ damage occurs. Causes of hypoxaemia can occur from the anaesthetic machine to the patient.

Causes of hypoxaemia in the anaesthetized patient

- Hypoxic gas mixture delivered to patient
- Disconnection of ventilator/anaesthetic circuit
- Airway obstruction
- Hypoventilation due to deep anaesthesia or opioid analgesics
- V/Q (ventilation/perfusion) mismatch, e.g. endobronchial intubation, pneumothorax, pneumonia, lung collapse
- Reduced cardiac output

Aspiration

With the loss of consciousness after induction of anaesthesia the patients' ability to protect their own airway is lost, and for this reason patients undergoing elective surgery are starved prior to anaesthesia.

Despite being nil by mouth it is impossible to guarantee the presence of an empty stomach in some patients. The factors which reduce gastric emptying include intra-abdominal pathologies, pain, opioid analgesia, alcohol, and pregnancy. In these patients special precautions have to be taken to avoid soiling the airway. The two principal methods are:

1. Avoid general anaesthesia and use a regional technique, e.g. subarachnoid block for a Caesarean section.

2. Use a rapid-sequence induction. The principle is to intubate the trachea as soon as possible after loss of consciousness. During the period between loss of consciousness and endotracheal intubation the airway is protected using cricoid pressure. To allow time to perform intubation without desaturating, the patient is preoxygenated; and to allow the patient to be woken up quickly if intubation is unsuccessful the patient is given a short-acting muscle relaxant, suxamethonium.

At the end of anaesthesia the patient is again at risk of aspiration until the airway reflexes are regained. Patients should be closely monitored during this period and nursed on their side once the endotracheal tube has been removed (extubated).

Anaesthetic diseases

These diseases are solely related to anaesthesia. They can cause problems postoperatively.

Malignant hyperthermia (MH)

This is an abnormal reaction to certain anaesthetic agents. It involves the uncoupling of metabolism and contraction of skeletal muscle, and manifests itself as hyperthermia, tachycardia, and hypercarbia. Treatment involves terminating surgery as soon as possible, removing the cause by switching to non-triggering agents, providing supportive therapy, and administering dantrolene. Patients should be monitored in an intensive care unit postoperatively as the syndrome can recur during the postoperative period.

It is possible to anaesthetize the patient in the future using agents that do not cause MH.

Suxamethonium apnoea

The major advantage of suxamethonium is that it delivers excellent intubating conditions quickly and spontaneous ventilation is restored within minutes. The offset of action is so rapid because it is hydrolysed *in vivo* by plasma cholinesterases. Several genetically determined abnormalities of the cholinesterase molecule can lead to prolonged action of suxamethonium. Suxamethonium apnoea presents as a prolonged neuromuscular blockade after the administration of suxamethonium. Treatment is directed at maintaining ventilation and anaesthesia whilst allowing the suxamethonium to be metabolized, albeit more slowly, by other cholinesterases.

Awareness

Awareness under anaesthesia is a common cause of preoperative anxiety. It occurs when a paralysed patient is insufficiently anaesthetized. The patient cannot communicate their awareness because they are paralysed. There is a spectrum of awareness from recalling voices, but not specific words, in theatre to being fully awake and in pain but unable to move.

Reduced concentrations of anaesthetic vapours can be used intentionally during hypotensive periods in theatre and unintentionally because of poor anaesthetic technique or equipment failure. Low concentrations of anaesthetic vapours have historically been used during Caesarean section under general anaesthesia, and it is for this reason that the incidence of awareness in this circumstance is so high. Scrupulous attention to detail, checking equipment, and the use of monitors of the concentration of anaesthetic vapours should all help to reduce the incidence of this problem. It is important that the whole operating team know that the patient may be more aware than usual in these circumstances.

Postoperative complications relating to anaesthesia

Trauma

Teeth and lips

Trauma to the teeth can occur during manipulation of the airway. Sound teeth can be chipped and loose teeth dislodged. Capped teeth are particularly at risk as they are less sturdy than native teeth. This is a problem both in terms of acceptability and the fact that the dislodged teeth can be aspirated into the bronchi and lungs producing atelectasis. Patients with unsound teeth should be counselled preoperatively and those with particularly loose teeth advised to visit a dentist before admission for elective surgery.

The nose, larynx, and pharynx

Laryngeal and pharyngeal trauma can occur at the same time as mouth trauma. Patients present with a sore throat during the postoperative period. In children, because of their proportionately smaller airways, laryngeal swelling secondary to airway trauma can cause significant airway obstruction requiring reintubation. Bleeding can occur from the nose during nasal intubation and during the passage of a nasopharyngeal airway or nasogastric tube.

Corneal abrasions

During anaesthesia the eyes can remain open. Without the moistening effects of tears the cornea can dry out and corneal abrasions occur. The eyes should be protected during anaesthesia using ointment and/or tape to keep them closed.

Nerve damage

Poor positioning of the patient can lead to damage to the brachial plexus and superficial nerves of the limbs. The upper arm should never be abducted further than 90 degrees, and the elbows (ulnar nerve) and legs in the lithotomy position (lateral peroneal nerve) should be padded to prevent damage. Failure to take measures to prevent superficial nerve damage may lead to litigation.

Respiratory complications

Airway obstruction

At the end of anaesthesia the muscle tone in the pharynx returns and patients begin to support their own airway. Patients should not be discharged from the recovery room until they can do this to the satisfaction of a trained member of staff. In addition, obstruction can occur at other levels in the respiratory system during the postoperative period. Nasal trauma or surgery can occlude the nose, requiring mouth-breathing. This can be a particular problem in young children who are obligate nose-breathers. Laryngeal spasm can occur in the postoperative period following extubation, and laryngeal oedema is a particular problem in children with small airways. Bronchospasm can occur following extubation.

Hypoventilation

Reduced breathing is a common occurrence in the postoperative period and can be due to reduced respiratory drive or peripheral factors leading to a reduced minute volume. Hypoventilation is a particular problem in the elderly and those patients with pre-existing chest disease. In normal respiration the alveoli are kept expanded by surfactant and occasional large 'sighing' breaths. Hypoventilation leads to alveolar collapse and hypoxaemia. Hypoventilation is often associated with a reduced ability to cough and clear bronchial secretions, which predisposes patients to postoperative chest infections.

Factors causing hypoventilation

- Central:
  - sedative premedicant drugs
  - anaesthetic agents
  - opioid analgesics
  - cerebrovascular event
- Peripheral factors:
  - residual neuromuscular blockade
  - pre-existing muscle disease
  - abdominal distention
  - abdominal pain
  - obesity

Residual neuromuscular blockade

Neuromuscular blockade is used to facilitate ventilation and to allow good surgical access during surgery. It should be reversed at the end of surgery using neostigmine if significant amounts of the drug are thought to remain in the body. Failure to reverse adequately results in hypoventilation due to muscle weakness.

Hypoxaemia

Hypoxaemia in the postoperative period can be due to hypoventilation (see above), ventilation perfusion (V/Q) mismatch, or increased oxygen utilization.

Causes of hypoxaemia

• V/Q mismatch:
  – collapse
  – consolidation
  – pulmonary oedema
  – pneumothorax
  – sepsis
  – pre-existing respiratory disease
• Increased oxygen utilization:
  – shivering
  – sepsis
  – malignant hyperthermia
  – convulsions

Postoperative hypoxaemia is often maximal on the third and fourth postoperative night. This corresponds with a high incidence of postoperative myocardial ischaemia (see below). The reason for this seems to be that there is a rebound increase in the incidence of rapid eye movement (REM) sleep and respiratory obstruction at this point. REM sleep is characteristically reduced or abolished in the first two or three postoperative nights.

Aspiration

Aspiration of lung contents may occur in the postoperative period or the manifestations of intraoperative aspiration may only become apparent during the postoperative period.

Soiling of the lung parenchyma with stomach contents causes a chemical pneumonitis with bronchospasm and hypoxaemia. The presence of food matter can also lead to collapse and pneumonia. Management is supportive with oxygen and respiratory support as required. Steps should also be taken to avoid further aspiration. If this occurred during the intraoperative period and the patient has fully regained consciousness then no further action is required to prevent aspiration in the absence of gastric outlet or intestinal obstruction. If the patient has a reduced level of consciousness then steps should be taken to protect the airway until consciousness is restored. This varies from nursing in the lateral position, so that any further regurgitation is directed away from the lungs, to airway protection with an endotracheal tube in the intensive care unit.

Cardiovascular complications

Hypotension

Postoperative hypotension is most commonly caused by hypovolaemia. In the young and fit, up to 40% of blood volume may be lost before any effect on blood pressure is seen. In the elderly, this figure is lower because of the reduced ability of the cardiovascular system to compensate.

Ideally the presence of hypovolaemia should be detected prior to hypotension developing. Tachycardia, reduced urine output, and thirst should all prompt the suspicion of hypovolaemia before the onset of hypotension. Regular and watchful nursing observation is the key to the early detection of hypovolaemia.

Evidence of bleeding or other fluid loss should be sought and treated before any thought is given to inotropic support. Fluid loss in the postoperative period is often occult. Drains may not drain and considerable quantities of fluid may be lost into the abdominal cavity postoperatively before any overt abdominal distention or other signs are noted. In addition, patients can be severely dehydrated preoperatively, and this should be corrected.

Myocardial dysfunction and altered vascular tone due to sepsis are the other two main causes of postoperative hypotension. Patients with postoperative hypotension should be nursed in a high-dependency area so that close monitoring of input/output and cardiovascular parameters can be performed. They should all receive high-flow oxygen. Invasive monitoring such as central venous pressure monitoring may be required.

Initial treatment in the absence of overt cardiovascular dysfunction should be with fluid. This should be given as a bolus of 250–500 ml of saline, colloid, or blood. Several fluid boluses may need to be given, and the need for further fluid should be assessed on the basis of the response to the previous challenge. Failure to respond to several fluid challenges should prompt a search for continuing blood loss or raise the possibility that sepsis/myocardial dysfunction is the cause of the hypotension.

Hypertension

Hypertension during the postoperative period increases myocardial oxygen requirement and should be avoided. It is usually caused by catecholamine release due to pain or anxiety. These should be treated before resorting to pharmacological means of controlling the blood pressure.

Myocardial infarction

Postoperative myocardial infarction is associated with a poor prognosis. It is more likely to occur in those patients with pre-existing cardiovascular disease, those undergoing emergency surgery, and those patients undergoing thoracic or intra-abdominal surgery. Its peak incidence is 3 days postoperatively. Although chest pain is the classical symptom, patients may present with shortness of breath, hypotension, or heart failure. A high index of suspicion is required to treat early.

Treatment of postoperative myocardial infarction

- Oxygen
- Intravenous opioid pain relief
- Aspirin

- Thrombolysis—may be inappropriate during the postoperative period; if so, then primary coronary angioplasty should be considered
- high-dependency or intensive therapy-unit (ITU) care

Postoperative MI complications

These include dysrhythmias with cardiac arrest, hypotension, heart failure, and pericardial tamponade (see Complications of cardiac surgery).

Pain

Pain is one of the major morbidities after both major and minor surgery. Pain is also associated with a number of untoward postoperative complications, which can be reduced or avoided with adequate pain relief. Catecholamine release occurs in response to pain during the postoperative period, this increases cardiac oxygen uptake and can precipitate myocardial ischaemia.

Hypoventilation relating to pain following abdominal surgery can lead to the retention of secretions, pulmonary collapse, and pneumonia. Physiotherapy and other manoeuvres aimed at reducing this (early mobilization) are hampered by pain. In addition, opioid pain relief suppresses the cough reflex and may even exacerbate this complication.

Treatment modalities
Simple analgesics

Paracetamol is largely without side-effects and is useful alone following minor surgery or later in the recovery stage of major surgery. In combination with codeine it is useful during intermediate surgery, and in combination with non-steroidal anti-inflammatory drugs (NSAIDs) it has been shown to reduce the amount of opioid analgesia required following major surgery.

NSAIDs

These can be used alone or in combination with simple analgesics following minor and intermediate surgery, and they have an opioid-sparing effect after major surgery. They should be used with caution in patients with previous gastric or duodenal ulceration, patients with renal failure, patients with asthma, and the elderly. NSAIDs can be given orally, rectally, intravenously, intramuscularly, and sublingually.

Opioids

Morphine is the mainstay of analgesia for major surgery. It is effective and safe when given in appropriate dosages. Several side-effects and complications do occur, however, and it is for this reason that other modes of analgesia are increasingly being used, either with or in place of morphine, to reduce these untoward effects.

Unwanted effects of morphine:

- Sedation
- Respiratory depression

* Depression of cough reflex
* Nausea and vomiting
* Itch
* Constipation and reduced gastric motility

Morphine can be delivered by intermittent injection or by continuous methods. Continuous infusion and patient-controlled analgesia systems (PCAs) have the advantage of more continuous morphine levels. However, following a change in the rate of infusion it takes several hours to reach equilibrium. For this reason, changing the rate is an inefficient way of achieving adequate pain relief. Giving opiates on demand gives poor pain relief between doses and is associated with the unwanted side-effects. It should be avoided if possible. However, adequate analgesia can be obtained using intravenous boluses titrated against patient response before PCAS or intravenous infusion are used to maintain analgesia, but this needs the presence of an acute pain team or strict agreed protocols.

Regional blockade

Local anaesthetics can be used with and without general anaesthesia. Used with a general anaesthetic they can provide analgesia during the immediate postoperative period, or for longer periods using an infusion of local anaesthetic via an indwelling catheter.

Maximum doses of local anaesthetic are:

* Lidocaine (lignocaine) (plain)   3 mg/kg
* Lidocaine (with adrenaline (epinephrine))   7 mg/kg
* Bupivacaine (plain or with adrenaline)   3 mg/kg
* Prilocaine   600 mg

Advantages and disadvantages of regional anaesthesia

Advantages	Disadvantages
Lack of sedation	Some blocks are unreliable
Complete analgesia possible	Patients may find numbness unpleasant
	Motor effect can be troubling
	Profound analgesia may mask compartment syndrome
	Hypotension with central blocks

Epidural analgesia

For major surgery epidural anaesthesia is increasingly considered to be the 'gold standard' method of achieving postoperative analgesia. It allows the possibility for patients undergoing major surgery to be without pain during the postoperative period and to achieve early mobilization with all its attendant benefits. In addition, there is increasing evidence that it prevents postoperative pulmonary complications and can improve gut function following abdominal surgery.

Site

For postoperative analgesia the epidural catheter should be placed at the intervertebral space corresponding to the highest dermatome of the scar. In practice, lumbar epidurals are used for lower limb and pelvic surgery, low thoracic for upper abdominal surgery, and higher thoracic for thoracic surgery.

Contraindications for epidural anaesthesia:

* Localized infection
* Fixed cardiac output state
* Clotting disorders
* Anticoagulants, including low molecular-weight heparin (LMWH) solutions used for epidural anaesthesia:
* Local anaesthetic solutions which give analgesia but also motor and vasomotor block;
* Opioids which give analgesia but can cause central respiratory depression;
* Mixtures, which combine the advantages of both and minimize the disadvantages, allowing a lower concentration of both.

Complications of epidural anaesthesia can be avoided by the use of an acute pain team and attention to siting, dose, and rate of administration. They include:

* Local
  - bleeding: leading to epidural haematoma and spinal cord compression,
  - infections: epidural abscess formation,
  - neurological sequelae: permanent neurological damage is rare;
* Cardiovascular
  - hypotension occurs due to vasodilatation or to a direct effect on the cardiac sympathetic fibres (T1–4);
* High block/total spinal
  - if the catheter migrates into the subarachnoid space a very high block can occur, causing respiratory depression and loss of consciousness;
* Postdural puncture headache
  - puncture of the dura with a 16-gauge needle causes severe headache in one-third of patients; they should be given fluids and simple analgesia, but if this fails to control the headache a 'blood patch' should be performed;
* Blood patch
  - 20 ml of the patient's own blood should be introduced into the epidural space, but should not be performed in the presence of pyrexia or sepsis; blood patching is effective in 50% of cases but may need to be repeated;

Postoperative nausea and vomiting

Many factors increase the risk of postoperative nausea and vomiting (PONV).

Causes of PONV

These include:

• Specific patient groups:	gynaecological, ENT, or gastrointestinal surgery
• Anaesthetic agents:	nitrous oxide, etomidate
• Other drugs:	metronidazole
• Movement:	causes disorientation
• Excessive early oral fluids:	can be avoided by administering IV fluids in theatre
• Opioid analgesics:	dose can be reduced using other treatment modalities

Treatment of PONV

Non-pharmacological methods can be employed, such as acupressure or the giving of fluids. Morphine can be avoided by using other methods of analgesia. Metoclopramide is a useful antiemetic but has been shown to be ineffective in 50% of trials. Cyclizine can cause sedation. Droperidol, ondansetron, and dexamethasone are increasingly useful for PONV but are expensive or have side-effects.

Due to the multifactorial nature of PONV and the multiple receptors involved in the chemoreceptor trigger zone, a combination approach is often used.

Hypothermia/shivering

Causes of hypothermia in theatre

- Vasodilatation causes increased loss from the skin
- Shivering abolished by general anaesthesia
- Cold environment
- Little clothing
- Evaporative losses during intra-abdominal surgery
- Infusion of cold fluids
- Cold/dry anaesthetic gases

Treatment

Hypothermia can be avoided by the use of a warm theatre, warm fluids, and warmed and humidified anaesthetic gases. The patients can be warmed with a warm air blanket (Bair Hugger). Exposed bowel should be covered to reduce fluid loss and cooling.

Hyperthermia

The causes of hyperthermia are sepsis, overwarming in theatre, and malignant hyperthermia.

Intensive care management of postoperative complications of organ failure

Intensive care is an area where patients with potentially remediable conditions and with potential incipient or actual organ failure can be managed. It provides advanced monitoring of organ function, treatment of organ failure, and 1:1 nursing care.

Postoperative admission to the intensive care unit can be elective (e.g. following major surgery for elective extubation) or immediately after surgery following an unexpected difficulty (e.g. after massive blood loss and consequent hypothermia, intraoperative cardiac instability). Patients can be admitted during the late postoperative period following the development of organ failure, or increasingly preoperatively for stabilization and optimization of cardiovascular/respiratory physiology before elective and emergency surgery.

Respiratory failure: pathophysiology, shunt, and dead space

These terms refer to ineffective ventilation or perfusion in the lung. In a shunt, pulmonary blood flow goes to areas of the lung that are not ventilated, e.g. a collapsed lung. In dead space, the volume of gas breathed is not in contact with respiratory mucosa, e.g. the trachea and major bronchi. Both are relative terms, and in real pathophysiology there are rarely any areas of lung tissue that correspond to these extremes.

The common causes of respiratory difficulty in the postoperative period are shunt and hypoventilation.

Type 1 vs. type 2 respiratory failure

In type 1 respiratory failure the basic pathology is usually a shunt. This results in hypoxia as deoxygenated blood is returned straight to the circulation reducing the PaO_2 by dilution.

Causes of postoperative respiratory failure

Type 1	Type 2
Collapse/atelectasis	Drugs: opioids, muscle relaxants
Consolidation	Airway obstruction
Pulmonary oedema	Chronic obstructive airways disease
Thromboembolism	Kyphoscoliosis
	Cerebral disease

In type 2 respiratory failure the problem is one of hypoventilation and hypercarbia. Hypoxia can be present, but is not always.

Effect of increasing the FiO_2

Increasing the fractional inspired oxygen (FiO_2) concentration improves hypoxia in type 1 respiratory failure. It will also increase the PaO_2 in type 2 failure but will have no effect on the hypercarbia. These patients need increased ventilation, either by removing the cause of their hypoventilation, stimulating their respiration pharmacologically, or by instituting respiratory support.

A small number of patients with longstanding chronic lung disease rely on hypoxia to stimulate their ventilation (in the majority of patients ventilation is stimulated by changes in CO_2 concentration). In these patients the administration of high FiO_2 will lead to gradual hypoventilation and worsening type 2 respiratory failure. This will not be shown by a change in pulse oximetry (SpO_2) until late, and so all patients with type 2 respiratory failure should have repeat blood gases taken after the administration of oxygen. Any deterioration in PCO_2 should prompt the stimulation of respiration either pharmacologically or mechanically.

The vast majority of hypoxic patients do not respond in this way. With the exception of the above minority of patients, all patients with respiratory failure should receive high-concentration oxygen.

Methods of delivering increased FiO_2

Device	FiO_2
Hudson mask	0.4 approx.
Venturi mask	0.24, 0.28, 0.35, 0.40, 0.60 accurate
Trauma mask	0.7 approx
Anaesthetic circuit with tight mask	1.0

Indications for the implementation of respiratory support

- Severe hypoxia despite supplemental oxygen
- Hypercarbia and respiratory acidosis
- Severe metabolic acidosis to control respiration and hyperventilate
- Exhaustion
- Airway control in the unconscious patient

Modes of ventilation

- **IPPV**—intermittent positive-pressure ventilation. Compulsory ventilation is often used immediately after instigation of ventilation. This does not allow the patient to initiate any breaths.
- **SIMV**—synchronized intermittent mandatory ventilation. This specifies the number of breaths that the patient must take per minute.

It synchronizes the ventilator with the patient's own respiratory effort. In the apnoeic patient SIMV functions as IPPV. It is used in conjunction with ASB during weaning.

* **ASB**—assisted spontaneous breathing. This relies on the patient to trigger ventilation and then assists with the delivery of the breath with positive pressure. This 'pressure support' can be reduced as weaning progresses.
* **CPAP**—continuous positive airway pressure. Can be used via a face mask or following intubation. It increases alveolar recruitment, and increases the functional residual capacity.
* **PEEP**—positive-end expiratory pressure. This functions similarly to CPAP in ventilated patients.
* **BIPAP**—biphasic positive airway pressure. Pressure and not volume determine the volume delivered. This is said to reduce the chance of barotrauma. This mode of ventilation is often used in patients with acute respiratory distress syndrome (ARDS) in combination with reversed-ratio ventilation.

Complications of mechanical ventilation

* Complications relating to intubation: failure to intubate, hypotension, hypertension, hypoxia
* Reduced cardiac output, particularly with high levels of PEEP
* Nosocomial infection
* Barotrauma: pneumothorax
* Respiratory muscle weakness

Sedation

Intensive care, and particularly mechanical ventilation, is distressing for patients and they need to be sedated. Commonly an opioid (morphine, fentanyl, or alfentanil) is combined with a sedative (midazolam or propofol). Some of these drugs can accumulate, which can contribute to difficulty in weaning.

Weaning/tracheostomy

Following short-term elective ventilation, weaning is usually a short process. The aim of weaning after long-term ventilation is to reduce sedation enough to allow spontaneous ventilation. The amount of support that the patient receives from the ventilator is then reduced until the patient can be extubated. Tracheostomy aids weaning by reducing the amount of sedation required.

Complications of tracheostomy

* Early
  – bleeding
  – hypoxia
  – malposition leading to mediastinitis

- – oesophageal and tracheal trauma
- – infection
- Late
  - – tracheal stenosis
  - – fistula formation

Types of tracheostomy

- Surgical tracheostomy is probably the safest in the presence of a large thick-set neck, palpable blood vessels, or bleeding disorder.
- Percutaneous tracheostomy can be performed in ITU without the need for surgical equipment or staff.
- The trachea is found by aspiration and can be confirmed by bronchoscopy.
- A guide wire is passed through the needle inserted in the trachea.
- The tract is widened either by dilatational forceps or sequential dilators.
- The tracheostomy is then advanced over the guide wire into the trachea.
- Bronchoscopy, capnography, or auscultation confirms the correct positioning.

Elective postoperative ventilation

Following anaesthesia the patient should be warm and cardiovascularly stable. Before extubation patients should be awake and able to protect their own airway. They should be fully reversed from neuromuscular blockade. In addition, they should not be severely acidotic.

If patients do not fulfil these criteria they should remain ventilated until they do. For this reason some patients are admitted to ITU postoperatively for elective extubation.

Cardiovascular failure

Physiology

The aim of the cardiovascular system is to provide adequate perfusion to vital organs. The presence of an adequate blood pressure or cardiac output alone does not ensure this. Both pressure and flow are required for effective organ perfusion.

Blood pressure equations

- Cardiac output = preload × contractility
- BP = cardiac output × systemic vascular resistance
- Oxygen delivery = cardiac output × oxygen content
- Oxygen content = SaO_2 (%) × Hb (g/dl) × 1.34

The control of circulation

This is based on:

- Baroreceptors, which sense pressure and respond to changes by reducing or increasing sympathetic outflow; and

- Stretch receptors, which respond to stretch in the capacitance vessels and respond by diuresis.

Classification of adrenoreceptors (see table)

Adrenoreceptor classification

Type	Site	Action
α_1	Vascular tissue	Vasoconstriction
α_2	Presynaptic	Central reduction in sympathetic drive
β_1	Heart	Increased contractility
β_2	Bronchial walls	Relaxation
	Muscle	Vasodilatation
	Vasculature	

Pathophysiology of hypotension (see table)

Pathophysiology of hypotension

	Primary abnormality	Compensatory changes	Treatment
Hypovolaemic	↓Preload	↑SVR and tachycardia	Fluid
Cardiogenic	↓Contractility	↑SVR and tachycardia	Contractability with inotropes
Septic	↓SVR	↑Cardiac output	↑SVR with vasoconstrictors

SVR, systemic vascular resistance.

Cardiovascular assessment

- Pulse—tachycardia is common in all forms of shock. It may be masked by β-blocking agents.
- Blood pressure—reduced in all forms of shock. It does not correlate with cardiac output. Remember that hypotension is a late sign of hypovolaemia in the young.
- Venous filling—raised jugular vein pressure (JVP) is a clinical marker of a raised central venous pressure (CVP)
- Urine output—in the absence of renal disease an adequate urine output implies reasonable organ perfusion.
- Other clinical signs implying circulatory failure:
  - peripheral vasoconstriction,
  - sweating,
  - confusion,
  - hyperventilation.

Cardiovascular monitoring

This should include:

* ECG—which gives information on cardiac rate and rhythm and can indicate the presence of myocardial ischaemia and other myocardial pathology.
* Non-invasive blood pressure monitoring—which can be unreliable in the mobile and anxious patient.
* Invasive blood pressure monitoring—is more reliable and gives beat-to-beat information. The arterial line can also be used for repeated analysis of blood gases.
* CVP—gives an indication of right heart filling pressures. Access to a central vein is also provided for the administration of inotropes.
* PAFC (pulmonary artery flotation catheter)—allows a number of cardiovascular parameters to be ascertained:
  - wedge pressure is an indication of left heart filling pressures;
  - cardiac output can be determined by thermodilution;
  - pulmonary artery oxygen saturation can be used to measure oxygen consumption;
  - multiple lumens are present that can be used for the infusion of drugs.
* Oesophageal Doppler—measures cardiac output and can give information about pre- and afterload. It is poorly tolerated without sedation and is usually reserved for ventilated patients.
* Echocardiography—gives information about the contractility of the heart and mechanical problems. Transthoracic echocardiography is difficult to perform in ventilated patients. The transoesophageal route gives better views and more information.

Treatment

Inotropes

Preload should be optimized before inotropes are used. Inotropes should be used only in a high-dependency area with ECG and preferably invasive blood pressure monitoring.

Effect of inotropes

Drug	Main site of action	Secondary effects	Effects on cardiovascular parameters
Adrenaline	β_1	α_1	+ve inotrope vasoconstrictor
Noradrenaline	α_1	β_1	vasoconstrictor +ve inotrope

(continued)

Effect of inotropes (*continued*)

Drug	Main site of action		Secondary effects	Effects on cardiovascular parameters
Dopamine	1. Dopamine		renal vasodilator	with increasing dose
	2. β_1		+ve inotrope	
	3. α_1		vasoconstrictor	
Dobutamine	β_1	β_2	+ve inotrope vasodilator	may cause hypotension if β_2 effects predominate
Milrinone	PDE inhibitor		+ve inotrope vasodilator	
Digoxin	Na^+/K^+–ATPase		+ve inotrope	

+ve, positive; PDE, phosphodiesterase.

Management of the hypotensive postoperative patient

A practical approach to the hypotensive postoperative patient includes:

* ensuring a patent airway and giving high flow oxygen;
* establishing a wide-bore intravenous access—16 G minimum;
* giving fluid boluses to optimize left ventricular filling;
* considering continued occult bleeding as a cause of the failure to respond to fluid therapy;
* considering high-dependency nursing and invasive cardiovascular monitoring;
* considering the causes of hypotension and appropriate treatment (e.g. sepsis and thromboembolism);
* only once preload is optimized or in the presence of life-threatening cardiovascular collapse should inotropes be used:
  – septic shock: noradrenaline or adrenaline
  – cardiogenic shock: dobutamine or adrenaline
  – pulmonary oedema and hypotension: consider vasodilators with inotropes.

Renal failure

Physiology of renal perfusion needs consideration. Renal perfusion involves 25% of cardiac output. Glomerular perfusion pressure is closely controlled by renal arteriolar tone. Prostaglandins are involved in arteriolar dilatation and care with NSAIDs is therefore needed. The vast majority of renal filtrate is reabsorbed.

Factors predisposing to postoperative renal dysfunction

* Preoperative renal dysfunction
* Surgery associated with major blood loss and fluid shifts
* Hypovolaemia
* Hypotension
* Sepsis
* Nephrotoxic drugs

Postoperative monitoring of renal function

Patients at risk of postoperative renal dysfunction should be closely monitored during the postoperative period. The most useful early indication of renal dysfunction is reduced urine output. Less than 0.5 ml/kg per h should be regarded as abnormal and acted upon.

Causes of reduced urine output

Common causes	Uncommon causes
Hypovolaemia	Established acute tubular necrosis
Obstruction of the bladder catheter	Renal vascular occlusion
	Obstruction of the renal tract
	Coincidental renal pathology (glomerulonephritis, etc.)

Management of reduced urine output

* Catheterize or ensure the bladder catheter is unblocked.
* Establish a wide-bore intravenous access.
* If hypotensive or evidence of sepsis/cardiovascular dysfunction give oxygen.
* Assess the patient's fluid status clinically and look for evidence of ongoing blood loss.
* Give fluid boluses to optimize left ventricular filling.
* Consider high-dependency nursing and invasive cardiovascular monitoring.
* If hypotensive with adequate preload give inotropes to restore mean arterial pressure.
* Consider furosemide (frusemide)/mannitol to convert low- to high-output renal failure.

Renal replacement therapy

Indications for renal replacement therapy are:

* worsening symptomatic uraemia
* fluid overload

- hyperkalaemia
- severe acidosis

Peritoneal dialysis

This involves the introduction of fluid into the peritoneal cavity, which equilibrates with the blood and results in the removal of K^+ and other unwanted metabolites. This method of dialysis is inefficient and is unlikely to provide effective renal replacement in the catabolic postoperative patient. It is often contraindicated after abdominal surgery.

Vascular access

High-flow vascular access is required for all other forms of dialysis and filtration. These carry the same risks as central lines.

Haemofiltration

Hydrostatic pressure forces plasma across a semipermeable membrane; the filtered fluid is replaced with a more physiological solution resulting in the removal of metabolites. This method of renal replacement requires almost continuous use to provide sufficient removal. It is, however, a reasonably cardiostable technique as the rapid fluid and electrolyte shifts seen with haemodialysis are not observed.

Haemodialysis

In this method of renal replacement, blood and dialysate equilibrate across a semipermeable membrane. This is a rapid method of renal replacement and is useful in the more mobile patient. Since haemodialysis requires its own specialized water supply, it cannot be used in all intensive care units.

Part 2
Complications after specific types of surgery

Chapter 11
Complications of gastrointestinal surgery

Infection

Deep infection: intra-abdominal abscess

Definition

This is an intra-abdominal collection of pus which may contain live and dead neutrophil leucocytes, live and dead bacteria, together with products of enzymatic tissue damage from bacterial exo- or endotoxins and proteases, cytokine release, and plasma. The sites of collection of pus include the subphrenic spaces, the subhepatic pouch, the paracolic gutters, the pelvis, between intestinal loops, or in the perinephric tissue (see figure).

Causes can be categorized as shown in the figure below.

Primary pathology

Where inflammatory peritoneal disease with or without uncomplicated surgery is followed by the development of an abscess. Typical examples include:

* acute appendicitis,
* acute diverticulitis,
* perforated peptic ulcer,
* suppurative salpingitis;

but there are many other examples.

Iatrogenic

When surgery for elective or emergency conditions has been complicated, leading to:

* contamination with spillage of intraluminal contents during elective or emergency intestinal and colonic resection;
* injury to the tail of the pancreas during splenectomy or surgery involving mobilization of the splenic flexure of the colon, resulting in the accumulation of initially enzyme-rich fluid in the left subhepatic space often followed by bacterial contamination;
* intraperitoneal haematoma becoming secondarily infected, for example a pelvic abscess, after right hemicolectomy;
* persistent seepage following an insecure omental patch applied to a perforated duodenal ulcer.

Predisposing factors
Coexistent disease

Particularly important components are impairment of the immune defence system (for example, a patient on steroids), the presence of metabolic

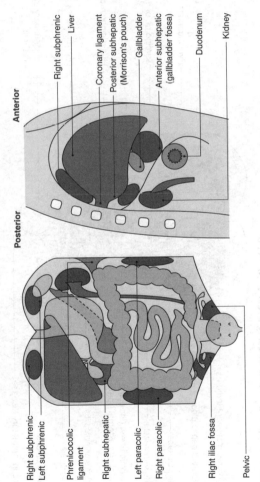

Anteroposterior sites of intra-abdominal abscesses

Right lateral sites of supracolic abscesses

Posterior   Anterior

Right subphrenic — Liver

Right subphrenic

Coronary ligament

Posterior subhepatic (Morrison's pouch)

Right subphrenic
Left subphrenic

Gallbladder

Phrenicocolic ligament

Anterior subhepatic (gallbladder fossa)

Right subhepatic

Duodenum

Left paracolic

Right paracolic

Kidney

Right iliac fossa

Pelvic

Abscess sites.

Intra-abdominal diseases causing abscess formation

Perforated malignant tumours

Perforated peptic ulcer

Biliary disease

Acute pancreatitis

Ischaemic bowel (including internal and external hernias)

Meckel's diverticulitis

Appendicitis

Crohn's disease

Pelvic inflammatory disease

Pyelonephritis

Carcinoma of the colon

Ureteric obstruction

Diverticulitis

Lower urinary tract infections

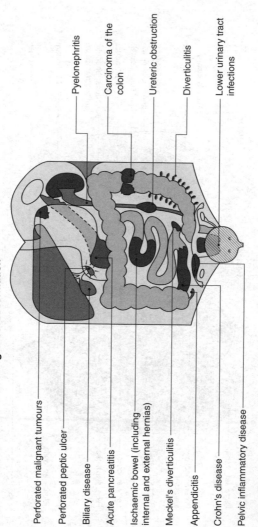

Causes of abscess formation.

diseases (such as diabetes mellitus), the elderly patient, the malnourished patient, and patients with extensive malignancy.

Site and nature of the pathology

Examples of this include: acute appendicitis complicated by local or general peritonitis leading to a pelvic or right iliac fossa collection of pus; perforated duodenal ulcer leading to a subhepatic or right paracolic collection; acute diverticulitis leading to a localized peritonitis and subsequent collection of pus in the left paracolic gutter.

Virulence and load of bacteria

For example, heavy contamination of the peritoneal cavity with colonic flora may lead to abscess formation. The organisms involved, in particular, are the Gram-negative aerobes such as *Escherichia coli* and anaerobic organisms including *Bacteroides*, *Enterococcus*, and *Clostridia* species.

Failure of therapeutic measures

When the surgeon finds general peritoneal contamination it is appropriate to wash out the area with normal saline or dilute aqueous antiseptic (such as chlorhexidine), with the aim of removing particulate material that would otherwise form a nidus for infection. Lack of care and thoroughness in this manoeuvre is a significant factor. The use of inappropriate antibiotics in relationship to the likely microorganisms at the time of surgery (the wrong empirical choice) or commencing the antibiotics too late are additional factors that increase the risk of an abscess developing. Surgery complicated by oozing and subsequent haematoma formation is another potent cause of therapeutic failure.

Presentation

General symptoms and signs include the patient feeling lethargic with anorexia and weight loss, often with nausea and generalized abdominal pain, and systemic features including tachycardia and pyrexia. The occurrence of SIRS (systemic inflammatory response syndrome) is usually readily definable and there may be signs of progression to single or multiple organ failure. Local symptoms and signs may include pain, tenderness, and swelling, together with altered visceral functions such as spurious diarrhoea, tenesmus, abdominal distension, vomiting, and frequency of micturition and strangury. Careful examination must include a general assessment and local inspection, looking for a tender swelling (and in this respect do not overlook the lumbar area where a perinephric or posterior-pointing subphrenic abscess may present). Since subphrenic abscesses may also cause a sympathetic pleural effusion, careful chest auscultation is essential. It is important to palpate gently and to include a digital rectal examination looking for the presence of mucus on the glove and a boggy swelling anteriorly, both of which indicate the likelihood of a pelvic abscess.

Timing

The inflammatory process leading to the formation of an abscess can be prolonged. In such cases, the postoperative course may initially appear to be satisfactory, but after an interval, varying from 5 to 20 days (although it may extend to many months), the patient's general condition deteriorates and a swinging, 'church spire', pyrexia develops. It is the development or progression of generalized signs that should alert the surgeon to the presence of an abscess.

Investigations

A full blood count, particularly white cell and differential counts, should be performed. It is also usual to send blood for electrolytes, urea, creatinine, and liver function tests, the latter being particularly relevant with regard to the level of albumin (which may reflect systemic inflammation and may fall in a precipitate manner) and also the presence or absence of enzymatic abnormalities (which may indicate a portal pyaemia). The coagulation profile should be checked, particularly as percutaneous or open drainage may need to be considered. Blood cultures may only be positive in 10% of cases but are a potent method for pathogen recognition.

Imaging includes ultrasound, which is inexpensive, relatively non-invasive, and can be done at the bedside, but is very operator-dependent and may be difficult to interpret during the postoperative period where there is much bowel gas. Where ultrasound is inconclusive but suspicion remains high, a contrast-enhanced computed tomography (CT) scan is usually the next investigation to consider. Although some reliance may be placed on the relatively non-invasive, isotope-labelled white cell scan, it is not as specific nor as sensitive. The advantage of both ultrasound and CT is that it enables the operator to not only locate but also to drain the collection under guidance. Most deep abscesses are now drained percutaneously in the radiology department, but an open operation may occasionally be required, particularly if the abscess is multiloculated or becomes chronic with a thick wall. It should be remembered that antibiotics will not penetrate into pus, but that antibiotic cover is important during manipulation when bacteria may be disseminated and also where there is an intra-abdominal phlegmon. ('Phlegmon' is a term used to define inflammatory tissue often with necrosis and some small multiple collections of microabscesses).

Deep infection: general peritonitis

As opposed to the process of localization with deep abscess formation, general peritonitis is fortunately a less frequent problem after abdominal surgery but is extremely serious. The presence of blood, bile, pancreatic juice, small intestinal or colonic contents, or urine, particularly if the leakage is persisting, will cause peritoneal irritation and the symptoms and signs of peritonitis.

Causes

+ An anastomotic leak;
+ Rupture of intra-abdominal abscess into the general peritoneal cavity, e.g. pelvic, subphrenic perianastomotic abscess;
+ Acute pancreatitis;
+ Acute cholecystitis (increased frequency in diabetic patients and those on total parenteral nutrition (TPN));
+ Perforated peptic or stress ulcer;
+ Mesenteric ischaemia (e.g. atrial fibrillation, cardiac failure).

Incidental causes

+ Acute appendicitis, acute cholecystitis, etc.

Predisposing factors, with particular reference to the commonest postoperative cause of a leaking anastomosis

+ Age (over 65 years);
+ Poor tissue perfusion, e.g. hypertension, cardiac failure;
+ Poor oxygenation, e.g. chronic obstructive pulmonary disease (COPD);
+ Malnutrition;
+ Immunocompromised patients (including immunocompromisation caused by medication), autoimmune disease (e.g. systemic lupus erythematosus (SLE));
+ Systemic disease, e.g. diabetes mellitus, renal failure;
+ Extensive malignancy.

Local factors include the site of anastomosis. For example, oesophageal and low rectal anastomoses are particularly prone to leak. Factors compromising anastomosis, such as the presence of peritonitis and poor blood supply, which may be related to systemic shock or local compromise because of tension on the anastomosis and poor technique

Presentation
Symptoms

These may often be masked by the absence of pain (e.g. patient on a ventilator, or a patient with an epidural or patient-controlled analgesia (PCA)). However, there are often general features, including failure to progress with a persistent tachycardia, pyrexia, and delay in return of gut function with abdominal distension, often with tenderness but not rigidity. High nasogastric aspiration and/or vomiting and the absence of flatus per rectum are all suggestive features. The clinician will be fully aware of the dangers of anastomotic leakage in certain situations and must be alert to the above features.

Diagnosis

Although often difficult, the experienced clinician will appreciate that the general signs and persistent abdominal distension with tenderness are of great concern. Laboratory features including an elevated WBC, often accompanied by electrolytic disturbance and particularly low albumin levels (less than 20 g/l) provide supporting evidence but are non-specific.

Imaging

The plain abdominal X-ray will show non-specific features such as distended loops of small bowel. However, there is often free gas from the original laparotomy in the peritoneum and therefore this test is often unhelpful.

Ultrasound may also be unhelpful due to the presence of gaseous distension in the intestines.

Contrast-enhanced CT may confirm a diagnosis with the demonstration of contrast leakage or suggest it by the presence of matted loops adjacent to the anastomosis indicative of the body's attempt to wall off the problem.

Treatment

Once the diagnosis is considered then the patient should be prepared for laparotomy with full resuscitation. If the patient is not already in an intensive therapy unit (ITU) or high-dependency unit (HDU), transfer preoperatively is advantageous.

Superficial infection: superficial surgical site infection

Predisposing factors—general

- Malnutrition;
- Immunocompromised patient (e.g. steroids, chemotherapy);
- Systemic disease, e.g. diabetes mellitus, chronic renal failure, jaundice;
- Widespread malignancy.

Local factors

- Primary pathology, e.g. presence of general peritonitis;
- Spillage of intestinal contents;
- Wound haematoma;
- Necrotic or foreign body in the wound.

Microbiology

The two commonest microorganism groups are:

- bowel flora, e.g. *E. coli*, *Bacteroides* species, *Streptococcus faecalis*, and *Enterococcus*, *Clostridia*, and *Proteus* species as well as *Pseudomonas aeruginosa*;

- staphylococci, including methicillin-resistant *Staphylococcus aureus* (MRSA) and *Staph. epidermidis*. This group becomes established when there has been a long preoperative stay due to skin colonization and is an example of hospital ward cross-infection. An outbreak of wound infection signals the need for extensive investigation to find the source of an MRSA epidemic, and for probable ward closure.

Presentation

General signs often include a persisting low-grade temperature. The patient may complain of persisting wound discomfort: examination may reveal surrounding erythema, swelling, and tension in the wound that subsequently becomes fluctuant and/or discharges pus.

Investigations

Pus should be taken for culture and sensitivity and it is appropriate to take blood cultures if the pyrexia is significant.

Treatment

Antibiotics are withheld unless there is spreading cellulitis. A particularly severe example is multiorgan failure with subcutaneous gangrene (the flesh-eating 'super-bug'). Multiple microorganisms, including anaerobic streptococci, are the cause of Meleney's gangrene of the abdominal wall or Fourniere's gangrene of the scrotum. These are the result of particularly virulent bacteria leading to spreading cellulitis and subcutaneous necrosis, often then progressing to myonecrosis, which, if left untreated will lead to death—it is more frequent in diabetic patients.

Spreading cellulitis can be treated with empirically appropriate antibiotic(s) for mixed gut flora or staphylococci; the regimen should be bacteriocidal in monotherapy or combination therapy to cover both anaerobic and aerobic organisms. An immediate Gram stain of the pus may provide useful additional guidance. Release of pus is essential, and tissue debridement of necrotic areas may need to be particularly extensive in cases of Meleney's or Fournier's gangrene.

Note—wound infection is a predisposing factor to wound dehiscence and in particular to the later development of an incisional hernia.

Anastomotic complications

These include:

- haemorrhage;
- perianastomotic abscess formation;
- leakage with resultant local general peritonitis;
- leakage with a low-output fistula of less than 500 ml/24 h, or a high-output fistula;
- recurrence of a primary pathology, e.g. carcinoma or Crohn's disease.

The technical points considered to be essential in avoiding anastomotic leakage are listed below:

- ensuring a good blood supply to the ends of the bowel to be joined,with particular reference to the way the mesentery in small- and large-intestinal anastomoses is handled so that the perpendicular branches from the arterial arcade are not compromised. It is also important to ensure that venous drainage is not impaired as this can lead to congestive ischaemia at the anastomosis.
- careful apposition using appropriate suture material and technique (absorbable suture such as Polydioxone used in a one-layer technique with sero-muscular suture). The diameter of the bowel ends should be as near equal as possible, and on occasions it is necessary to 'fishtail' the smaller diameter of the bowel to be anastomosed by cutting along the antimesenteric border.
- the avoidance of tension by appropriate mobilization. Where stapling devices are used instead of sutures, the surgeon must be familiar with the particular type of instruments and their application.

Complications at specific anastomosis sites

Oesophogastric anastomosis

Leakage from the anastomosis, which causes a very high mortality rate, is usually due to a combination of factors, such as poor blood supply, friable tissue, the use of too small a staple gun, or poor suture technique and tension. Bleeding during the immediate postoperative period may occur from the suture line or from a failure to secure one of many vessels ligated in the procedure. The presence of reflux of gastric acid or bile may lead to oesophagitis and, on occasion, chronic (anaemia) or acute blood loss from frank ulceration.

Gastrojejunal anastomosis

- Bleeding (usually on the gastric side of an anastomosis), is one of the commoner complications after stapling using the gastrointestinal anastomosis gun (GIA);

- Poor drainage in the postoperative period with a persistent nasogastric aspirate;
- Intussusception where the efferent loop intussuscepts into the gastric remnant causing obstruction (gangrene may occur);
- Volvulus at the anastomosis;
- A stomal ulcer which may cause haematemesis or melaena; may perforate leading to general peritonitis; may heal and lead to stenosis.

Small intestinal anastomosis

- Bleeding presenting as shock or/and intra-abdominal pain, anaemia, fullness or a mass near the site of operation, or melaena if it is intraluminal;
- Leakage presents as general peritonitis or as a local mass associated with ileus which then discharges as a fistula through the wound; there is usually a severe systemic response with SIRS;
- Failure to securely close the mesentery, leading to herniation and obstruction;
- Stenosis due to poor blood supply or recurrence of the primary problem, e.g. Crohn's disease.

Large intestinal anastomosis (after right hemicolectomy, etc.)

- Bleeding tends to be persisting bright blood passed per rectum, or if it is intra-abdominal or intrapelvic a mass associated with anaemia, which may subsequently lead to an abscess or stricture;
- Leakage, perianastomotic collection, local or general peritonitis, fistula;
- Stricture following leakage or technical fault.

Investigations and management of anastomotic complications

Bleeding

Requires urgent assessment of clotting and, according to the general state of the patient, may require blood transfusion and energetic correction of clotting disorders. When intraperitoneal bleeding persists, laparotomy is mandatory. Where bleeding is intraluminal (for example, after gastrojejunostomy or oesophagogastrojejunotomy) or if stress ulceration is suspected, then upper GI endoscopy is appropriate and may allow bleeding to be controlled with adrenaline (epinephrine) injection, diathermy, fibrin injection, or sclerotherapy. Sometimes arteriography can also be a vital help, particularly when the patient becomes systemically compromised, indicating continuous bleeding, and when the site of bleeding is not clear. In this situation, identification of the bleeding site is possible and embolization may be useful for its control. Isotope scanning is not appropriate for investigating acute postoperative haemorrhage.

Leakage

The two major problems following failure of anastomosis in the alimentary tract are ensuing sepsis and interference with intestinal function. Important points in management include:

+ Measures to control the effect of systemic infection and avoidance of multiorgan dysfunction by adequate and expeditious resuscitation; in particular, those involving protection of renal function and the use of appropriate antibiotics. This usually requires transfer of the patient to a high-dependency unit or intensive care unit, with particular emphasis on improving the cardiac output and circulatory state which may require a central venous line, an arterial line, and occasionally a Swan–Ganz catheter. This enables the appropriate inotropic support, e.g. noradrenaline (norepinephrine), dobutamine, and dopamine to be monitored. Cardiac irregularities may also require control. Respiratory function must be maximized to combat tissue anoxia, and in this respect a mini-tracheostomy with or without ventilatory support may be indicated. Renal dysfunction is initially an injury to the tubules following a reduction in renal plasma flow. Good fluid perfusion with adequate oxygenation and control of sepsis are the basic principles of management. The value of dopamine in a renal dosage is debatable; but when used in a circulatory support capacity it is important to carefully monitor the circulatory volume, bearing in mind that in sepsis the capacity is often increased due to vasodilatation. Overexpansion can often result in hyponatraemia and a fall in osmolality due to dilution of the plasma proteins, both of which further impair renal function. Antibiotic therapy is essential for the control of sepsis and the appropriate effective bactericidal antibiotic should be chosen, which should not be the same as that used in surgical prophylaxis. Third-generation cephalosporins, the newer penicillins, meropenem, imipenem, and tazobactam are important and are given based on local policies. Fungal superinfection must be guarded against and regular swabs are required (skin, upper airways, urine, blood, and any other lesion or discharge).

+ Local control of sepsis may require drainage, either by using a percutaneous route or by re-operation.

+ Diversion of the intestinal stream may be needed, for example the use of a loop ileostomy for a leaking right hemicolectomy or more distal anastomosis. On occasion, stenting may be possible—this is particularly referable to an oesophageal leak or a low anterior resection rectal leak.

+ Nutrition may be either enteral (preferably) with a feeding jejunostomy or parenteral (TPN). Sometimes the surgeon has the foresight to establish a feeding jejunostomy at the time of surgery, for example at radical oesophageal gastric or colonic surgery. The enteral route may not be appropriate where there is widespread intra-abdominal sepsis, fistulation, or ileus with impaired motility and reduced reabsorption.

Parenteral nutritional feeding should be through a dedicated tunnelled central line. The enteral feed should be made up in the pharmacy under sterile conditions—peripheral vein feeding is feasible, but is usually only a temporary measure prior to the establishment of the full TPN and dedicated feeding line.

The advantage of the enteral route is that it is more efficient, avoids entry-site sepsis, and maintains the intestinal barrier function against translocation. Provided sterile-manufactured enteral feed is used, bacterial enteritis is uncommon although the faeces tend to be unformed—this can be improved with the addition of fibre.

Parenteral nutrition is less efficient and suffers particularly from the associated problem of line sepsis—a dedicated feeding team has proved to be the best way of reducing sepsis. Advice should be taken with regard to the calorific value, protein content, and the particular requirements of the patient, particularly when there is established renal or hepatic failure together. Attention to trace elements is important. There has been a tendency in the past to provide too high a calorie intake which is poorly utilized in the presence of sepsis.

* Recurrent intra-abdominal abscess. Wherever possible percutaneous drainage is advisable, but sometimes, if it is multilocular, this cannot be successful and operation is required. Ultrasound evaluation, although relatively non-invasive and applicable to the ITU or HDU patient, is subjective and is made more difficult to interpret if there is ileus with gaseous distension of the intestines. CT scanning with intravenous or alimentary tract opacification is helpful and is not precluded provided the patient is haemodynamically stable, even if they are requiring ventilation. Isotope scanning is now less used because of its poor sensitivity and specificity. The medical team must be aware of the cumulative dose of irradiation with respect to serial CT scans.

* Established fistula: the management of which will depend on a number of factors:
  - high- or low-volume output (low volume = less than 500ml/24h);
  - the nature of the contents: proximal jejunal fistulas or duodenal fistulas containing high electrolyte and high enzyme contents are very challenging and there may be multiple exit points on the abdominal wall, often through a wound, that lead to increased collection difficulties and the risk of skin excoriation and digestion;
  - the underlying disease process;
  - the degree of continuity or lack of continuity of the bowel or viscus involved;
  - the presence or absence of distal obstruction.

When the patient has been resuscitated, stabilized, and nutritional requirements met, attention must be paid to the satisfactory collection of the fistula fluid. In this respect, the assistance of a stoma therapist is invaluable. It is often helpful with a high-output fistula to analyse the electrolyte content and replace accordingly. There is evidence that subcutaneous octeotride can reduce the volume of pancreatic, biliary, and duodenal secretions. Investigations of the alimentary tract present the radiologist with difficulties because of the presence of either ileus or the diluting effect of accumulated intestinal secretions. Barium cannot be used because it is toxic. CT scanning is helpful and a fistulogram can, on occasions, provide useful information. There is often associated sepsis and when SIRS and the multiorgan dysfunction syndrome (MODS) are present then aggressive antibiotic therapy is appropriate. Improved drainage can sometimes be achieved under radiological control. Definitive surgery should not be undertaken in the presence of uncontrolled sepsis.

Visceral injury

Open operation

Injury may occur because of the difficulty of the surgery for extensive complex disease such as multiple adhesions, Crohn's disease, or a resectable malignancy involving the adjacent viscera, or because of inadvertent iatrogenic injury. It is simplest to consider the various intra-abdominal organs and structures separately, highlighting when they are at particular risk. In some situations management is relatively straightforward with complications which may not be clinically significant, whereas in others they may lead to mortality, including death in the operating theatre.

Surgery to specific organs and structures
Spleen

The spleen is at risk of capsular tear during gastric resection, pancreatic surgery and mobilization of the splenic flexure of the colon. Inadvertent traction on adhesions results in tearing of the splenic capsule, and when small this may be controlled by diathermy using blunt forceps or the application of a haemostatic agent such as Surgicel, with or without suture. The application of an absorbable net, made, for example, of polyglactin, placed over a more seriously damaged spleen together with haemostatic agents may be needed, although this is more appropriate to traumatic rupture. On occasions, splenectomy for uncontrolled splenic bleeding is required, with or without implantation of splenic tissue into the layers of omentum to encourage development of splenunculi (which do not fully restore immunocompetence), but this may subsequently lead to adhesions. The asplenic patient should be nationally registered, requires immunization against capsulated organisms (*Pneumococcus*, *Haemophilus*, and *Meningococcus* spp.) and should take oral phenoxymethylpenicillin (penicillin V) 500 mg twice daily for a minimum of 2 years. Overwhelming postsplenectomy infection is much less common in adults than in children.

Late presentation of intraoperative injury to the spleen also occurs. It is recognized when a patient presents with discomfort in the upper abdomen and either a haemoperitoneum or a perisplenic collection (seen on ultrasound) and a falling haemoglobin level. Surgery is usually required.

Liver

Minor injury is not uncommon and may occur during cholecystectomy with tearing of the liver capsule around the gallbladder bed. This is usually well controlled with diathermy and the surgeon should not forget the value of hot-packing an oozing surface area of the liver, waiting, and then precisely controlling the individual bleeding points with diathermy.

The application of Surgicel can also be useful, particularly in the oozing gallbladder bed. In this situation Surgicel is applied with a hot swab placed over it and left there for 2–3 minutes, the swab can be removed later without disturbing the Surgicel. More major bleeding may require buttress suturing with a special blunt liver needle. Sutures are initially applied beside the bleeding area and then the effective control sutures are inserted at right angles. The use of the buttress sutures prevents the suture tearing the capsule and liver tissue when the knot is tightened. It is useful to apply Surgicel or another haemostatic agent to the bleeding area when the sutures are tightened.

Late complications of liver injury include perihepatic collections of blood and/or bile which usually require ultrasound-guided percutaneous drainage. If the injury is deeper than had been initially suspected, persistent bleeding or persistent bile leak may present as a recurring perihepatic collection. Arterial bleeding can be effectively controlled by embolization of the appropriate hepatic branch. Management of a leaking bile duct radicle involves both adequate drainage of the perihepatic collection and percutaneous transhepatic stenting.

Oesophageal injury

This may occur during vagotomy for duodenal ulcer disease—an operation in decline following the introduction of effective medical treatment—or during hiatus hernia repair. Significant reflux oesophagitis is often accompanied by perioesophagitis, or ulceration and dense perioesophageal tissues, resulting in difficult mobilization of the oesophagus in the hiatus of the diaphragm. This is a very serious life-threatening complication. The oesophagus should always be inspected after it has been manipulated, since the best opportunity for the patient's survival is to identify the injury and either repair it by direct suture or with a patch involving the utilization of the proximal gastric wall, or by resection. The particular danger is leakage of contaminated gastric fluid into the supra- or subdiaphragmatic spaces producing either an empyema or subphrenic abscess, or—most serious of all—mediastinitis.

Small bowel

This is probably the most frequent abdominal viscus to be injured during surgery, particularly during mobilization/division of adhesions relating to previous pathology or, most commonly, previous surgery. While exploring the abdomen the small bowel may be entered or the seromuscular or seromuscular mucosal layers torn. Unless the injury leaves a very ragged segment of bowel (requiring resection) this can usually be repaired by careful suture technique. Another cause of small-bowel complications is a damaged blood supply: One of the most serious situations follows compromise of either the superior mesenteric vein or artery, most frequently after a high tie of the ileocolic artery during right hemicolectomy to remove enlarged lymph nodes. The resulting ischaemia may require extensive resection and result in the short bowel-syndrome. Ischaemic small bowel may be difficult to recognize in the immediate postoperative period and may only be considered with the development of serious sepsis.

Small-bowel adhesions are fibrinous in the early phase following peritonitis or handling. These usually resolve, but may organize into fibrous bands either in sheets or string-like bands. The latter are the more serious because they permit a volvulus or internal herniation to occur, so that the blood supply of the involved intestine may become compromised. The topic of adhesions is presented later.

Large bowel

The most serious complication is compromise of the blood supply leading to anastomotic breakdown. Management depends on the extent and severity—if small, no more than antibiotics and control of the faecal fistula with a stoma bag may be required. More severe compromise requires systemic antibiotics, with re-operation and peritoneal lavage, and diversion of the faecal stream and drainage. Sometimes stenting the leaking colonic anastomosis may be possible, but this technique is still in its infancy. When there is complete anastomotic breakdown with a non-viable gut, the patient is in life-threatening danger of sepsis-induced MODS, which requires resuscitation on ITU with intravenous antibiotics and early return to theatre with further bowel resection, establishment of a proximal stoma, and peritoneal toilet. The abdominal wound may be either closed in its muscular layers leaving the superficial tissues open, or laparostomy may be required where the abdomen is left open, after drainage of the sepsis; the whole abdomen being treated as if it was the abscess cavity. When the sepsis has subsided, reinspection is a relatively simple matter and at that stage insertion of a mesh may be decided upon, since primary wound closure is neither possible nor desirable.

Pancreas

The types of operation that may be associated with postsurgical acute pancreatitis include: cholecystectomy and common bile duct exploration, particularly if the sphincter of Oddi is aggressively dilated or traumatized during stone extraction; or when a limb of a T-tube runs across the sphincter into the duodenum; or when a transduodenal sphincteroplasty is undertaken with failure to identify and thus protect the pancreatic duct orifice from inclusion in the sphincteroplasty suture line. Partial gastrectomy, particularly for a penetrating ulcer, risks pancreatic damage. The base of the benign ulcer should be left *in situ*, since excision will undoubtedly damage pancreatic acini and ducts with the risk of leak. Damage to a significant first-order or main pancreatic duct results in a peripancreatic collection which becomes an abscess or a pancreatic fistula. Colonic resection including transverse colectomy, left hemicolectomy, and total colectomy may also result in postoperative pancreatitis. Splenectomy may cause trauma to the tail of the pancreas with leakage of pancreatic enzymes producing, most commonly, a subphrenic abscess or if a drain is *in situ*, a pancreatic fistula.

Management of visceral injury

Pancreas

A high index of suspicion is essential after biliary, gastric, or colonic surgery when there is undue postoperative pain associated with tachycardia, poor urine output, and very significantly upper abdominal tenderness which should indicate the need to measure the plasma amylase. Once a diagnosis of acute pancreatitis has been made, accurate fluid replacement with careful electrolyte balance and a dedicated central intravenous line for parenteral nutrition is unusually required, ideally on an HDU. It is good practice to assess severity using a scoring system such as APACHE II, Ranson or Glasgow—the latter is probably the most useful for postoperative pancreatitis. The presence of these factors indicates a severe disease:

- On admission (immediately postop):
  - age > 55 years
  - WBC > 15×10^9/l
  - blood glucose > 10 mmol/l (in non-diabetic patients)
  - serum urea > 16 mmol/l
  - PaO_2 < 9 kPa
- Within 48 hours:
  - serum calcium < 2.0 mmol/l
  - serum albumin < 32 g/l
  - LDH > 600 units/l (LDH, lactate dehydrogenase)
  - AST > 600 units/l (AST, aspartate aminotransferase)

The mortality associated with acute pancreatitis is high. The patient should be stepped up to ITU care when the pancreatitis is judged to be severe. Imaging with contrast-enhanced CT should be considered in conjunction with the patient's circulatory and respiratory state to assess the extent of any pancreatic necrosis.

A pancreatic fistula can lead to serious excoriation of the skin and subcutaneous tissue—the help of a stoma therapist to produce a reliable collection system, thus enabling accurate volume monitoring and good skin protection, is essential.

Ureter and bladder

These viscera may be injured during gynaecological and colorectal surgery. The presence of extensive neoplasia increases the risk. Recognition of the injury at the time of surgery allows immediate repair of the ureter, usually incorporating a pigtail stent, which can subsequently be removed cystoscopically or radiologically. Injuries of the bladder base are particularly serious and in the female may lead to persistent incontinence, sometimes with a cystovaginal fistula. Failure to recognize ureteric injury leads to extravasation and abscess formation. Effective control may need partial resection and anastomosis of the ureter. Sometimes control may be achieved by insertion of a stent radiologically. If there is division with shortening, then anastomosis of the proximal ureter to the bladder using a Boari flap reconstruction may be required.

Major vessels, especially pelvic veins and presacral veins, may be subject to injury when there is extensive local malignant or inflammatory disease involving the rectum primarily and the female genital tract secondarily. Major venous haemorrhage is particularly difficult to control and the patient may die on the operating table.

Minimally invasive surgery

General

Visceral injury and complications

These may occur at a number of stages. Insertion of a Verres needle to create the pneumoperitoneum may, particularly in the presence of adhesions, enter the small or large intestine, traumatize mesenteric vessels, or, indeed, even the aorta or vena cava. Use of the blunt Hasan cannula technique may overcome this. A carbon dioxide embolus may occur if it is not appreciated that the Verres needle is in a vessel, or at a later stage when there is a large exposed visceral area, e.g. the gallbladder bed, where a venous tributary is exposed to the positive pressure within the abdominal cavity. Insertion of the ports may result in injury to the same organs described above with, in addition, damage to the liver. There are some dramatic instances described of ports that have been inserted through the liver, entering the diaphragmatic surface, and exiting posteriorly.

The most frequent laparoscopic procedures in general surgery include:

• diagnostic laparoscopy for acute abdominal pain, particularly in the female in the childbearing phase of life;

• staging laparoscopy in malignant disease, particularly gastric, distal oesophageal, and pancreatic carcinomas;

• therapeutic laparoscopic repair of hiatus hernia;

• and, most frequently of all, laparoscopic cholecystectomy.

Bleeding

This may occur from the abdominal wall muscles, such as the superior epigastric when the port for cholecystectomy is placed too far laterally in an attempt to avoid the falciform ligament, or from the other ports when a muscular branch is injured. This may lead to a painful local haematoma or sometimes significant anaemia with extensive extravasation. Bleeding from an intra-abdominal injury is a much more serious consequence. This may be due to the Verres needle or port entering a major vessel and requires instant laparotomy, which may require help from an experienced vascular surgeon. If the mesenteric vessels are injured this may not only cause a mesenteric haematoma but also compromise blood supply to the gut. In laparoscopic cholecystectomy, bleeding may occur from the cystic artery, gallbladder bed, or a mistaken hepatic artery, the latter being a serious consequence needing intervention.

Specific visceral damage

The anatomical structures may be mistaken during laparoscopic cholecystectomy and laparoscopic repair of hiatus hernia. With reference to laparoscopic cholecystectomy, the bile duct may be clipped, cut, or a segment resected. Extensive use of coagulation diathermy may result in ischaemia of the bile duct wall with bile leakage that can lead to a subhepatic collection, or a biliary fistula if there is a drain. The degree of damage varies enormously and treatment may range from early and simple removal of the clips to major duct repair (the French connection with a hepaticojejunostomy Roux-en-Y) usually to the confluence or left hepatic duct. Occasionally it is necessary, where damage is very extensive and the confluence itself is seriously damaged, to perform anastomosis to the segment III duct. There may rarely be major duct and vascular injury combined, either to the hepatic artery or portal vein, and in this situation liver transplantation may need to be considered. Laparoscopic repair of a hiatus hernia may be associated with injury to the spleen or to the oesophagus itself (which is usually due to the surgeon dissecting in the wrong plane or the overuse of diathermy). Dysphagia may be due to overtightening of the sutures or a perioesophageal haematoma, and failure of the repair may be due to the sutures being inadequate.

Organ-specific complications

Oesophagus

Complications may follow upper GI endoscopy, particularly those including therapeutic measures such as negotiation or dilatation of a stricture, dilatation of an achalasic segment, or laser resection of tumours. Complications range from inhalation of oesophageal contents, bleeding, and perforation, the latter can often be treated by conservative measures—nil orally, parenteral nutrition, antibiotics, and sometimes stenting.

Surgical complications may follow surgery for oesophageal reflux and hiatus hernia, oesophageal resection, and surgical treatment of achalasia (cardiomyotomy). Injury to the wall or failure of an anastomosis leads to the leakage of oesophageal and gastric contents into the mediastinum and pleural cavity with the rapid onset of SIRS and multiorgan failure, particularly pulmonary and renal. Oesophageal anastomoses are particularly prone to leakage because the anastomoses are technically difficult, and the absence of peritoneal covering to the oesophagus with the rather friable oesophageal musculature means that the sutures rely for much of their tensile strength on the mucosa and submucosa. There is a high mortality and often the patient's reserve to withstand this complication is reduced because they are elderly, may be malnourished, and often have coexistent COPD. Prevention of these serious complications is obviously most important but, although the advent of a fistula is managed along the lines already described, a particular problem is that the fistula track is indirect and may result in the pooling of secretions within the pleural cavity and the mediastinum.

Reflux and regurgitation are common sequels when the lower physiological gastro-oesophageal sphincter is compromised or excised, as in a resection. It is important in this situation to prevent inhalation by nasogastric aspiration with the use of prokinetics such as metoclopramide or domperidone and acid reduction (H_2 receptor antagonists or polyphosphoinositides (PPIs)). Later on, the simple measure of sleeping propped up (this is most easily and reliably achieved using a V-shaped pillow since ordinary pillows result in the patient rolling off), and raising the head of the bed—but this is uncomfortable to both patients and their partners and is often abandoned. Reflux of bile-stained fluid can quite rapidly lead to stenosis of the anastomosis with ulceration and subsequent fibrosis, and to a very severe grade-IV haemorrhagic oesophagitis.

Debilitated patients (including those who have had major oesophageal surgery) with complications are at risk from superinfection, particularly after prolonged antibiotic use. Favourite sites for fungal infection in the thorax are the lungs and pharynx—particularly frequent is oesophageal candidiasis, which should be considered when a patient complains of painful dysphagia.

Stomach

Elective surgery for peptic ulcer is now relatively rare. The majority of ulcers are related to *Helicobacter pylori* infection or the ingestion of non-steroidal anti-inflammatory drugs (NSAIDs). However, the healing of some ulcers is resistant to helicobacter eradication therapy or withdrawal of some NSAIDs. Surgery should therefore be directed towards the complications of peptic ulceration induced by such agents as steroids or NSAIDs (i.e. bleeding, perforation, or gastric outlet obstruction due to stenosis). It is recognized that these complications of the disease process can occur in the absence of any clearly demarcated aetiological factor. Thus, the operations of vagotomy and pyloroplasty, or vagotomy and drainage, or selective or highly selective vagotomy are now almost confined to the history books.

Major surgery is either palliative or curative for gastric malignancy (most frequently adenocarcinoma but also lymphoma). When the lesion is resectable this amounts to a radical upper or lower, or total gastrectomy combined with a lymphadenectomy and occasionally adjacent distal pancreatic or colonic resection. Potentially this major surgery can lead to a large number of intraoperative, early, intermediate, and late specific complications.

Intraoperative complications

Extensive disease may result in complications of bleeding or visceral injury, e.g. to the pancreas or mesocolon, or transverse colon and the spleen. Recognition of the injury and appropriate repair should be carried out. Pancreatic injury may cause postoperative pancreatitis, interference with the blood supply to the colon may require resection, splenic injury may respond, if small, to diathermy control, splenorrhaphy, but splenectomy may be required.

Early complications

- **Bleeding**—is most frequently from the gastric side of the suture line. It often settles spontaneously but may require re-operation with under-running. Lavage with chilled saline with or without adrenaline is no longer favoured. Intraperitoneal bleeding may be due to a slipped ligature, which is a technical error, or an unrecognized splenic injury.

- **Acute pancreatitis**—is often severe and may lead to SIRS and MODS.

- **Anastomotic failure**—is most frequently seen:
  - at oesophageal anastomosis, **or**
  - in the Polya-type gastrectomy with duodenal stump dehiscence, mortality is high. Resuscitation is required in intensive care, followed by

laparotomy and establishment of controlled drainage, particularly of the duodenal stump. The opportunity for effective resuturing is not usually an option. A feeding jejunostomy should be established if not already done.

Intermediate complications

+ **Dysphagia**—is often due to dysfunction and subsequent oedema and in the later situation fibrosis at the oesophageal anastomosis. This is causally related to bile reflux which is a common sequel after gastric resection. It is treated by prokinetics and mucosal protective agents (such as sucralphate).

+ **Anastomostic hold-up**—is a particular problem after gastrojejunal anastomosis and its aetiology is often unclear. There may be a dramatic obstruction due to retrograde intussusception or volvulus at the site of the anastomosis, but more often endoscopy will show that the anastomosis is quite patent. The hold up will usually settle with time; the presence of a feeding jejunostomy, created at the time of surgery, usually overcomes this effectively, since it offers a route for feeding and also the return of some or all of the clean aspirated contents from the gastric remnant.

Late complications

Generally gastric resection results in very considerable physiological changes, and for the ease of reading these will be classified as follows:

+ **Loss of appetite and postprandial fullness**—due to a reduced or absent gastric reservoir, the patient may need to take very frequent, small meals. Bile regurgitation produces a gastritis in the stomach remnant or oesophagitis, further reducing appetite.

+ **Weight loss**—is commonly due to decreased food intake, sometimes impaired absorption, and on occasions concomitant disease is highlighted, such as pancreatic insufficiency or a malabsorption syndrome, such as gluten enteropathy. It may also be related to recurrence of the original disease, stomal ulceration, or pulmonary disease—there is an increased risk of tuberculosis in these patients.

+ **Altered bowel habit, looseness, and diarrhoea**—is a complication of division of the vagus nerve, which is common to many of these operations. The patient may suffer from severe episodic watery diarrhoea and associated with considerable urgency. It is unpredictable and therefore difficult to control with standard medications such as imodium or codeine phosphate. It usually reduces in severity and frequency with time.

+ **Nausea and vomiting**—is often due to the highly irritant, bile reflux. Avoidance of fatty meals, which reduce upper gastrointestinal motility is helpful, as well as the specific medications already mentioned. The aetiology of bile vomiting in the post-Polya gastrectomy patient follows stimulation of the biliary and pancreatic juices, when food enters the stomach, which flow into the afferent loop forming a layer over the food. The patient then vomits pure bile and pancreatic juice.

- **Dumping**—this may be early or late and is very characteristic of the Polya-type partial gastrectomy. Early dumping is due to the rapid egress of hyperosmolar stomach contents into the small bowel, thereby producing distension with outpouring of fluid into the lumen of the small bowel. The patient feels very unwell, nauseated, faint, and sweaty and wishes to lie down. There are also audible borborygmi and sometimes colic. It settles spontaneously in 1–2 hours and can be prevented or reduced in severity by the patient avoiding hyperosmolar foods and taking fluid at a time separate from food. It eases with time.

- **Late dumping**—is characterized by the patient feeling cold, clammy, sweaty and unwell some 2 hours after a meal. It is due to the absorption of a large amount of carbohydrate from the proximal small intestine, with a resulting excessive response of insulin secretion from the pancreas giving a temporary hypoglycaemia. It is relieved by ingestion of carbohydrate in the form of a glucose drink or sweet.

- **Nutrition**—in addition to weight loss there are specific deficiencies, particularly of iron and vitamin B_{12}. A total gastrectomy patient always requires injections of vitamin B_{12} every 3 months.

- **Stomal ulceration**—recurrent or stomal ulceration tends to develop on the jejunal side of a gastric anastomosis and may present with complications including bleeding, with haematemesis or melaena, perforation with general peritonitis, and less commonly with stenosis of the stoma. Bleeding may be managed conservatively by endoscopic injection therapy and blood transfusion. It is usual to give protein-pump inhibitors and full eradication therapy for *Helicobacter* spp. if confirmed by testing. Avoidance of NSAIDs is mandatory. Perforation requires surgery and, depending on the state of the patient, involves either patching of the perforation or taking down and redoing the anastomosis. The latter is a major procedure in an ill patient. Stenosis can resolved with balloon dilatation and PPI and/or helicobacter eradication therapy, but it may require surgery.

- **Recurrence of carcinoma**—unfortunately, this is not infrequent in the Western world and tends to present as a lymph node mass with secondary involvement of the stomach remnant. A predisposing factor to recurrence in the stomach remnant itself is extensive intestinal metaplasia. Patients who have had a long-standing partial gastrectomy for duodenal ulcer disease are at an increased risk of developing an adenocarcinoma in the gastric remnant.

- **General complications** such as abdominal wall dehiscence and incisional hernia—are more frequent following the upper midline incision, or at the centre point of a roof-top incision if the latter has been used for extensive gastric resection. The thoracoabdominal approach is often complicated by discomfort at the costal margin, intercostal neuralgia, but less commonly by herniation.

Biliary tract

General comments

The detection of abnormal liver function tests postoperatively, irrespective of the type of surgery, must always be taken seriously. An elevated bilirubin may have prehepatic, hepatic, and posthepatic causes. Prehepatic causes are associated with normal enzyme levels and after surgery may relate to either haemolysis or possibly to an exacerbation of abnormal bilirubin transport rate mechanisms, e.g. Gilbert's syndrome. Elevation of AST and alanine aminotransferase (ALT) indicate hepatocellular damage and may often be associated with a low albumin level due to synthesis problems. Aetiology may be divided into two broad categories: drug-related and infection. The former often produce a mixed picture of abnormal liver function tests (LFTs) with elevation of AST, ALT, and alkaline phosphatase, indicating both hepatocellular damage and cholestasis. The other broad group, infective causes, may be of viral or bacterial aetiology—particularly important is the transmission of hepatitis C and hepatitis B; Epstein–Barr virus (EBV) and cytomegalo inclusion virus (CMV) are of special concern in immunocompromised patients. Established bacterial infections (as in severe cholangitis or intrahepatic abscesses) cause the AST and ALT levels to rise and to remain elevated, as well as a rise in the alkaline phosphate level. If the infecting microorganism is identified as a virus, the help of a hepatologist should be enlisted to define treatment and prognosis accurately since the occurrence of hepatitic C infection may lead to chronic active hepatitis and cirrhosis (with an increased incidence of hepatocellular carcinoma) or the patient may become a carrier. With regard to bacterial infection affecting the liver, through portal pyaemia, severe pelvic inflammatory disease (caused by *Chlamydia* spp.), appendicitis, or diverticulitis are well-recognized causes.

Cholestasis is characterized by an elevation of alkaline phosphatase. It has a number of causes which may be divided into intrahepatic and extrahepatic. Many drugs can cause cholestasis and often just simple withdrawal will result in improvement and resolution. Mechanical obstruction is often accompanied by cholangitis which may progress to multiple liver abscesses. Intraluminal biliary tract obstruction is most commonly related to calculous disease with the responsible bacteria being typically bowel flora, although anaerobes are uncommon. Intramural causes include a benign stricture (which may follow surgical trauma) or a primary malignancy (usually cholangiocarcinoma). Calculi and benign strictures are characteristically associated with Charcot's triad: namely, jaundice, pain, and rigors. The management of septic cholestasis requires precise diagnosis. Laboratory tests should include liver function tests and clotting studies, it is also advisable to carry out full viral and autoantibody screens, then high-quality imaging, including ultrasound and MR cholangiography.

Specific biliary complications

Laparoscopic cholecystectomy has now superseded the open route as the operation of choice, although surgeons should not regard it as a dishonour or failure to have to convert to the open procedure (in approximately 10% of operations). Patient safety is paramount since significant bile duct injury is never associated with a normal life expectancy.

Laparoscopic/open cholecystectomy

Bleeding

The cystic artery may not be identified or may not be adequately ligated or clipped during the process of cholecystectomy. In a difficult dissection it may be traumatized or it may be disrupted and the proximal end will recoil, not bleeding during the operation but producing a secondary haemorrhage necessitating the patient's return for re-operation. More frequently there is oozing from the gallbladder bed, particularly where the cholecystectomy has been done in the presence of acute inflammation, and this may lead to a subhepatic haematoma which may in turn become infected.

Subhepatic collection

This is not uncommon after laparoscopic and open cholecystectomy and, interestingly, the use of drains has not been shown to significantly reduce its incidence. A collection of bile, blood, and lymph in the gallbladder fossa and subhepatic pouch is likely to become infected as the presence of stone disease is always associated with bacteria. It is more likely during cholecystectomy for acute inflammation or when there are many adhesions, or fibrosis, when the dissection strays deep to the gallbladder bed and there is more likely to be oozing from the liver. Occasionally the duct of Luschka (a small biliary ductule that enters the gallbladder directly from the right hepatic lobe through the gallbladder bed) may be divided.

The collection may lead to the patient becoming unwell; often having gone home, they are readmitted with pyrexia, commonly mild jaundice, intense nausea, and discomfort or pain. The patient should be assessed with blood tests including blood cultures, given appropriate antibiotics if systemically unwell, and then imaged using ultrasound. If a collection is identified it can usually be treated by percutaneous aspiration. A more serious cause of a subhepatic collection occurs when it is associated with injury to the bile ducts. This can be due to diathermy injury with subsequent necrosis of an area of the duct wall, failure to secure the cystic duct by double ligature or clipping, laceration of a bile duct during cholecystectomy, or, indeed, division of the bile duct with or without resection where the proximal end of either the left hepatic, right hepatic, or common hepatic ducts drain directly into the subhepatic area.

The key to management is resuscitation, control of infection by taking appropriate cultures (including blood cultures) and starting on broad-spectrum antibiotics, and then imaging using ultrasound, magnetic resonance (MR) cholangiography, or endoscopic retrograde cholangiopancreatography (ERCP) as appropriate (see later).

Cholangitis

Cholangitis is an ascending infection of the biliary tree, usually bacterial, and the more commonly involved organisms include *E. coli* and *Streptococcus*, *Klebsiella*, *Enterococcus*, *Staphylococcus*, and *Proteus* species, and less commonly *Pseudomonas* spp. and the Gram-negative anaerobic bacteria, such as *Bacteroides* species. Occasionally, clostridial species may be involved, particularly in diabetic patients.

Patients present as being unwell, and this can be a life-threatening condition with high pyrexia, rigors, pain, and jaundice. Liver function tests are characterized by elevated bilirubin, AST, and alkaline phosphatase, although the extent of the elevation is usually more marked in respect of alkaline phosphatase. In the elderly patient, renal function is threatened.

Treatment involves energetic resuscitation and the appropriate antibiotics followed by intense investigation. Causes include: residual or recurrent common bile duct stones, or a benign stricture from previous stone disease. Stones may cause ulceration of the bile duct and surgical removal may lead to healing by fibrosis but, more commonly, stricture relates to surgical injury during cholecystectomy. Changes in liver function tests are characterized by raised bilirubin, AST, and particularly alkaline phosphatase levels. If the obstruction and infection persist then vitamin K absorption will be impaired and the INR or prothrombin time become prolonged. Following control of sepsis and identification of the cause, residual or recurrent stones can often be treated by endoscopic sphincterotomy without resort to open exploration. Leakage from the cystic duct, due to a slipped ligature or clip, can be treated by ERCP, endoscopic sphincterotomy (ES), and insertion of a stent. Stricture of the bile duct (post-traumatic benign fibrous stricture) may initially be treated by balloon dilatation and insertion of a stent. However, definitive surgery is usually required unless the patient is very unfit, otherwise recurrent cholangitis with the development of sludge and possibly calculi in the distal biliary tree is common. Bile duct reconstruction is a major intervention which should be undertaken by a specialist. Residual or recurrent bile duct stones may present: with jaundice during the early postoperative phase; with persistent high-volume bile drainage with a T-tube if the bile duct has been explored by supraduodenal choledochostomy; or with a persistent biliary fistula if the bile duct has been primarily sutured or the T-tube removed without ensuring adequate flow of contrast medium into the duodenum. This may also be seen after endoscopic sphincterotomy where the endoscopist has been unable to clear the bile ducts of calculi, or has accepted that the stones cannot be removed on the first occasion in the expectation that they may pass spontaneously. In the elderly patient where there are multiple stones, it may be accepted that these are left *in situ* and a stent is then inserted to promote good biliary flow. The surgeon should always be aware that the retrieval of one bile duct stone necessitates a very careful look for further stones—it is well documented that residual calculi most frequently occur in the situation where, at the primary operation, a number of stones have been extracted from the bile duct.

Alternative treatments for residual as opposed to recurrent stones exist for the patient who has undergone open exploration via the supraduodenal route with insertion of a T-tube. If the stone lies between the point of insertion of a T-tube into the bile duct and sphincter there are two alternatives: either ERCP and endoscopic sphincterotomy; or flushing through the T-tube, which must be done under careful pressure control and antibiotic cover, otherwise serious sepsis may ensue. If this methods fails and ERCP either fails or is considered to be inappropriate, then the patient and surgeon must wait for 6 weeks for the fibrous track around the T-tube to mature. At that stage after cholangiography and reconfirmation of the presence of residual stones, the T-tube is extracted and by means of a steerable basket catheter the stone can be extracted under radiological guidance (the Burhenne method). Flexible choledochoscopy and extraction under direct vision are alternatives to the basket method. After removal of the stone a catheter is inserted down the T-tube tract to maintain patency and a further cholangiography is taken to confirm the absence of any residual calculi and the free flow of contrast into the duodenum. The catheter can then be removed.

Bile duct injuries

In view of the large number of anatomical variations in this area, together with the very varied pathology, any surgeon in carrying out cholecystectomy must be alert of the dangers of biliary injury. If it occurs, the optimum results are gained by recognition at the time of surgery and by enlisting the help of a specialist biliary surgeon or transferring the patient to a specialist unit if the injury is extensive. Where the injury is not recognized at the time of surgery, the patient is likely to present with septic complications, i.e. a biliary fistula, bile leak with subhepatic collection, or cholangitis. The therapeutic principles in such cases are the control of sepsis with drainage of any collection, antibiotic cover, full investigation to establish the nature of the injury and its severity, and referral for appropriate treatment. The results of the first repair should give the best opportunity for a satisfactory long-term result. After a bile duct repair, the patient should have regular follow-ups with liver function tests and, if appropriate, imaging for at least 10 years. It is always important to define if there has been associated vascular injury and in this respect MRI scans are very helpful.

Cholecystoduodenostomy and choledochoduodenostomy

Cholecystduodenostomy is an operation that is now less commonly performed for bypassing malignancy—less invasive alternatives include insertion of a stent: ideally by the endoscopic route, but if necessary by the percutaneous or combined approach. Choledochoduodenostomy is utilized when it is not possible to be certain that the bile duct has been cleared of calculi or when there is a distal stricture considered unsuitable for excisional surgery, whether malignant or benign, by a direct approach with a transduodenal strictureplasty. Apart from anastomotic leakage, which is relatively rare, a specific complication is known as the 'sump' syndrome in which the patient has discomfort and infection arising from residual calculi stacking up in the distal bile duct. In addition, cholangitis may occur where the stoma has stenosed—it should be made at least 2 cm wide to allow free egress of bile and ingress of duodenal contents.

Pancreas

Pancreatic surgery for benign or malignant disease is major and carries significant risks. The more common procedures increasingly carried out in selected centres with high expertise in patient selection, regular practice of this difficult surgery, and intensive postoperative care include:

* resection of the head;
* pancreatic duodenectomy with preservation of the pylorus in benign disease and for most carcinomas of the distal bile duct and ampulla;
* distal pancreatectomy;
* total pancreatectomy;
* lateral pancreaticojejunostomy for the chain of leaking chronic pancreatitis (Frey operation);

Lesser procedures include:

* cystojejunostomy or cystogastrostomy for true or pseudo cysts; and
* transduodenal local resection of ampullary carcinoma with reimplantantion of the biliary and pancreatic ducts.

Intraoperative complications

* Visceral injury, especially blood vessels, e.g. portal vein haemorrhage;
* Technical difficulties with anastomosis:
  - *pancreatic*—the duct may be small leading to difficulty in suturing to the jejunal loop, or the suture to the pancreatic parenchyma may cut out resulting in an insecure pancreaticojejunostomy;
  - *biliary*—if the bile duct is small it may cause obstruction, cholangitis, and stenosis;
  - *duodenal*—if the blood supply to the retained duodenum is precarious, the anastomosis may fail, leak, be slow to 'open up', or stenose.

Early postoperative period

Elderly, jaundiced patients undergoing prolonged operation with significant fluid loss and hypothermia, are predisposed to suboptimal circulatory function, and renal failure is not infrequent. Where persisting lung disease (COAD, chronic obstructive airways disease) is significant, there is a risk of:

+ respiratory failure;
+ anastomotic leak;
+ ileus—a feeding jejunostomy allows effective feeding utilizing a small section of jejunum;
+ pancreatitis (acute).

Intermediate postoperative period

Commonly:

+ septic complications particularly affecting the lung and pleural space; and
+ intra-abdominal (subphrenic, paracolic) complications.

Or less commonly:

+ cholangitis (obstruction at the anastomosis), and
+ wound infection (predisposing to incisional hernia).

Experience of the surgeon and his team together with an appropriately experienced radiologist both pre- and postoperatively and access to an ITU all help to reduce the surgical risks of pancreatic resection.

Late complications

+ Incisional hernia
+ Obstruction
+ Weight loss
+ Steatorrhoea
+ Malabsorption
+ Recurrent cholangitis
+ Recurrence of primary pathology, e.g. carcinoma of the head of the pancreas
+ Progression of primary disease, e.g. chronic pancreatitis (patients who continue to drink alcohol)
+ Diabetes mellitus

Patient follow-up is important during the early years.

Small bowel

The majority of small-bowel operations are resections, although bypass or stricture-plasty, particularly for Crohn's disease, are also performed. The complications of a small-bowel resection may be summarized as:

- obstruction;
- leakage;
- bleeding;
- malabsorption of specific elements (e.g. vitamin B_{12})—if the terminal ileum has been resected or if there has been a massive resection there will be malabsorption leading to weight loss with steatorrhoea; stenosis of the anastomosis, or blind loops with bypasses, lead to bacterial colonization and this may lead to malabsorption;
- recurrence of the original pathology—this is perhaps most typically seen with Crohn's disease.

Obstruction

Obstruction of the small intestines may be classified as:

- partial or complete
- acute or chronic
- associated with loss of viability

Adhesions

This is one of the most unpredictable postoperative complications in terms of morbidity and mortality. Adhesions may arise as a result of the primary pathology, e.g. acute appendicitis with peritonitis, or as a result of surgery (minimally invasive surgery carries an advantage over open surgery in this respect).

Preventive measures

- Prompt treatment
- At operation, avoid glove powder and leaving debris or necrotic tissue (e.g. distal to a ligature)

Clinical presentation
Acute small-bowel obstruction

Patients present with vomiting and pain—the more proximal the site of the obstruction, the more prominent the vomiting and dehydration and the less marked pain (colic). There is an absence of passage of flatus.

Adhesions produce obstruction by a string-like band(s) causing simple end obstruction, or by trapping a small-bowel loop, or by causing a volvulus.

Initial management is the relief of pain, fluid replacement intra-venously to restore urine output, and nasogastric decompression to relieve repeated vomiting (and prevent inhalation) and aid natural resolution of the problem.

When should surgery be undertaken?

Laparotomy and the relief of obstruction is indicated for bowel with an impaired blood supply (arterial or venous) and for established ischaemia—the decision is based on careful clinical management.

1. Is the pain *continuous* with exacerbation of colic?
2. Is there persisting tachycardia/or pyrexia (despite adequate conservative treatment)?
3. Is there persisting local or general tenderness or guarding (rigidity in the presence of suspected adhesion obstruction is an absolute indication for surgery after appropriate intensive resuscitation)?

Recurrent small-bowel obstruction

Repeated admission for conservative treatment which is satisfactory in the short term sometimes requires surgical intervention with adhesiolysis and sometimes insertion of a long enteral tube (the Aberdeen or Jones tube).

Adhesion are frequently considered to be a cause of recurring mild or chronic abdominal pain. The evidence for this is weak and often division of adhesions (currently using laparoscopic methods) does not guarantee relief of symptoms.

Postoperative intestinal leakage

Leakage can either present as general peritonitis or either fistulation to the wound or down a drain site. Intestinal leakage requires transfer of the patient to the intensive care unit because they are usually desperately ill with signs of general peritonitis, SIRS, and at risk of MODS. Following a period of resuscitation and appropriate antibiotic therapy, they should be transferred to theatre for laparotomy with cleansing of the peritoneum, during which a decision has to be made whether the anastomosis can be redone or whether it is safer to bring out both ends to the surface (exteriorization). Of course, if the anastomosis is proximal this will lead to a very high-output jejunostomy, which itself creates considerable management problems both from the high volume to be collected satisfactorily into an appliance and also from the point of nutrition and electrolyte and fluid balance.

Fistulas in the small bowel may be high or low output. A low output is where the volume per 24 hours is less than 500 ml—this is usually neither associated with fluid and electrolyte balance problems nor nutritional deficiencies. However, because the track is often indirect there may be considerable septic problems. A high-output fistula is associated with the loss of significant volumes of fluid and electrolytes, poor nutrition, and skin excoriation due to the enzymatic activity of the proximal small bowel and fluid containing, as it does, pancreatic and duodenal enzymes. For the high-output fistula there are important principles of management:

1. **Adequate fluid and electrolyte replacement**—is facilitated by accurate collection of the fistula fluid together with analysis of the electrolyte content.

2. **Nutrition**—the enteral route is often precluded; in fact, one of the principles is to rest the intestinal tract and thus total parenteral nutrition through a tunnelled dedicated central line catheter is appropriate.

3. **Control of sepsis**—this is a combination of appropriate antibiotic therapy and the securing of direct drainage. Establishing the extent and nature of the fistula requires identification of the site of distal obstruction, whether the bowel is healthy at that point or is involved with a disease process such as Crohn's disease or cancer, and whether the bowel anastomosis is still in continuity. Lack of bowel continuity and distal obstruction indicate that the fistula cannot be expected to close spontaneously. It is important to ensure that the distal small bowel and colon do not become blocked with inspissated faecal material.

Surgery for a fistula should not be undertaken in the malnourished septic patient and requires an experienced gastrointestinal surgeon. The principles of defining the fistula or fistulas, excising diseased bowel, performing a good anastomosis with precision and lack of tension, and ensuring that there is no distal obstruction are critical. In the attempt to reduce the volume of a high-output fistula, pharmacological agents have been tried (e.g. somatostatin), with reduction of acid secretion either by intravenous H_2-antagonists (e.g. ranitidine) or if small amount of fluids can be tolerated, by oral PPIs.

Where there is extensive disease (e.g. caused by irradiation or Crohn's disease) with severe sepsis, then it may be better to establish two formal ends of bowel—either ileostomy or jejunostomy with the proximal end (which is the functional end), and by bringing up the distal end as a 'mucous fistula'. This will allow time for continued resuscitation, resolution of sepsis, and surgery under more auspicious conditions.

Bleeding

Bleeding after small-bowel surgery may occur in the mesentery or from a mesenteric vessel into the peritoneum producing a haemoperitoneum (most of these lead to abdominal pain and collapse and usually indicate if significant laparotomy). Most commonly, bleeding from the anastomosis usually presents as melaena and frequently settles spontaneously, although transfusion may be required and on occasions re-laparotomy with revision of the anastomosis.

Malabsorption

Short-bowel syndrome

This may arise where recurrent surgery is performed (e.g. for Crohn's disease) or where a massive small-bowel resection is undertaken because of severe injury such as ischaemia or irradiation. If anastomosis has been done it can be expected that, given time, there will be adaptation and proliferation of the small-bowel villi leading to improved absorption; however, in the early stages severe electrolyte and fluid loss with malabsorption and malnutrition are evident. This is an indication for total parenteral nutrition and, eventually, home parenteral nutrition—where the patient will be taught how to carry out overnight feeding, with limited oral fluids being permitted, and occasionally a small amount of liquid diet which is often elemental in the first instance. Attempts to control the diarrhoea involve prescribing high doses of codeine phosphate and loperamide. Acid reduction is essential. These patients are best managed in nutritional units and can expect a reasonable quality of independent life.

Complications of colorectal surgery

Complications after minor proctological procedures

Fissure *in ano*

Sphincter stretch

This is no longer recognized as a first-line operation due to risk of **incontinence**. The incontinence risk is higher in the older age group, particularly multigravidae.

Sphincterotomy

Complications:

- the incontinence risk must be discussed when taking consent, as slightly altered control of faeces is initially not unusual but it should settle after a few weeks;
- abscess, which may need drainage;
- new fissure at sphincterotomy site;
- bleeding, which rarely may need surgical intervention if packing is ineffective.

Fistula *in ano*

- Laying open:
  - haemorrhage;
  - failure of open wound to heal;
  - incontinence if there is suprasphincteric involvement which is not recognized;
  - perianal soreness is inevitable.
- Seton, if fistula is suprasphincteric:
  - causes discomfort and irritability;
  - leads to infection with recurrent abscesses, discharge of pus, and occasionally systemic sepsis;
  - means that the risk of incontinence remains.

Incontinence may require surgical intervention with specialist repair or occasionally a proximal stoma.

Anal polyp excision

Usually this is not painful and it carries a low risk of complications. A full thickness, overgenerous excision may cause haemorrhage or lead to infection.

Haemorrhoids

Banding

- Extreme pain results if the band is too distal, and the patient may need to be admitted to hospital for opiate therapy or removal of the band;
- Haemorrhage—minor is inevitable, major is rare and requires surgery if packing is ineffective;
- Anorectal abscess;
- Fissure.

Injection

- Urological complications may occur if anterior injection is too deep haematuria, haemospermia, or dysuria;
- An abscess which requires drainage;
- Necrosis of the area if overstrong phenol is inadvertently used (use 5% phenol in oil).

Operation

Haemorrhoidectomy

May result in:

- abscess and sepsis (rare);
- soreness;
- urinary retention which needs catheterization;
- difficult bowel evacuation because of severe pain;
- incontinence—do not damage the sphincter;
- anal stenosis—too much skin taken, skin bridges must be adequate; reconstruction or proximal stoma may be required if it is severe, but it usually responds to dilatation.

Abscess

Incision and drainage are usually complication free, but:

- there is the risk of not recognizing an underlying fistula—further abscesses or sepsis, or failure to heal;
- there may be underlying unrecognized disease (as in all proctological operations), such as Crohn's disease, which relates to poor results and requires intervention; if in doubt take a biopsy at first operation.

Complication of endoscopic procedures

Colonoscopy

Endoscopy of the colon may be diagnostic or therapeutic; obviously the complication rate is higher where operative procedures are performed. These days it is usual for the procedure to be diagnostic with a view to it being operative if necessary—biopsy, polyp removal, injection of haemorrhagic areas may be necessary.

Specific complications are unusual (< 1% risk):

- **bowel perforation**—usually occurs at polypectomy, although it may occur due to pressure during a diagnostic procedure, particularly in patients with inflammatory bowel disease. The perforation may be total—giving peritonitis—or incomplete—causing local inflammation which may lead to abscess formation. Treatment may need to be operative but it can be expectant (abscesses may be drained by interventional radiology), particularly as the bowel should be empty of faeces. **Beware** the risk of faecal peritonitis and its severe sequelae which may be life-threatening. Suspicion and anticipation are the key, with an early decision for operation.

- **bleeding**—usually settles. Any coagulopathy needs attention but the need for surgical intervention is rare.

Rigid sigmoidoscopy

Although this is unusual to cause complications, bleeding after biopsy of a tumour can be seen. Similarly, bowel perforation is possible, albeit rare.

Stoma formation

Stomas may be necessary for temporary faecal diversion to cover anastomoses and minimize the complications of leak, or as an emergency procedure after bowel perforation which may be primary or a postoperative complication. Permanent stomas are usually performed when there is no adequate bowel distal to the stoma (such as abdominoperineal (A/P) excision for cancer).

Loop stomas when total bowel continuity is only partially disrupted are normally used only as a temporary measure, whereas end stomas are generally used for permanency—but sometimes they can be a temporary measure (e.g. Hartman's operation). It should be noted that a temporary stoma in certain circumstances may have to become permanent, either due to other complications or the patient's general condition not safely allowing further surgery.

The complications of both loop and end stomas are similar, However, loop stomas have the added complication that it is possible, but unusual, that the faecal stream may not be totally diverted and may continue down the bowel.

- The stomas formed are:
  - loop ileostomy—usual covering stoma after a distal colonic anastomosis;
  - end ileostomy;
  - caecostomy—rarely performed now;
  - loop transverse colostomy—was the conventional covering stoma for anterior resection, now rarely used due to high prolapse risk and difficulty in managing a 'wet colostomy';
  - loop sigmoid colostomy;

- end colostomy;
- double-barrelled colostomy (Paul Mikulicz).
- Usual practice for stoma formation is:
  - loop ileostomy
  - end ileostomy
  - loop distal colostomy
  - end distal colostomy

Rarely, high small-bowel stomas are necessary with the inherent problems of high output and fluid and nutritional balance difficulties.

Specific complications of stomas

- **Necrosis**—due to poor blood supply, and is a technical error in the stoma formation. However, beware the obese abdomen and short mesocolon that may cause great difficulty in stoma formation without tension. Necrosis may be superficial and not require surgical intervention, it can be recognized by insertion of a small test tube into the stoma.
- **Retraction**—again a technical error due to not mobilizing the bowel to come out to the surface well enough. It is usually minimal and self-correcting but may need refashioning.
- **Peristomal abscess**—less common than might be expected.
- **Stenosis**—a late result of ischaemia and retraction. May require refashioning if dilatation fails.
- **Prolapse**—a late complication that may cause great concern. Common after right transverse loop colostomy and almost always requires surgical intervention.
- **Parastomal hernia**—may be a difficult problem and may be hard to repair. Surgical intervention is critical when there is bowel obstruction in the hernia.

Major colorectal surgery

Colonic resections are undertaken for cancer, diverticular disease, inflammatory bowel disease, and ischaemic bowel disease. The major surgery of the colon and rectum must involve ensuring an adequate blood supply to the bowel remaining, and most complications result from not ensuring this. Specific complications such as anastomotic failure and sepsis may be life-threatening and in no small way contribute to the mortality (about 5%) of these procedures. Anticipation and early recognition with surgical intervention are the key to successful management.

Where excision of cancer for curative intent is undertaken, great care must be taken to ensure that bowel used for the anastomosis is viable. Some operations are more liable to anastomotic complications than others: low anterior resection is particularly vulnerable, due to the risk of loss of blood supply to the bowel deep in the pelvis and anastomosis with the distal rectum. The splenic flexure has a similar anatomical predisposition to poor blood supply. If the bowel ends are clearly not viable prior to anastomosis they must be refashioned.

Wound infection and, to a lesser extent, intraperitoneal sepsis are recognized complications. Antibiotic prophylaxis and adequate bowel preparation have been shown to be effective. It is negligent not to use antibiotic prophylaxis for colonic resections.

After colonic resection there are risks of:

- haemorrhage;
- infection—wound and intraperitoneal;
- anastomotic dehiscence;
- wound dehiscence.

Moreover, myocardial and pulmonary complications, while being more general as opposed to specific complications, are common in what is an older group of patients often with significant comorbidity.

Specific operations and their complication risks
Right hemicolectomy

This includes extended right hemicolectomy with resection of the colon and caecum to the descending or upper sigmoid colon, usually from obstructing cancer. This extended operation is more likely to cause specific complications of:

- wound infection;
- anastomotic dehiscence—this is relatively unusual as long as there is no obstruction in the colon distal to the anastomosis; this complication presents as an intra-abdominal abscess, a fistula, or peritonitis;
- anastomotic bleeding (rare);
- postoperative bowel frequency and minor incontinence is more common after the extended operation.

Left hemicolectomy

Once surgery involves the left colon the risk and incidence of complications increases. This operation may be performed for cancer, diverticular disease, or more rarely inflammatory bowel disease (e.g. Crohn's disease) and should entail anastomosing the transverse colon to the upper rectum. It is essential that the resection should be to the rectosigmoid junction at least, because if this is left below a suture line it acts as a physiological sphincter and can cause enough distal obstruction to provoke an anastomotic leak.

- **Learning point**: make sure there is no anastomosis just proximal to the rectosigmoid junction.

Complications are more common, and similarly are:

- infection—wound and intraperitoneal;
- suture line dehiscence (with fistula abscess or peritonitis);

- wound dehiscence usually presenting late as an incisional hernia— while a burst abdomen should be totally preventable with modern techniques it is still occasionally seen;
- postoperative ileus—obstruction that may be related to a subclinical leak;
- neurological complications (see later);
- suture line recurrence of cancer.

High anterior resection

From a complication perspective, this procedure is similar to left hemicolectomy.

Low anterior resection

In this operation the rectum itself is mobilized in the pelvis, in the case of cancer, with a mesorectal excision. This brings in a whole host of other potential problems and complications. A total mesenteric excision with a distal anastomosis, while necessary for cancer cure, increases the risk of complications. Avoidance of anastomotic tension by full splenic flexure mobilization helps to reduce anastomotic breakdown.

The anastomosis is usually stapled, but can be sutured, and is much more at risk of breakdown—clinical leak rates may be as high as 5–10%; occult leak rates are much higher if this is sought with a water-soluble contrast enema. Identification of leaks by digital or endoscopic examination may worsen anastomotic disruption.

As before, the complications are:

- wound infection;
- intraperitoneal sepsis and pelvis sepsis, which may lead to SIRS and MODS with a high mortality;
- anastomotic dehiscence causing peritonitis, faecal fistula, or peritonitis;
- ileus—obstruction,

In a very low anterior resection with a distal rectal anastomosis and total mesenteric excision a colopouch may diminish the risk of anastomotic complications overall. However, necrosis of the pouch may also occur and can be a life-threatening complication requiring urgent difficult salvage surgery.

Late complications:

- incontinence of faeces following anal sphincter damage at surgery (sphincter stretch and stapler passage) or too distal an anastomosis;
- tenesmus or loss of sensation of full rectum (due to low anastomosis and usually self-limiting)—if difficult to manage and not self-limiting a permanent stoma may be required;
- small-bowel obstruction due to adhesions or cancer recurrence.

Abdominoperineal excision of the rectum

There is less risk in this operation than with low anterior resection as there is no anastomosis. However, there is a perineal wound which leads to the pelvic space and this wound may be slow in healing. Occasionally the perineal wound has to be packed if haemostasis of the pelvic space is imperfect. Wound infection (abdomen or perineum) is the commonest complication.

The end colostomy in the left iliac fossa may become ischaemic (and may later be stenotic) and may be the site of a parastomal hernia or, rarely, prolapse. Refashioning by surgery may be needed.

Proctocolectomy

Usually undertaken for inflammatory bowel disease but may be used for polyposis syndromes. The end ileostomy has similar complications to colostomy and the perineal wound may well be a problem if the operation is performed for Crohn's disease, particularly when the anus is involved. Some patients may be left with a permanent unhealed perineal wound.

Pouch surgery

This is usually undertaken for ulcerative colitis but is also used for familial adenomatous polyposis when, in both instances, proctocolectomy is also performed. Proctocolectomy with ileoanal pouch has become the standard operation for ulcerative colitis, provided the patient accepts the potential for specific problems. It is occasionally performed for Crohn's colitis, but in these circumstances there is a higher risk of ileitis or pouchitis.

The complications, except those specifically involving the pouch which will be listed separately, are similar to those of the other colonic resections.

Although the ileal pouch and anastomosis does have a risk of anastomotic breakdown, the ileum has a superior blood supply to the colon and these problems are less frequent than after low anterior resection.

The pouch itself is liable to 'pouchitis', which can cause chronic ill health and unacceptable diarrhoea in patients who, even if they are considered to have a good result, have a median daily bowel frequency of 4–5 times/day.

Pouchitis was initially found in the 'continent' Koch pouches. It may well be a form of inflammatory bowel disease as it is much less common in patients who have familial adenomatous polyposis. In patients with ileoanal pouches pouchitis may be a single episode, be recurrent, or become chronic. It may persuade the patient to return to ileostomy life, after medical therapy has been tried.

Rectal prolapse

- Any rectopexy suture may lead to perianorectal infection if the bowel is inadvertently breached.
- Rectopexy with a mesh has a further increased risk of local infection as a large foreign body is left behind. Usually these are complication-free; but the surgeon must be wary of a suture passing into the bowel lumen and contaminating the field, with the attendant risk of infection which may need excision of the mesh.
- Resection rectopexy is the operation of choice because there should be a low complication rate, although the bowel is opened. Antibiotic prophylaxis should lessen this risk.

Late complications after major colorectal surgery

- Incisional hernia;
- Anastomotic stricture—usually in the more distal rectal anastomoses, although cancer recurrence at the suture line can also cause this;
- Stoma problems:
  - stenosis,
  - hernia;
- Neurological problems:
  - urinary incontinence,
  - sexual impotence and retrograde ejaculation.

To avoid these distressing neurological sequelae, it is mandatory when performing this surgery to avoid injuring the autonomic nerves over the anterior surface of the distal aorta and in the pelvis posterior to the mesorectum, as long as this is not incompatible with a curative resection if the surgery is being performed for cancer.

Laparoscopic colorectal surgery

Laparoscopic surgery is being performed for both benign and malignant disease. When laparoscopic colorectal resections are performed for cancer there have been many reports of port-site recurrence. This procedure is still under review and should only be performed as part of a controlled trial, according to the National Institute for Clinical Excellence (NICE) guidelines.

However, there is no such restriction on laparoscopic surgery for benign disease. In particular, surgery for rectal prolapse lends itself to this approach and laparoscopic rectopexy and resection rectopexy are performed in some centres as the procedure of choice. Colorectal anastomosis to reverse a Hartman's procedure also has its advocates for the laparoscopic technique.

The complications of these procedures are the complications of laparoscopy plus the complications of the operation when done by the open method, although they are reportedly less common.

Chapter 12
Complications of peripheral vascular surgery

Complications of infrainguinal bypass grafting

Infrainguinal bypass is a common operation with approximately 5–6000 performed annually within the UK. Indications for surgery include short-distance claudication, critical limb ischaemia, and acute lower limb ischaemia, with the type of bypass depending on the level and extent of the peripheral vascular disease. Infrainguinal reconstruction includes femoropopliteal (above or below the knee), femorocrural (tibial or peroneal vessels), and popliteal-crural or -pedal. An autologous long saphenous vein is used as the conduit of choice as it is resistant to infection and has superior patency rates. It can be used *in situ*, after the passage of a valvulotome, or it can be reversed. A prosthetic bypass conduit (polytetrafluoroethylene (PTFE) or Dacron) can be used as an alternative if an autologous vein is not available.

Early complications

By definition these occur within 30 days of surgery.

Graft related

Graft thrombosis is the principal cause of graft failure in the early postoperative period, and is usually related to a technical problem with the graft or an 'inappropriate' procedure being performed.

Technical problems

- Poor quality vein—diseased or small calibre (<3 mm);
- Residual valve cusps affect the *in situ* venous conduit following inadequate valve stripping with the valvulotome;
- Poor anastomotic technique;
- Kinking of the bypass.

Inappropriate procedure

Poor inflow—an aortoiliac stenosis merits an inflow procedure being performed first (i.e. angioplasty, stent, bypass). Poor run-off. Poor outflow from the graft adversely affects patency. Additionally, prosthetic graft thrombosis can occur as a primary event with no underlying technical problem, which is due to the inherent thrombogenicity of the PTFE conduit.

Treatment

Graft thrombosis

This results in lower limb ischaemia which may threaten limb viability. Ischaemia may be acute or more profound than the pre-existing ischaemic state because collaterals are damaged during bypass grafting. It requires urgent return to theatre for graft thrombectomy. On-table thrombolysis may be used and a completion angiogram taken before definitive repair to any technical graft problem (e.g. vein patch angioplasty or graft replacement). The urgency of surgery is very high in vein grafts, which should ideally involve a return to theatre within 6 h. Endothelial damage after this period means that graft salvage or prolonged patency is unlikely and the graft will require replacement. After 28 days, percutaneous catheter thrombolysis is an option followed by treatment to any underlying technical problem. In the absence of an underlying graft defect consideration should be given to warfarinization.

Graft infection

Although graft infection can present in the early postoperative period, it usually presents between 1 and 6 months postoperatively.

Compartment syndrome

This can complicate revascularization of the acutely ischaemic lower limb. It is of particular concern if the viability of the lower limb is threatened with signs of progressive ischaemia being present (i.e. paraesthesiae, partial paresis, and muscle tenderness). Reperfusion of ischaemic muscle causes capillary leak and swelling and a rise in the intracompartmental pressure (normally <30 mmHg in a normotensive patient). Venous outflow is obstructed, causing oedema and a rise in interstitial pressure. Congestion within the capillary bed occurs and reduced transcapillary diffusion causes ischaemia at a cellular level. A vicious cycle is thus established with progressive swelling, a rise in intracompartmental pressure (ICP), and cellular ischaemia. In the terminal phase, compartmental pressures can exceed systolic blood pressure, peripheral pulses are lost, and limb loss is the likely outcome.

Clinical features include pain which is disproportionate to physical signs, muscle tenderness, pain on passive extension, and hypoaesthesia in the distribution of peripheral nerves running through the comparment. In the leg, early signs include paraesthesia in the first web space and an inability to dorsiflex the foot as a result of deep peroneal nerve ischaemia.

An intracompartmental pressure of >30–50 mmHg, measured by a needle pressure transducer is diagnostic of the compartment syndrome and immediate 4-compartment fasciotomies should be performed through a medial and lateral incision. These should extend from just below the upper tibial plateau to the malleolar level. A delay in treatment can lead to irreversible nerve damage, and muscle necrosis with subsequent healing by fibrosis will result in a Volkmann's ischaemic contracture.

General

Mortality rates

Vascular disease is a generalized disorder, which also affects the coronary arteries and cerebral circulation. Acute myocardial infarction (AMI) and stroke account for the majority of deaths complicating surgery. An estimated 30-day mortality of around 2–3% exists for elective surgery within the UK. Mortality is higher in the critically ischaemic patient and those with acute ischaemia. An embolus is more dangerous than a thrombosis because of underlying arrhythmias or AMI.

Wound infection

Particularly the groin wound in the obese, diabetics, and those on oral steroids. This is a particularly dangerous situation in the presence of prosthetic graft material, which is highly susceptible to infection. Methicillin-resistant *Staphylococcus aureus* (MRSA) is increasingly implicated in the aetiology of wound and graft infection postoperatively. Pre-existing colonization may increase an individual's risk to this, and as a result many units perform an MRSA screen (i.e. nose, groin, axilla, perineum, and open wounds) on admission to hospital. Aggressive eradication should take place before surgery and includes the use of nasal Bactroban (mupirocin) or Naseptin (mupirocin and chlorhexidine). Skin carriage can be treated with antiseptic bathing in chlorhexidine or povidone-iodine and hexachlorophene powder can be used in the groin and axillas. All treatment should be for 5 days and swabs repeated to ensure eradication. Otherwise patients should have as short a time as possible before their surgery to prevent colonization with MRSA.

Treatment of wound infection—patients should be started on intravenous antibiotics and the wound redressed on a daily basis and observed. Every effort should be made to ensure adequate nutrition, including the use of oral vitamin supplements.

Skin flap necrosis

This can occur in the leg if the skin flaps are undermined when harvesting the long saphenous vein (LSV). Can also result from infection.

Skin flares

In the case of *in situ* grafting an untied side branch of the LSV may result in an arteriovenous fistula. As the fistula matures, the skin becomes reddened and eventually necroses.

Treatment—AV fistulas can be identified on an early duplex scan. They should be marked on the skin and can be ligated under local anaesthesia.

Lymphocele formation

Damage to the afferent lymphatics or lymph nodes during groin dissection can result in a local collection of lymph. If aspirated they tend to reaccumulate. 90% resolve spontaneously, although this may take many months. Lymphatic leaks can be managed by placing a stoma bag over the wound. In the majority of cases they settle on conservative treatment. In those cases where the leaks persist, re-exploration of the groin with visualization and ligation of the leak and or a sartorius muscle flap may be undertaken.

Wound haematoma

This can result from anastomotic bleeding, bleeding from where the graft is tunnelled or from branches of the long saphenous vein if inadequately ligated.

Treatment—the majority of wound haematomas resolve spontaneously. In those where the graft is compromised the haematoma should be evacuated. Other indications for evacuation and drainage include infection.

Reperfusion syndrome

Re-vascularization of a non-viable acutely ischaemic lower limb (characterized by paraesthesiae, complete paresis, muscle turgor, and fixed mottled pigmentation) can result in the release of toxic anaerobic metabolites from infarcted muscle in to the systemic circulation. Subsequent acidosis and hyperkalaemia results in myocardial depression and fatal arrhythmias. Rhabdomyolysis results in myoglobinuria, which is a potent cause of acute renal failure (ARF). Myoglobin contains iron, and this is the likely cause of tubular damage rather than mechanical blockage of the tubules.

Treatment of myoglobinuria—(in conjunction with a nephrologist):

1. Correct hypovolaemia (injured muscle sequestrates massive amounts of fluid).
2. Ensure clearance of haem proteins from circulation; solute diuresis using mannitol (e.g. 30 ml/h) and maintenance of a urine pH >6.5 using sodium bicarbonate.
3. Limit haem protein cytotoxicity; the role of desferrioxamine is unclear.
4. Hypocalcaemia may occur and patients require calcium infusion.
5. Treatment should be continued until myoglobinuria disappears.
6. Established oliguric renal failure requires formal renal support.

Primary amputation

This is performed for the non-viable limb. In profound acute ischaemia white cell activation can precipitate a systemic inflammatory response with the release of cytokines, free radicals, prostaglandins, kinins, and nitric oxide resulting in a generalized vasodilatory state with leak from major capillary beds. Multiorgan dysfunction syndrome (MODS) may ensue with adult respiratory distress syndrome (ARDS), ARF, high-output septic shock, disseminated intravascular coagulation (DIC), stress ulceration, and ileus.

Intermediate complications

These characteristically occur between 1 and 12 months postoperatively. During this period there are three main causes of graft failure: graft stenosis, graft infection, and false aneurysm—these will be discussed in turn.

Graft stenosis

It is well established that 25–30% of all infrainguinal grafts develop a narrowing within the first 12 months of surgery. Such stenoses are responsible for 80% of all graft thromboses.

Vein grafts

Re-endothelialization of a venous conduit occurs within 2–4 weeks. Subjecting the vein to arterial pressures, however, results in the development of myointimal hyperplasia. This occurs between 1 and 12 months postoperatively and is characterized by smooth muscle migration from media to intima, smooth muscle proliferation, and the deposition of extracellular matrix. In focal areas this can cause a localized vein graft stenosis (VGS) in the body of a vein graft or perianastomotic areas. The causes or mechanisms governing the development of VGS are not understood but are likely to relate to both local and systemic factors.

Local factors implicated in the development of VGS

- Mechanical trauma to endothelium during surgery—includes clamp damage, rough handling, and excessive distension of reversed saphenous vein. In the case of *in situ* bypass grafting, the passage of the valvotome produces endothelial damage.

- Thermal injury to the endothelium—a prolonged warm ischaemic time may predispose to VGS.

- The use of a poor quality vein or diseased vein (periadventitial fibrosis, varicosities, venous blebs), small-calibre vein (<3 mm), or composite vein is likely to predispose to VGS. Valvotomy sites have shown no correlation with the site of stenosis.

- Low shear stress—the development of areas of turbulence and vortices in perianastomotic areas are associated with low shear stress and are implicated in both the development of VGS and prosthetic graft stenosis.

Systemic factors

Elevated plasma fibrinogen, fibrinopeptides, Von Willebrand's factor, lipoprotein A, and cigarette smoking are thought to be associated with the development of graft stenosis. An aberrant vascular smooth muscle response, assayed in cell culture, has been postulated as the cause.

Prosthetic grafts

Endothelization within prosthetic grafts does not take place in humans and the vein grafts become lined with proteinaceous material composed mainly of fibrin (neointima). In the absence of an endothelial monolayer the luminal surface is thrombogenic, and primary thrombosis can occur below the threshold thrombotic velocity even in the absence of a stenosis. The ingrowth of pannus consisting of smooth muscle and endothelial cells occurs only within 1–2 cm from the ends of the graft. These perianastomotic

areas are prone to the development of myointimal hyperplasia with stenosis and risk of graft failure.

Duplex surveillance

Because of the 25–30% risk of stenosis within 12 months, many centres
undertake a duplex surveillance programme. Scans are performed 1, 3, 6, 9,
and 12 months postoperatively. Detection of a stenosis allows a relatively
simple intervention in the form of angioplasty, open patch angioplasty, or
an interposition graft to prevent graft failure. Graft failure carries a 50%
risk of limb loss with consequent financial cost and loss in quality of life to
the patient. Duplex has been shown to improve the assisted primary
patency rates of vein grafts, but this does not necessarily correlate with
limb salvage or quality of life.

Treatment of graft stenosis

Graft stenosis in anastomotic regions are best treated by direct surgical
intervention with patching or graft replacement. Those in the body of the
graft can be treated by balloon angioplasty in the first instance. If this fails,
surgery in the form of vein patch angioplasty or direct graft replacement
maintains graft patency. Angioplasty should be avoided within the first
28 days and at anastomotic sites.

Graft infection

Prosthetic graft infection is a well-recognized and feared complication
of vascular surgery, with an overall incidence of around 2% (ranging
between 1% and 6% in published series) for prosthetic grafts. More
recently, MRSA has been identified as a causative agent in secondary haemorrhage from vein grafts. It commonly presents with localized signs of
cellulitis, a seropurulent discharge or sinus formation, or non-specific
systemic manifestations including pyrexia and general malaise. The patient
is often bacteraemic or septicaemic with a raised neutrophil count and
inflammatory markers (SIRS, systemic inflammatory response syndrome).
Anastomotic false aneurysms are associated with infection and anastomotic secondary haemorrhage is common. Mycotic aneurysm of the native
vessels, septic emboli, or other forms of metastatic infection are less
common sequelae. Vein grafts are more resistant to infection, although
in situ grafts are at risk if the overlying skin breaks down. Vein graft infection tends to present with anastomotic secondary haemorrhage which can
be life-threatening. Infection usually takes place at the time of graft implantation, although any subsequent source of bacteraemia is a potential risk.
The most commonly isolated pathogenic organism is *Staphylococcus aureus*,
but *Staph. epidermidis*, pseudomonads, *Escherichia coli*, and *Klebsiella* and
Salmonella spp. can be isolated. One worrying trend over the past few years
is the emergence of methicillin-resistant *Staphylococcus aureus* (MRSA) as a
common pathogen in nosocomial graft infection. The proportion of graft
infections caused by MRSA is increasing, with some centres reporting as
much as a 2–40% increase over the past 5 years.

Treatment—in the case of secondary haemorrhage resuscitation should be commenced and the patient transferred urgently to theatre for graft ligation, when the native artery is oversewn or vein patched and the surrounding area debrided of any necrotic material. Distal revascularization may be attempted using vein, but only through a non-infected site to a more distal patent vessel. In those patients with a non-viable leg, primary amputation should be performed. This may need to be considered to preserve life in catastrophic haemorrhage.

False aneurysm formation

False aneurysm formation is a recognized complication of vascular surgery with an overall incidence of 2–3% after femoral anastomosis (including aortofemoral grafts). After arterial reconstruction, false aneurysm formation usually involves the anastomosis and is related to the use of prosthetic material, infection, delayed fracture of suture material/graft, or poor surgical technique. Patients may be asymptomatic or present with pain, swelling, or haemorrhage.

Ultrasound is used in the diagnosis of false aneurysm. Surgical intervention should be considered once the aneurysm becomes symptomatic or exceeds 3 cm. Prior to surgery the patient should undergo an arteriogram to define the local vascular anatomy. Surgical options include direct graft replacement or patching of the defect.

Late complications—after 12 months

Features

+ **Disease progression**—extension of the atherosclerotic disease in either the inflow or run-off to an infrainguinal graft is the commonest cause of graft failure in this period. It typically occurs after 2 years. Angioplasty or surgery may be used to maintain the patency of the graft.

+ **Anastomotic false aneurysm formation**—covert infection or delayed fracture of the suture or Dacron graft material means that anastomotic false aneurysm formation can present many years after graft implantation. Once a false aneurysm exceeds 3 cm in diameter or the patient develops symptoms then intra-arterial digital subtraction arteriography (iaDSA) and direct surgical repair is indicated.

+ **True aneurysms**—affecting the body of vein grafts have been reported. These are likely to result from transmural ischaemia or trauma incurred at the time of vein harvesting. They have the potential to rupture, thrombose, or embolize with subsequent graft failure. True aneurysms are best repaired using an interposition vein graft.

+ **Accelerated atherosclerosis**—of vein graft affects the body of vein grafts 3–5 years postimplantation. It has been demonstrated in up to 15% of femoropopliteal vein grafts and can be distinguished from spontaneous atherosclerosis by its greater cellularity and lipid content. It is a potential source of graft failure.

Outcome

Following infrainguinal reconstruction, outcome can be measured in terms of graft patency, limb salvage in the critically ischaemic, and quality of life. Graft patency as such does not necessarily correlate with limb salvage or quality of life. Overall approximate 5-year primary patency rates are shown in the table below.

Bypass conduit	Vein	PTFE	PTFE with cuff or patch
Above knee femoropopliteal bypass	65–70% (80% at 2 years)	55–65% (80% at 2 years)	
Below knee femoropopliteal bypass	50%	20 to 30%	Up to 57% at 3 years
Femorodistal bypass	25%	10%	Up to 55% at 2 years claimed

In addition to the development of graft stenoses many other local factors influence primary graft patency including the level of distal anastomosis, type of bypass conduit (both illustrated in the above table), distal run-off, indication for bypass (claudicants can expect better patency rates than the critically ischaemic), ankle brachial-pressure index (ABPI), and the quality of the vessel used for the distal anastomosis.

Duplex surveillance of vein grafts has shown to be a sensitive method of detecting graft stenoses. It allows easy intervention (i.e. angioplasty, open patch plasty, or interposition graft) to prevent graft failure and this is known as 'assisted primary patency'.

The use of adjunctive anastomotic techniques for PTFE bypasses—the long-term patency rates for PTFE below the knee are inferior to those for veins (see above table). Many explanations for this have been proposed. The mismatch in compliance between graft and native artery, iatrogenic injury from anastomotic suturing, and low shear stress at the heel and toe are thought to induce myointimal hyperplasia and stenosis at the distal anastomosis.

Complications of abdominal aortic surgery

Abdominal aortic reconstruction is undertaken for both aneurysmal and occlusive disease.

Complications of elective aortic aneurysm surgery

An artery is aneurysmal when there is a 50% increase in the diameter of the wall, or when the diameter of the aorta exceeds 3 cm. Aneurysms primarily affect elderly males and have a 5% prevalence in males between the ages of 65 and 74 years.

Elective repair for large aneurysms is undertaken when the risk of death from rupture outweighs the risks of elective surgery. In the UK this has been undertaken when the aneurysm measures 6 cm. At 6 cm the risk of rupture at 1 year is around 25%, and less than 5 cm is around 5%. Aneurysms less than 5.5 cm in diameter should be managed by duplex ultrasound surveillance.

Symptomatic aneurysms, or those rapidly expanding (i.e. >1 cm per year), have a high risk of rupture and should also be repaired. Conventional repair involves a transperitoneal approach to the infrarenal aorta and has a number of complications.

Intraoperative complications

- Damage of adjacent structures—complications from the transperitoneal approach to the abdominal aorta include inadvertent enterotomy, particularly in the presence of adhesions from previous surgery:
- Damage to the left renal vein—can complicate dissection of the aneurysm neck, it may need to be controlled and ligated for juxtarenal aneurysms. In the case of ligation there is an increased risk of progressive deterioration in renal function.
- The 4th part of the duodenum—may also be damaged at this stage of the procedure, with a subsequent risk of graft infection or aortoduodenal fistulation. This is most commonly seen with inflammatory aneurysms.
- Damage to the left ureter—can take place with the risk of subsequent ureteric obstruction, urinoma formation, or urinary fistula.

All the above injuries are of particular concern when repairing inflammatory aneurysms where the left renal vein, duodenum, or left ureter can be incorporated in to the periaortitis process.

In the case of an inflammatory aneurysm there is often a place for ureteric stent insertion to allow direct visualization of the ureters during surgery.

• Primary haemorrhage—intraoperative bleeding is a hazard even in elective repair and is usually related to inadvertent damage to the left renal vein, lumbar arteries, or iliac veins. Back bleeding may occur from the lumbar arteries or the inferior mesenteric artery (IMA) when the aneurysm sac is opened.

Early complications—less than 30 days

Mortality

The 30-day mortality for elective aneurysm repair in teaching hospitals in the UK has been estimated at 5–10%. This may be an underestimation.

The risk factors for aneurysm development are similar to atherosclerosis (i.e. male, hypertension, smoking, diabetes, and familial risk), consequently at least 25% of patients have associated generalized atherosclerotic disease. Cardiac events account for 70% of all fatalities in the early postoperative period. Risk to the individual patient rises sharply with age or the presence of ischaemic heart disease, chronic obstructive pulmonary disease (COPD), and renal impairment. The decision to operate is therefore based on the patient's physiological versus chronological age. Mortality is largely related to aortic cross-clamping and the transperitoneal approach to the aorta. Aortic cross-clamping is associated with a rise in left ventricular end-diastolic pressure causing subendocardial ischaemia. This can precipitate arrhythmias or progress to AMI. Prolonged clamping is associated with an ischaemia-reperfusion syndrome which can result in MODS. The transperitoneal approach itself is associated with postoperative wound pain, cardiorespiratory depression, and gastrointestinal failure.

Specific

Reactionary haemorrhage

Bleeding in the immediate postoperative period can be a result of technical problems (e.g. anastomotic, lumbar and inferior mesenteric arteries, or coagulopathy. Coagulopathic bleeding problems are well recognized even after the repair of elective infrarenal aneurysms. Volume-expansion products, massive blood transfusion, acidosis, anticoagulant therapy, cell salvage, and clamp times have all been implicated. Hypothermia has been shown to inhibit the coagulatory cascade, activate the fibrinolytic cascade, and induce platelet dysfunction.

Retroperitoneal haematoma

Closure of the peritoneum over the aortic graft provides a degree of tamponade. Blood can accumulate in the retroperitoneum, however, and reabsorption can cause derangement of liver function tests or clinical jaundice. Haematoma also represents a potential source of infection and is implicated in the development of multiorgan failure.

Acute ischaemic colitis

The overall incidence of left-sided colonic ischaemia is 2% after elective aortic surgery. This can rise, however, up to 12% following emergency aneurysm repair. The blood supply to the left colon is from the left colic branch of the inferior mesenteric artery. Collateral supply is from the middle colic branch of the superior mesenteric artery and the superior haemorrhoidal branches of the internal iliac artery. If the collateral supply is poor then ligation of the IMA during reconstruction can result in ischaemic colitis. In practice, if the colon looks dusky and ischaemic during surgery then the IMA should be reimplanted. Ischaemic colitis presents with a pyrexia and bloody diarrhoea. Transmural ischaemia may progress to colonic infarction with perforation/faecal peritonitis with consequent acidosis, sepsis, and cardiovascular collapse. This is more likely to occur following emergency abdominal aortic aneurysmectomy (AAA) surgery. Ischaemia confers a 40–50% mortality, which rises to over 90% if the ischaemia is transmural. Sigmoid tonometry has been advocated as a method of early detection of colonic ischaemia, but remains a research tool.

Femoral or popliteal embolus

During elective repair the iliac arteries are clamped before the proximal clamp is applied to avoid distal embolization of an atheromatous plaque or thrombus. Large emboli can result in acute lower limb ischaemia. When the clamps are released the common femoral arteries in the groin are compressed to allow potential emboli to pass in to the internal iliac system, which has minimal clinical consequence.

Rare complications

- 'Trash foot'—cholesterol and platelet emboli can result in multiple small cutaneous infarcts to the feet.
- Graft occlusion—thrombosis of the graft in the early postoperative period is rare.
- Paraplegia—spinal cord ischaemia can result from a combination of intraoperative hypotension, prolonged clamp times, the division of arteries supplying the spinal cord, and ischaemic-reperfusion injury. It complicates only 0.2% of elective abdominal aneurysm repairs but this rises to 2% for emergency repairs.

General
Cardiac events

These are responsible for the majority of early postoperative fatalities, due to AMI and arrhythmias as outlined above. Pre-existing cardiac disease—including AMI within 6 months, unstable angina, complex arrhythmias, two- or three-vessel coronary artery disease (CAD), or congestive cardiac failure—grossly elevate operative mortality rates and should be regarded as absolute contraindications to open surgery. Patients with ischaemic heart disease who have undergone coronary revascularization can expect a normal operative mortality rate. There is now evidence to support the use of β-blockade during the perioperative period in patients with CAD. It is important to avoid anaemia and hypo- and hyperkalaemia in patients with CAD as this may precipitate cardiac events.

Stroke

Intraoperative hypotension in a generalized arteriopath carries a risk of stroke. This can be related to internal carotid artery (ICA) disease or to cerebrovascular disease. Carotid endarterectomy should only be undertaken in symptomatic patients with a known significant ICA stenosis (i.e. >70%).

Complications relating to the transperitoneal approach

- Ileus—excessive handling, cooling, and desiccation of the intestines as well as leakage of blood within the peritoneal cavity can all cause a delay in the return of gastric, colonic, and small intestinal function. The use of a self-retaining retractor may well avoid some of these problems, especially if the bowel is kept within the abdominal cavity. Gastroparesis, small-bowel ileus, and colonic pseudo-obstruction can all complicate aneurysm surgery.

- Hypothermia—is common following aneurysm repair. Prophylactic measures such as the use of warmed blood products and a warming device (e.g. Bair Hugger®) should be employed. Hypothermia is likely to play a key role in the pathogenesis of postoperative coagulopathy.

- Acute pancreatitis—this is a rare consequence of blunt injury to the pancreas (e.g. retractor-related) during mobilization of the aneurysm neck.

Wound complications

A full-length, midline incision or transverse incision is used to gain access to the infrarenal aorta. Infection, superficial disruption, full-thickness dehiscence, with or without a burst abdomen, are well documented complications in the early postoperative period. The use of a transverse abdominal incision may be associated with less postoperative wound pain, pulmonary complications, and a reduced incidence of incisional herniation. For those patients undergoing aortobifemoral reconstruction similar complications can occur in the groin, as well as the formation of lymphoceles.

Respiratory failure

Postoperative wound pain is common and results in a reduced respiratory excursion with a drop in functional residual capacity. Reduced ability to cough results in mucus plugging; in combination, these factors cause basal atelectasis and chest infection may supervene. This necessitates the prophylactic use of optimal pain control (usually epidural anaesthetic) and intensive physiotherapy. Acute respiratory distress syndrome (ARDS) may occur, but more commonly complicates the repair of ruptured aneurysms. All patients should be seen by the physiotherapist prior to surgery. Patients should be regularly monitored by a pulse oximeter and treated by increasing the inspired oxygen concentration.

Deep venous thrombosis

Prophylactic doses of subcutaneous low molecular-weight heparin (e.g. Clexane 20 mg) are given at night, thus avoiding any problems with the epidural insertion. In general, the use of anti-thromboembolism disease (TED) stockings should be avoided in patients with significant peripheral vascular disease.

Intermediate and late complications

Graft infection is a feared complication of aneurysm surgery with a reported incidence of between 1 and 3%, it is associated with a mortality rate of 50%. Most infections probably occur at the time of implantation, although haematogenous spread (i.e. bacteraemia) is a potential source. Erosion of a graft can occur into adjacent viscera. Aortoduodenal fistulas may present insidiously with anaemia, a pyrexia, and raised inflammatory markers or acutely with catastrophic upper gastrointestinal bleeding (haematemesis or melaena). Aortoenteric fistulas may present similarly. Aortocaval fistulas result in venous hypertension, bilateral leg oedema, a wide pulse pressure, and possible cardiac failure. All carry a dismal prognosis and it is therefore important to ensure adequate closure of the peritoneum to reduce the risk of fistulation.

Treatment
Infected aortic grafts

These usually require excision and revascularization by extra-anatomical axillobifemoral grafting to avoid infected tissue planes. Others have advocated *in situ* replacement with rifampicin-bonded grafts and omental flaps.

Conservative management with graft preservation, local antibiotic irrigation via a catheter, and an omental flap is less commonly practised. In all cases, prolonged antibiotics should be given for 6–12 weeks. Secondary aortoduodenal fistula requires fistula excision, graft excision with oversewing of the aortic stump, and axillobifemoral reconstruction. Mortality rates are 80 to 90%.

Graft occlusion

Patency rates for suprainguinal reconstruction are excellent and exceed 90% at 5 years. Myointimal hyperplasia and progressive atherosclerotic disease may occur and result in re-stenosis or thrombosis.

Anastomotic false aneurysm

This affects up to 3% of aortic reconstructions and in particular the femoral anastomosis of aortobifemoral grafts.

Erectile dysfunction

Such dysfunction can occur as a result of damage to the preaortic nervi erigentes during dissection of the aneurysm sac.

Infrarenal aorta

This can be exposed using a retroperitoneal approach, which has the potential advantages of less intraoperative fluid losses, reduced postoperative ileus, less haemodynamic stresses, reduced postoperative wound pain, and subsequent pulmonary complications.

Complications of emergency AAA surgery

Emergency repair is undertaken for patients with a ruptured or leaking aneurysm. This should be distinguished from patients undergoing 'urgent' operations who present with pain but who have no evidence of leak on CT scan or operatively. Such patients have a higher operative mortality rate (around 10%) than true elective aneurysms.

• Mortality—the overall mortality of patients with ruptured or leaking abdominal aortic aneurysms is around 80%. Around 50% of patients reach hospital and most series show that the 30-day mortality rate for these patients is 50%.

• Intraoperative haemorrhage—technical problems in gaining control of the neck of the aneurysm can lead to rapid exsanguination and death on the operating table. Reactive haemorrhage postoperatively is also commonplace and is often related to coagulopathies (as outlined above). On their return to the intensive care unit (ICU), patients will usually have profound clotting abnormalities including thrombocytopenia and/or disseminated intravascular coagulation (DIC).

• Of patients surviving the first 24 hours on the ICU, the morbidity rate exceeds 50%. The majority of deaths in the 30-day postoperative period are due to the development of a multiorgan dysfunction syndrome.

• The systemic inflammatory response syndrome (SIRS), sepsis, and multiorgan dysfunction syndrome (MODS).

Patients who undergo emergency aneurysm repair for leaking or ruptured abdominal aortic aneurysm can anticipate a very high mortality rate even following a technically successful repair. The combined insult of hypotension, massive blood loss, ischaemic-reperfusion injury, and extravasation of blood into the retroperitoneum or peritoneal cavity results in neutrophil activation and the release of inflammatory mediators (cytokines, prostaglandins, free radicles, kinins, nitric oxide, and bacterial endotoxin). In turn, these can precipitate a response that mimics sepsis. SIRS is characterized by a hyperdynamic circulation with vasodilatation and capillary leak. Despite an increase in cardiac output, this may be abnormally distributed with reduced perfusion to the kidneys and gut, or increased cardiac output may not meet the increased oxygen requirements of end organs thereby resulting in ischaemia. Multiorgan dysfunction syndrome is likely to ensue, this carries a poor prognosis with a 40%, 60%, and 98% mortality for one-, two-, and three-system failure, respectively.

Manifestations of MODS

Respiratory failure

Adult respiratory distress syndrome (ARDS) is the pulmonary manifestation of MODS and is characterized by profound hypoxaemia, non-cardiogenic pulmonary oedema, reduced pulmonary compliance, and ventilation–perfusion mismatch. Standard intermittent positive-pressure ventilation may not be adequate to maintain oxygenation, so that inverse inspiratory:expiratory ratio ventilation, pressure-controlled ventilation, or nitric oxide therapy may be required. Nosocomial pneumonia, barotrauma, and oxygen toxicity may contribute to respiratory failure.

Cardiovascular failure

The hyperdynamic circulation is characterized by vasodilatation and a compensatory increase in cardiac output to maintain blood pressure. Inotropes and vasopressors are required.

Renal failure

Some 70% of all patients undergoing emergency repair develop acute renal failure. This is often due to a combination of factors:

• Prerenal—intraoperative hypovolaemic shock or postoperative septic shock can result in renal hypoperfusion and acute tubular necrosis. Inotropes and vasopressors may further reduce renal perfusion. Surgical factors may contribute, including a supra- or juxtarenal clamp site and ligation of the left renal vein when gaining proximal control.

• Renal—nephrotoxic drugs (aminoglycosides, non-steroidal anti-inflammatory drugs (NSAIDs)), haemoglobinuria, myoglobulinuria, and renal artery stenosis can all add to the renal insult. Surgical factors such as a supra- or juxtarenal clamp site or ligation of the left renal vein are also risk factors.

Disseminated intravascular coagulation (DIC)

Volume-expansion products, massive blood transfusion, hypothermia, acidosis, anticoagulants, and a suprarenal clamp site are all implicated in the development of DIC. It is characterized by a consumption coagulopathy with platelet aggregation and activation of the coagulation and fibrinolytic cascades. The end result is microvascular thrombosis, resulting in end-organ ischaemia and contributing to MODS, and enhanced fibrinolytic activity resulting in uncontrolled bleeding. In all these case the use of a cell-salvage system may reduce the need for homologous blood. Blood products—including packed cells, fresh-frozen plasma, and cryoprecipitate—are required as well as vitamin K.

Gastrointestinal failure

Shunting of blood away from the gut in SIRS can damage the integrity of the gut's mucosal barrier, allowing the translocation of bacteria and endo-toxins in to the systemic circulation. These may contribute to SIRS/MODS. Stress ulceration is another consequence of reduced blood flow to the gut. Early enteral feeding is therefore important to prevent these complications, as well as to provide nutritional support to help meet the patients' increased metabolic requirements.

Complications of endovascular aneurysm repair (EVAR)

Endovascular aneurysm repair was first undertaken in 1990 and since then aortic stent grafts have rapidly developed. Tube grafts, aorto-uni-iliac grafts are available in modular and non-modular form. The graft may be fully stented or incorporate stents only at its extremities. Stents are placed via a transfemoral or transiliac route, usually under general anaesthesia. As stents are deployed intraluminally the transperitoneal approach to the aorta and aortic cross-clamping are avoided, thus reducing the physiological insult to the patient. Reduced morbidity and mortality rates, reduced postoperative pain (and the complications relating to prolonged immobilization), and reduced hospital stay (most patients only require to stay for 2–3 days postoperatively) are potential benefits of this approach.

- EVAR 1 is a current study comparing open to endovascular repair in patients less than 60 years and in stages ASA I–III (ASA, American Society of Anesthesiologists).
- EVAR 2 is comparing endovascular repair to conservative management in those unfit for open surgery (ASA IV).

Additionally, endovascular repair is highly dependent upon aneurysm morphology and the calibre and tortuosity of the iliac arteries/distal aorta. Only 5% of aneurysms are treatable with a tube graft, 40% with a bifurcated graft, and up to 66% with an aorto-uni-iliac graft (the latter require occlusion of the contralateral iliac system and a femorofemoral crossover procedure).

Early complications (less than 30 days)

Primary success rates of EVAR (graft implantation without conversion to open surgery) now average around 90% in most major centres.

Mortality

The 30-day mortality for EVAR is around 3% in ASA I–III. Most early postoperative deaths are related to cardiac events. There is little data, however, about those unfit for surgery (i.e. ASA IV). Open repair for those with severe cardiorespiratory or renal disease carries upwards of a 40% mortality and it is hoped that EVAR will offer more favourable results. Stent deployment under local or regional anaesthetic may be of benefit in these cases.

Local vascular complications
Primary endoleak

This complication is specific to aneurysm repair and implies a failure to exclude the aneurysm sac from the circulation. Primary endoleak occurs from the time of surgery and rates lie between 5% and 44% of reported series. A recent meta-analysis showed an overall incidence of 17%. Around 50% of these settle spontaneously and leaks from the distal graft tend to follow a more benign course. In the presence of a persisting endoleak, aneurysm expansion occurs in 86% of patients and the risk of aneurysm rupture persists.

- Classification of endoleaks:
  - Type I: related to the proximal or distal graft;
  - Type II: due to retrograde flow from collaterals;
  - Type III: due to fabric tears, graft disintegration, or graft limb disconnection;
  - Type IV: graft porosity allowing flow through the graft wall.

Radiological treatment may require proximal or distal extension cuffs or embolization of collaterals. If this fails to settle leaks then laparotomy and proximal banding or open repair may be required.

Distal embolization of atheromatous plaque
This can occur during stent deployment and require femoral embolectomy.

Microembolization
Microembolization may occur resulting in 'trash phenomena' to the feet. Massive microembolization resulting from endoluminal manipulation within the aneurysm sac has been reported and can involve the renal, visceral, and lower limb arteries. It is associated with the SIRS and carries a poor prognosis.

Stent migration
Inadequate fixation of the proximal stent can allow early stent migration with the risk of graft thrombosis or graft limb dislocation.

Damage to native iliac arteries during deployment
The iliac arteries must be of reasonable calibre (>6 mm) and non-tortuous to allow successful stent deployment. Deployment carries a risk of intimal dissection and flaps, embolization of atheromatous plaque, thrombosis, rupture, and false aneurysm formation. In some cases the iliac artery may need to be replaced.

Renal artery occlusion
This is a rare but potential risk of EVAR and is caused by the proximal stent impinging on the renal artery ostia. Recent series have demonstrated no adverse effects on renal function when an uncovered stent is deployed across the origins of the renal arteries, although the long-term effect is unknown.

General complications
- Renal impairment—occurs in 25% of patients. This may be related to intravenous contrast, renal artery emboli, or stent deployment across the origins of the renal arteries.

- Back pain—is a common occurrence following stent deployment.
- Wound complications in the groin—local wound infection occurs in 1% of patients. This is of particular significance if an aorto-uni-iliac stent has been used with a femorofemoral crossover graft, which is at risk of graft infection lying within the subcutaneous tissues.
- Pyrexia of unknown origin.

Intermediate and late complications of EVAR—after 30 days

Despite results in the early postoperative period being acceptable, the incidence of stent failure in the intermediate period lies at around 25% and in the long-term is largely unknown.

- Secondary endoleak—continued development of perigraft flow (secondary endoleak) is well documented and recent meta-analysis suggests that it occurs in 7% of all patients. It can occur many months after implantation, and for this reason duplex or CT surveillance of all aortic stent grafts is required.
- Aneurysm sac shrinkage—recent data has shown that aneurysm sacs distort and shorten with time. This can result in subsequent distortion or kinking of the graft with possible graft thrombosis. Limb dislodgement may occur with the risk of developing secondary endoleak or graft limb thrombosis.
- Stent migration—ongoing expansion of the aortic neck can allow late migration of the stent, precipitating graft or graft limb thrombosis and disconnection of the graft limbs.
- Graft limb occlusion—thrombosis of a graft limb can result from stent migration, stent distortion, or from progression of atherosclerotic disease in the iliac segment.
- Femoral false aneurysm—can complicate the transfemoral approach required for stent deployment.

Complications of surgery for aortoiliac occlusive disease

Aortoiliac segment occlusive disease is associated with a 70% 10-year mortality rate, due largely to atherothrombotic vascular events (i.e. acute myocardial infarction and stroke). Suprainguinal reconstruction can be anatomical or extra-anatomical, this surgery generally carries higher rates of morbidity and mortality than endovascular techniques and should be reserved for when the latter are not feasible. Suprainguinal reconstruction is largely performed for critical ischaemia, but can be considered in the short-distance claudicant who is fit.

Anatomical

Aortobifemoral bypass

This can be performed for aortic occlusive disease or bilateral iliac disease. A transperitoneal approach is required, and aortic cross-clamping and morbidity and mortality are parallel with elective aortic aneurysm repair. The 5% mortality rate rises in the presence of cardiorespiratory or renal disease. Long-term patency rates are excellent with a 90% 5-year patency.

Iliofemoral bypass

This can be used for unilateral iliac occlusion. It can be performed as a unilateral procedure or as a crossover. It avoids the use of a transperitoneal approach and consequently has a 3% mortality rate. Patency rates are also good with around 80% patent at 5 years.

Extra-anatomical

Extra-anatomical reconstruction can be considered for the presence of intraperitoneal sepsis or for a patient with significant medical comorbidity (i.e. severe cardiorespiratory or renal impairment) requiring aortoiliac reconstruction. The avoidance of aortic cross-clamping and a transperitoneal approach to the aorta reduces operative morbidity and mortality. Patency rates are less favourable however.

Axillobifemoral bypass

Axillobifemoral bypass can be used for aortic occlusion, bilateral iliac segment disease, or following the removal of an infected aortic graft. Mortality lies at around 3% and patency between 58 and 93% at 1 year.

Specific complications

- Graft occlusion—the use of long segments of PTFE and lower flow mean patency rates are worse than aortofemoral grafting. External

compression of the subcutaneously tunnelled graft has also been implicated in the cause of graft thrombosis, which may be related to body
posture during sleep. *In situ* thrombosis of the axillary artery has also
been reported.

- Anastomotic haemorrhage is usually related to graft infection or false
  aneurysm formation. If the axillary anastomosis is performed too laterally, however, it will be under tension and when the arm is fully
  abducted may be disrupted.
- Brachial artery embolus.
- Damage to the lower routes of the brachial plexus.
- Femorofemoral crossover is used for unilateral iliac occlusion as an
  alternative to aortoiliac reconstruction. Mortality is around 2% and
  patency rates of up to 70% at 5 years are possible.

Complications of thoracoabdominal aneurysm repair

Aneurysms involving the suprarenal part of the aorta are traditionally classified as thoracoabdominal aneurysms (TAA). The Crawford classification is as follows:

- Type I: majority of descending aorta and proximal abdominal aorta;
- Type II: majority of descending aorta and majority of abdominal aorta;
- Type III: distal descending aorta and majority of abdominal aorta;
- Type IV: majority of abdominal aorta including visceral artery origins.

TAAs are usually due to medial degenerative disease or chronic dissection. Back pain is more commonly present than in AAA and acute or worsening pain may precede rupture or intramural dissection.

For repair the patient is positioned on their right side and the aorta is accessed through a midline abdominal incision extended through the costal margin and along the 7/8th rib for the lower thoracic aorta or 4/5th rib for the upper. The abdominal aorta is approached retroperitoneally following medial visceral rotation of the colon, spleen, and pancreas. Intercostal and visceral arteries usually require reimplantation.

The operative mortality is high and ranges from 10 to 35%. The majority of early postoperative deaths are due to cardiac problems and coagulopathy, whereas late deaths are largely related to the development of MODS.

Managed conservatively alone, only 25% of patients with a thoracoabdominal aneurysm survive 2 years, due to rupture. As a result, those patients who are fit (i.e. without significant cardiorespiratory or renal impairment) should be offered surgery.

Complications are similar to those encountered during AAA surgery. There are, however some specific points to be aware of:

- Bleeding and coagulopathy—reactive haemorrhage is a major problem following TAA repair and can be due to technical problems or coagulopathy. 8% of all patients undergoing thoracoabdominal aneurysm repair require emergency re-exploration and these account for 26% of early postoperative deaths in this subgroup. Prolonged supracoeliac clamp times are implicated in the development of DIC, and it has been shown on an animal model that the development of DIC is related to occlusion of the superior mesenteric artery (versus coeliac). Ischaemia-reperfusion has been shown to alter small-bowel permeability with loss of the mucosal barrier. Bacterial translocation, endotoxaemia, acidosis, and hyperkalaemia within the mesenteric effluent have all been implicated in the development of DIC but the mechanism remains unclear. This ischaemic-reperfusion injury has implications in the development of MODS.

♦ Paraplegia—the incidence of paraplegia is around 20% following TAA repair (ranging from 4 to 30% in reported series) and results from spinal cord ischaemia. The main determinants of ischaemia are the extent of the aneurysm (highest in Crawford type II aneurysms), clamp times, hypotension, and intercostal reattachment. Division of intercostal or upper lumbar vessels, which may supply the artery of Adamkiewicz, can result in spinal cord damage. To minimize this risk, reconstruction should be performed as quickly as possible (i.e. the 'clamp and go' technique) or sequential clamping may be employed. More recent developments for spinal cord protection include CSF drainage, hypothermia, partial left heart bypass, selective visceral artery perfusion, and circulatory hypothermic arrest.

♦ Respiratory failure is a major source of morbidity postoperatively with an incidence of over 20%. The insertion of a double-lumen endotracheal tube is required to allow collapse of the left lung to facilitate aneurysm repair. Pulmonary collapse and postoperative pain following combined thoracotomy and laparotomy can result in atelectasis and sputum retention with consequent suprainfection. Postoperatively, these patients are managed on the intensive care unit where prophylactic thoracic epidural, chest physiotherapy, and oxygen therapy are routinely used. A mini-tracheostomy may be inserted and suction employed in those with sputum retention. Prolonged postoperative ventilation requires formal tracheostomy to facilitate weaning.

♦ Complications relating to visceral ischaemic-reperfusion injury. The use of a supracoeliac clamp site means that most intra-abdominal viscera are subject to a ischaemic-reperfusion injury and this is implicated in the development of acute renal failure, DIC, and SIRS/MODS.

♦ Specific complications relating to thoracotomy:
  - *haemothorax*—although the chest is routinely drained, a haemothorax can result if this is not adequate. Suprainfection can result in a pleural empyema. This requires antibiotics, chest tube drainage, or surgical drainage if these measures fail.
  - *supraventricular dysrhythmias*—atrial fibrillation can occur 2–5 days postoperatively. Prophylactic digoxin or amiodarone is used in some centres.

Complications of carotid endarterectomy (CEA)

Stroke is the third commonest cause of death in the UK with an annual incidence of 2 per 1000 population. 80% of strokes are ischaemic in origin and around 50% of these have significant internal carotid artery (ICA) disease. Trials have demonstrated a clear benefit in long-term stroke reduction using carotid endarterectomy plus best medical treatment versus best medical treatment alone in patients with carotid territory symptoms and a severe ICA stenosis (>70%).

This group of patients represent the majority of patients considered for CEA in the UK. To achieve the 6- to 10-fold reduction in the long-term risk of stroke (or a 75% reduction in relative risk of stroke at 2 to 3 years), the combined perioperative stroke and mortality rate must be below 6% and stroke rate below 3–5%. In the UK, carotid surgery is performed under both general anaesthesia and cervical block with local anaesthetic infiltration.

Early complications (less than 30 days)

General

Mortality

The 30-day mortality rate for CEA is around 1.5–2%. The risk, however, rises in the presence of ischaemic heart disease. Around 1% of perioperative deaths are due to stroke and a similar number due to cardiac events.

Stroke

The overall stroke rate in the early postoperative period ranges from 2.4 to 6.9% in reported series. The majority of all early postoperative strokes (2–3%) are due to intraoperative emboli. Early stroke can be classified as operative if the patient awakes from general anaesthesia with a new neurological deficit. These are usually caused by emboli thrown off during dissection of the carotid arteries, cross-clamping, shunting, and restoration of blood flow. Surgical technique can clearly affect this and care must be taken to minimize the risks by carefully ensuring a complete endarterectomy, tacking down the distal intima, irrigating with heparinized saline to remove particulate debris, back bleeding the ICA first to remove air and debris and restoring flow to the external carotid artery first.

Intraoperative strokes

Intraoperative cerebral hypoperfusion can result in cerebral ischaemia and irreversible neurological deficit. Patients with a pre-existing neurological deficit or those with a haemodynamically significant contralateral ICA disease are particularly at risk from fluctuations in cerebral perfusion pressure.

The use of a Javid, Sundht, or Pruit shunt, from the common carotid to internal carotid artery, can protect against ischaemia. Some surgeons shunt routinely, whilst others shunt selectively for an ICA stump pressure of <50 mmHg (this may bear little relation to cerebral blood flow in the presence of anatomical abnormalities or stenoses to the circle of Willis) or for a 50% drop in middle cerebral artery blood flow velocity on transcranial Doppler. The most sensitive means of evaluating ischaemia directly is to perform the operation under local anaesthetic and shunt if the patient develops neurological symptoms. There is little that can be done for operative strokes.

Postoperative strokes

These usually occur within 6 h of surgery. They are often related to thrombosis and/or embolism from the endarterectomy site. This can be confirmed on duplex and merits re-operation with thrombectomy as this may improve the neurological deficit. Cochrane meta-analysis has shown the use of a carotid patch (versus primary closure of the carotid artery) may reduce the risk of thrombotic stroke. Haemorrhagic stroke may also occur and is related to aspirin, heparin, and uncontrolled hypertension.

Blood pressure changes

The aetiology of blood pressures changes around the time of carotid surgery are not completely understood. Intraoperative hypotension and bradycardia are likely to arise as a consequence of stimulation of the carotid sinus. This is a bulge in the origin of the ICA containing baroreceptors in its wall. Its function concerns haemostatic reflexes and the control of blood pressure. Stimulation during surgery can produce reflex bradycardia and hypotension and for this reason the nerve to the carotid sinus (a branch of IX) should be blocked by local anaesthetic infiltration if there are problems during the anaesthetic.

Postoperative hypertension

This is a major problem with a reported incidence of up to 66%. It may be related to devascularization of the carotid sinus nerve or to effects of the local anaesthetic wearing off. It is associated with myocardial infarction and the development of the hyperperfusion syndrome (see below), and for these reasons it is vital that blood pressure is well controlled.

Hyperperfusion syndrome

Increased cerebral perfusion to the ipsilateral cortex is well documented following CEA and may be caused by a loss of cerebral autoregulation. The cerebral hyperperfusion syndrome is associated with uncontrolled postoperative hypertension. In extreme circumstances it can result in seizures, confusion, and cerebral haemorrhage.

Bleeding and haematoma

The use of aspirin and systemic heparin result in an incidence of 0.7–1.5% of cervical haematoma. Many surgeons use a small, sealed suction drain as a consequence.

False aneurysm formation

This can complicate haematoma formation if suture line bleeding continues. The incidence ranges from 0.1 to 0.6%.

Infection

Wound infection following carotid surgery is rare (0.1%). If a synthetic carotid patch is used this may become infected with potential secondary haemorrhage or false aneurysm formation.

Venous carotid patch dehiscence

Occurs in up to 0.5% of patients, resulting in potentially catastrophic secondary haemorrhage. This is more common if the distal long saphenous vein is used as the patch material.

Cranial nerve injuries

These are relatively common with an incidence of 2–7% and include:

* Glossopharyngeal (IX) and vagus nerves (X)—7%. Both nerves lie in close proximity to the carotid bifurcation and are thus at risk. Injury is rarely permanent and is usually manifest by changes in swallowing around the time of surgery. In those patients with difficulty in swallowing a speech therapist should be involved in their management.
* Hypoglossal nerve (XII)—6%. This nerves crosses anteriorly to the carotid bifurcation and injury will result in deviation of the tongue to the side of the injury.
* Mandibular and cervical branches of the facial nerve (VII)—2%. The mandibular and cervical branches can be damaged by the skin incision along the anterior border of sternomastoid that extends up to the angle of the mandible. Neuropraxia may result from excessive retraction.
* Transverse cervical nerve. This is routinely damaged when the skin incision is along the anterior border of sternomastoid. Male patients particularly need to be warned because of the risk of shaving injuries!

Immediate and late complications

Carotid re-stenosis

The incidence of carotid re-stenosis (>50%) lies around 13%, although the pathological mechanisms governing this are not known. It is more common in women, and there is some evidence to suggest that patching the carotid artery in women may affect this incidence. The majority of patients are asymptomatic and for this reason duplex surveillance is not routinely employed during the follow-up period. The overall risk of stroke relating to an internal carotid endarterectomy site is 1% per annum and re-operation is necessary in between 1 and 3.6% of all patients.

Chapter 13
Complications after cardiopulmonary surgery

Complications after cardiac surgery

The increased number, variety, and complexity of cardiac surgical procedures have increased the potential for surgical complications. The use of cardiopulmonary bypass and planned intraoperative cardiac ischaemia present a range of potential complications specific to cardiac surgery.

Whilst it is usual for postoperative cardiac patients to be looked after in an ITU-like environment, the vast majority recover from surgery normally, requiring little more than a few hours assisted ventilation and invasive haemodynamic monitoring. The majority of postoperative problems do not required complicated management, and very few require surgical intervention.

The most common complications of cardiac operations may be considered as:

- complications involving the heart; and
- complications involving other organ systems.

Complications involving the heart

Low cardiac output

A low cardiac output state occurs in approximately 20% of patients who undergo cardiac surgery and is defined as a cardiac index <2.0 l/min per m².

The clinical manifestations are poor peripheral perfusion, urine output, and oxygenation as well as metabolic acidosis.

Happiness is warm toes and a full urine bag

(Prof. G. H. Smith, 1980)

Causes of low cardiac output:

- Reduced preload (e.g. hypovolaemia, cardiac tamponade, tension pneumothorax)
- Decreased myocardial contractility (e.g. pre-existing impaired cardiac function, acute myocardial ischaemia, hypoxia, acidosis)
- Increased afterload (e.g. vasoconstriction, fluid overload)
- Cardiac arrhythmias

Assessment of a low postoperative cardiac output includes physical examination with chest X-ray, ECG, and measurement of urine output and mediastinal drainage.

Invasive haemodynamic monitoring involves measurement of arterial blood pressure, right atrial pressure with arterial blood gases, electrolytes, and haematocrit. The use of a pulmonary artery (PA) catheter should be considered to determine left-sided filling pressures, cardiac output, systemic vascular resistance, and mixed venous oxygen saturation.

Management

Should:

+ optimize preload (left atrial pressure of 15–18 mmHg);
+ optimize heart rate and rhythm (heart rate of 90–100 beats/min and consider the use of temporary pacing);
+ improve cardiac contractility with inotropic drugs;
+ reduce afterload, using vasodilators;
+ correct anaemia and acidosis;
+ include assisted ventilation with adequate oxygen delivery;
+ use mechanical circulatory support with intra-aortic balloon counter-pulsation to decrease myocardial oxygen demand and improve coronary perfusion;

Circulatory assist devices to provide flow for supporting the systemic or pulmonary circulation can be used as a bridge to transplantation.

Arrhythmias

These are common after cardiac surgery.

Supraventricular arrhythmias (especially atrial fibrillation) occur in 10–40% of patients and usually within 1–3 days of surgery.

Causes

These include:

+ hypo- or hyperkalaemia
+ pre-existing arrhythmias
+ myocardial ischaemia
+ hypoxia, acidosis
+ surgical trauma

Assessment requires 12-lead ECG and measurement of serum electrolytes (especially potassium) and arterial blood gases to judge the respiratory status, with assessment of haemodynamic compromise and hence the degree of urgency of any intervention that may be necessary.

Management

+ Correct possible causes (such as hypokalaemia or hypoxia).
+ Supraventricular tachycardia or atrial fibrillation requires amiodarone, digoxin, or DC cardioversion.
+ Bradycardia or conduction disturbance may need atrial, ventricular, or sequential pacing.

- Ventricular fibrillation, tachycardia, or other life-threatening arrhythmias require DC cardioversion.

Perioperative myocardial infarction

The incidence is between 3 and 5%.

Causes

These include incomplete intraoperative myocardial protection, incomplete myocardial revascularization, embolic occlusion or thrombosis of a native vessel or a new graft, or coronary artery or conduit spasm.

Diagnosis

The diagnosis is based on ECG, creatine kinase, and membrane-bound creatine kinase (CK-MB) fraction, Troponin T assay, and wall motion abnormalities determined by echocardiography.

Management

This will depend on the nature of presentation. Salvage of potentially viable myocardium may be possible with further surgery or by PTCA. Otherwise supportive management is required, as with non-perioperative infarction.

Postoperative pericardial tamponade

This is related to persistent mediastinal bleeding. Cardiac output reduces progressively and the right atrial pressure rises. Tamponade can be difficult to distinguish from myocardial failure but diagnosis is usually clinical: chest X-ray and transthoracic echocardiography often fail to confirm the diagnosis, but transoesophageal echo is extremely useful in difficult situations.

Treatment requires transfer to the operating room for re-exploration, relief of tamponade and haemostasis.

Complications involving other organ systems

Renal insufficiency

Up to 15% of patients develop some evidence of renal dysfunction following cardiac surgery. The causes are preoperative problems (renal impairment, nephrotoxins, etc.) or hypoperfusion associated with cardiopulmonary bypass, low cardiac output syndrome, or hypotension.

Diagnosis is made on oliguria (urine output <0.5 ml/kg per h) and elevated serum urea and creatinine.

Management

- Ensure adequate position of the urine catheter.
- Optimize preload.
- Optimize cardiac output.
- Start 'renal' dose of dopamine (3 μg/kg per min), which is conventional but increasingly questioned.
- Use a diuretic once the cardiac output is adequate (furosemide (frusemide) or bumetanide as a bolus or continuous infusion).
- Haemodialysis or ultrafiltration is required in established renal failure, volume overload, hyperkalaemia, acidosis, or uraemia.

Gastrointestinal tract complications

These may occur independently or as part of multisystem failure following cardiopulmonary bypass. The mechanism is either reduced perfusion due to low cardiac output or abnormal perfusion on cardiopulmonary bypass.

Main complications

- Gastrointestinal bleeding, which is often preceded by a history of gastritis or previous ulcer disease and H_2-antagonists generally used for prophylaxis. Endoscopy is required for diagnosis and treatment and coagulopathy needs correction.
- Mesenteric ischaemia and infarction, which presents with a severely ill patient showing any combination of ileus, sepsis, acidosis, diarrhoea, bleeding, renal failure, low or even high cardiac output. The treatment is laparotomy and bowel resection (and occasionally successful embolectomy) but it has a poor prognosis.
- Biliary complications.
- Pancreatitis.

+ Liver dysfunction, commonly seen in relation to multisystem organ failure and sepsis.

Haematological complications

Some 3–5% of patients require re-exploration for bleeding after heart surgery. The causes being 'surgical' bleeding (in two-thirds of cases) and a coagulopathy (in the rest), usually caused by the extracorporeal circuit (related to heparin, platelet damage and dysfunction, fibrinolysis, and depletion of coagulation factors).

Management requires control of hypertension and the giving of blood products (protamine, platelets, fresh-frozen plasma, cryoprecipitate), according to coagulation studies.

Re-exploration is indicated if bleeding is:

+ >500 ml in the first hour;
+ 400 ml/h during each of the next 2 h;
+ 300 ml/h in the first 3 h;
+ 1000 ml total in the first 4 h.

Infectious complications

Prophylactic antibiotics are given for the first 24 hours postoperatively.

Most common infections

Sternal wound infections

This can be either superficial or deep (mediastinitis).

Risk factors include: diabetes, obesity, chronic obstructive pulmonary disease (COPD), and low cardiac output.

Sternal wound infections present with fever, purulent drainage, leucocytosis, and there may be sternal dehiscence when mediastinitis is present.

Management requires antibiotics and local drainage. Sternal dehiscence and mediastinitis require re-operation, debridement, and irrigation. Sternal reconstruction may be required with muscle or omental flaps.

Leg wound infections

The risk factors include poor peripheral perfusion, tissue oedema, obesity, diabetes, and poor surgical technique. They are a common cause of prolonged postoperative morbidity.

Suction drains may help to reduce the incidence, but management involves antibiotics and leg elevation. Debridement and reconstruction may occasionally be necessary.

Pneumonia

Some degree of lung collapse is common after cardiac surgery, hence analgesia, respiratory exercises, and physiotherapy are crucial.

Diagnosis is based on purulent sputum, cough, fever, and leucocytosis. The sputum culture may reveal a positive growth of a microorganism.

There is infiltrate or lobar shadowing on chest X-ray and management is based on antibiotics and physiotherapy.

Neurological complications

The incidence of a major neurological complication is less than 1%, but less severe neuropsychological problems may occur in up to 25% of patients.

Neurological complications include:

+ focal neurological deficit or stroke;
+ neuropsychological disturbance: confusion, agitation, disorientation, depression, personality changes;
+ peripheral nerve injury: caused by sternal retraction;
+ phrenic nerve palsy: left internal thoracic artery dissection, cold injury to the phrenic nerve.

Major neurological deficits have risk factors in the history of a past stroke, in older age, and if there is calcification of the aorta.

Causes

Include:

+ cerebral hypoperfusion with low perioperative perfusion pressure, and significant carotid stenosis;
+ emboli to the brain from intracardiac thrombus, atherosclerotic aorta, or air embolism;
+ intracerebral bleeding due to vascular malformation or hypertension and anticoagulation.

Assessment

Requires a neurological examination, CT scan, and carotid Doppler ultrasound.

Management

Involves the use of heparin, if there is no evidence of intracerebral bleeding, and the management of intracranial pressure and early physiotherapy and rehabilitation.

Pulmonary complications

Risk factors include smoking, COPD, obesity, and old age.

The causes of acute respiratory failure include:

+ atelectasis, pneumothorax, pleural effusion;
+ pulmonary oedema;
+ pneumonia, bronchospasm;
+ prolonged mechanical ventilation.

Assessment requires a physical examination, with attention to the presence of air entry or wheeze. Position of the endotracheal (ET) tube should be checked on chest X-ray. Arterial blood gases should be measured and checked with ventilator settings.

Management

Requires identifiable problems (sedation, analgesia, pleural drainage) to be treated with optimization of cardiac output and ventilator settings (positive end-expiratory pressure (PEEP), fractional concentration of oxygen in inspired gas (FiO_2)). Bronchodilators and diuretics may be necessary.

Other respiratory complications

Include:

- pneumothorax
- pneumonia
- atelectasis
- bronchospasm
- adult respiratory distress syndrome (ARDS)
- chronic respiratory failure

Complications after pulmonary surgery

Persistent air leak

This may develop from the lung parenchyma or a major airways stump. Air leak through the chest drains is the obvious sign.

Management

Includes:

- checking drainage unit for leaks;
- a chest X-ray to visualize lung expansion and position of chest drains;
- addition of suction.

If the lung is fully expanded the majority of air leaks will seal spontaneously. Obstruction of major airways with sputum will prevent full expansion, so physiotherapy and bronchial suction may be required. If air leak persist for more than 2 weeks, consider pleurodesis. Massive air leaks require bronchoscopy and possible re-exploration.

Atelectasis

This follows retained secretions and/or hypoventilation due to pain.

Management

Includes:

- physiotherapy
- adequate analgesia
- adequate pleural drainage.
- bronchoscopy
- minitracheostomy

Arrhythmias

The most common are supraventricular tachycardias, mainly atrial fibrillation. These are treated with digoxin or amiodarone and correction of hypokalaemia and hypoxia.

Respiratory failure

Risk factors include patients with borderline lung function, infection of the remaining lung parenchyma, atelectasis, and fluid overload.

Failure is managed by:

- treating the specific cause (fluid restriction, antibiotics, etc.);
- control of bronchial secretions;
- mechanical ventilation if necessary.

Bronchopleural fistula

This is more common after pneumonectomy and can be acute or chronic (defined as >2 weeks after surgery). It presents with fever and cough with fluid or blood or respiratory failure. An alteration in fluid level in pneumonectomy space may be seen on chest X-ray.

The cause is a residual tumour in the bronchial stump or poor surgical technique with failure to close a bronchial stump adequately or ischaemia or infection of a bronchial stump.

Management

Requires:

- pleural drainage
- bronchoscopy
- antibiotics
- consideration of re-operation

Empyema

This forms in a persistent intrapleural space after pulmonary resection and presents with fever, pleural effusion, and an air–fluid level on chest X-ray. Purulent pleural fluid is obtained on aspiration which usually cultures upper respiratory tract organisms or *Staphylococcus* spp.

Management

Requires:

- chest tube insertion;
- antibiotics according to sensitivity;
- decortication (removal of the empyema membrane).

Chapter 14
Complications of thoracic outlet decompression and transthoracic endoscopic sympathectomy

Complications of thoracic outlet decompression

Thoracic outlet decompression may be performed for thoracic outlet syndrome (TOS) following failure of conservative management. TOS presents with neurogenic symptoms in 95% of cases and arterial or venous in the other 5%. Decompression, in the absence of an obvious cause or for venous symptoms, involves first rib resection performed via a transaxillary approach. Alternatively, a supraclavicular approach may be used, which allows excision of cervical ribs, division of fibrous bands, scalenectomy, and treatment of an underlying vascular lesion (e.g. arterial stenosis, poststenotic dilatation, or aneurysm). This approach provides good exposure in revision surgery. The infraclavicular approach is less popular. The supraclavicular fossa and thoracic outlet contain many vital neurovascular structures and decompression is a technically demanding procedure requiring specialized instruments. Complications include:

- **Tears in the pleura**—are relatively common, occurring in up to 50% of series using a supraclavicular approach. Pneumothorax can be aspirated with a catheter and the defect sutured if recognized intraoperatively. If not, then postoperative pneumothorax may result in up to 13% of patients. Small ones may resolve spontaneously but larger require a chest tube.

- **Haemothorax**—occurs in 1% of cases. These should be treated by a chest drain.

- **Lymphatic damage**—minor lymphatic injury complicates up to 13% of cases and results in small amounts of lymph leakage from the wound or lymphocele development. Major lymphatic injury is far less common and can result in a chylous fistula or chylothorax. This includes injury to the thoracic duct on the left side as it turns laterally at the transverse process of C7 to enter the innominate vein.

- **Injury to major vessels**—occurs in 2% of cases including the subclavian, axillary, internal mammary, and superior intercostal vessels. Uncontrollable haemorrhage using an axillary approach may be difficult to deal with and require conversion to a supraclavicular approach or division of the clavicle.

- **Nerve injuries**—most postoperative nerve injuries are transient neuropraxias due to operative irritation or traction. Nerves at specific risk include:

  - phrenic nerve which runs down the anterior border of scalenus anterior. Transient paralysis occurs in up to 8% of patients following a supraclavicular approach, usually manifested as an elevated hemidiaphragm on the postoperative chest radiograph;

- long thoracic nerve of Bell (nerve to serratus anterior)—can be damaged in up to 8% of cases, either via the supraclavicular or transaxillary approach. Winging of the scapula results.
- vagus and recurrent laryngeal nerves—these cross anteriorly to the subclavian artery. Damage can result with postoperative problems of deglutination and hoarseness of the voice in up to 2% of patients.
- intercostobrachial nerve—this can be damaged or may have to be sacrificed during a transaxillary approach. This gives rise to numbness along the medial aspect of the upper arm.
- brachial plexus—injury to the brachial plexus effects 3% of patients. The trunks and divisions of the brachial plexus are prone to injury as they emerge through the interval between the anterior and middle scalene muscles. Usually this is transient and results in paraesthesia or weakness in the arm.

- **Pain syndrome**—some patients suffer from burning pain and increased sympathetic tone postprocedure. This may be akin to a sympathetic dystrophy.
- **Recurrent symptoms**—90% of procedures result in primary success with an improvement of symptoms. There is a 20% recurrence rate by 18 months and a 30% recurrence in the long term. This does not seem to be affected by which procedure were performed initially (i.e. first rib resection, scalenectomy, or cervical rib resection). Re-operation with a different procedure from that used initially carries a 40 to 50% chance of success. Recurrence is usually related to fibrotic scarring at the site of a previous excision impinging on the thoracic outlet.

Complications of transthoracic endoscopic sympathectomy

Cervical sympathectomy is indicated where ablation of the sympathetic nerve supply to the upper limb is required. This is most commonly for palmar and axillary hyperhidrosis, but also reflex sympathetic dystrophy, thrombangitis obliterans (Buerger's disease), selected patients with Raynaud's syndrome, and non-reconstructable critical ischaemia of the hand. Cervical, transaxillary, or transthoracic approaches have traditionally been used but these have been largely superseded by the endoscopic transthoracic approach. This is because of reduced trauma to the patient, reduced postoperative pain and respiratory complications, and technical ease for the surgeon. Bilateral procedures can be performed at the same sitting and a more rapid recovery is feasible. The operation is performed under general anaesthesia with a double-lumen endotracheal tube and involves the diathermy ablation of T2 and T3 sympathetic thoracic ganglia for palmar symptoms. T4 and T5 may be selectively ablated for axillary hyperhidrosis.

Intraoperative complications

• Risk of oxygen desaturation with one lung ventilation.

Postoperative complications

• **Pneumothorax**—this occurs in 5% of patients. Routine chest drainage is not required as inflation of the lung can be directly visualized with the thoracoscope and the pleura sutured. A chest radiograph is taken in the recovery room to exclude this complication and a further film the following morning. Air leak can occur from inadequate port-site closure or a small puncture to the lung itself. When performing a bilateral procedure many surgeons insert a drain in to the first side to prevent tension pneumothorax when the second side is done.

• **Surgical emphysema**—a small number of patients develop this around the chest wall and neck as a result of air leak.

• **Haemothorax**—loss of blood into the pleural cavity can occur from damage to the intercostal, pleural, and internal mammary vessels. If not recognized during the procedure this can result in haemothorax formation and may require a chest tube.

• **Pain**—many patients experience postoperative periscapular and port-site related pain, which can be reduced by the use of local infiltration at the end of the procedure. The incidence and severity of pain is substantially reduced compared to the open procedure and consequently the respiratory complications of atelectasis and chest infection are reduced.

- **Intraoperative damage to intrathoracic structures**— injury can occur during the procedure to the lungs, heart, great vessels, etc. These complications may be higher when using a Verres' needle to insufflate carbon dioxide before trocar insertion.

- **Horner's syndrome**—this occurs in 1% of patients and is due to inadvertent damage to the stellate ganglion with the diathermy probe. This is usually transient and 0.5% are present at 6 weeks and 0.1% present at 6 months.

- **Compensatory hyperhidrosis**—occurs in up to 25% of patients and usually involves the trunk. Its aetiology is not clear, but destruction of the T4 ganglion in addition to T2 and T3 is associated with an increased incidence. Similarly, postgustatory sweating can also occur.

- **Intercostobrachial neuralgia**—this can result from damage to the intercostobrachial nerve when the port-site in the midaxillary line, 4th intercostal space is made. This results in paraesthesia or dysaesthesia on the medial aspect of the upper arm.

- **Recurrent symptoms**—long-term recurrence occurs in around 6% of patients. Re-operation using the endoscopic route is usually feasible, although pleural adhesions can hinder the procedure.

Chapter 15
Complications of interventional vascular radiology

Complications of interventional vascular radiology

Vascular interventional radiology plays an increasingly common role in the management of patients with vascular disease. Procedures may be diagnostic or therapeutic and include those discussed in this chapter.

Diagnostic arteriography

Intra-arterial digital subtraction angiography (IADSA)

Intra-arterial digital subtraction angiography (IADSA)

Diagnostic arteriography

Arteriography remains the 'gold standard' for obtaining accurate anatomical information about the vascular tree.

Intra-arterial digital subtraction angiography (iaDSA)

Angiographic assessment involves percutaneous catheterization of an artery, injection of contrast and acquisition of radiographic images. Most routine angiography is performed under local anaesthesia via a retrograde femoral arterial puncture. Alternative access points are the brachial and radial arteries. The popliteal and axillary arteries are seldom used. The incidence of serious iatrogenic injuries is around 1%.

Intravenous digital subtraction angiography (ivDSA)

Involves the passage of a catheter into the right atrium, usually via an antecubital vein or the femoral vein. The complications of direct arterial puncture are avoided but image quality is poor. The high contrast load exacerbates problems of nephrotoxicity and cardiac failure. It is usually undertaken in patients with difficult arterial access or as a diagnostic procedure prior to thrombolysis.

Contrast venography

This is now rarely performed, having been superseded by non-invasive duplex imaging. Ascending venography involves the application of a tourniquet around the ankle and injection of contrast in to the dorsal veins of the foot. It can be used to demonstrate occlusion of the deep system, post-thrombotic narrowing, or perforator incompetence. Descending venography involves the injection of contrast into the femoral vein to look for deep venous incompetence. Complications include local thrombophlebitis, deep venous thrombosis, contrast reactions, and complications arising from the puncture site.

Balloon angioplasty

Balloon angioplasty

Percutaneous transluminal angioplasty (PTA) is an established method of treating arterial stenoses/occlusions in short-distance claudicants and in critical limb ischaemia. It involves arterial catheterization, performed under local anaesthetic. The diseased arterial segment is traversed using a guide-wire under fluoroscopic control, a balloon catheter is inflated causing longitudinal plaque fissuring and consequent luminal gain.

PTA is commonly used within the peripheral vascular tree—the more distal the procedure the worse the primary success rate and higher the complication rate. The coronary, renal, subclavian, and carotid arteries are all amenable to angioplasty.

Angioplasty is a relatively safe procedure with a mortality rate of less than 1%. The incidence of serious complications lies around 5%.

Intravascular stents

Intravascular stents are used for the treatment of atherosclerotic arterial stenoses or occlusions. Deployment may be indicated in critically ischaemic patients or in those with short-distance claudication. They may also be used in the treatment of aortoiliac aneurysms and for malignant vascular compression (e.g. superior vena cava) if conventional palliative treatment has failed.

Stents are metallic and can be balloon-expandable (e.g. Palmaz) or self-expanding (e.g. Wallstent, memotherm stent). They are inserted percutaneously, via a transfemoral route, under local anaesthetic.

In the arterial tree, stent deployment is the treatment of choice for long-segment occlusive disease of the aortoiliac segment and in renal artery ostial lesions. Stents can also be used for primary angioplasty failure as a result of elastic recoil, a residual pressure gradient, or flow-limiting intimal dissection. The presence of heavy calcification, eccentric plaque, or a high risk of distal embolization reduces the chance of primary success with angioplasty and may be an indication for stenting.

Complications

All interventional vascular radiological procedures, including angiography, angioplasty, and stenting, involve similar techniques and thus share a number of common complications.

Early complications

Often manifested immediately, they include those arising from the arterial puncture site, intervention site, or remote complications.

Complications at the puncture site

These are the most common of all complications.

Minor bruising

Some cutaneous bruising occurs in most patients and is of no clinical importance.

Groin haematoma

Usually results from inadequate haemostasis and is immediately apparent. Haematoma is more likely in obese and anticoagulated patients.

Management: monitor the patient's pulse and BP closely. Ensure that the haematoma is not expanding, draw a line around its border, and observe frequently for an increase in size. If there is enlargement seek a vascular surgical opinion. Conservative management is often all that is required, but the patient should be told that the lump may well persist for several months. A few patients have continued bleeding and they should be actively resuscitated and have the puncture site surgically explored.

False aneurysm (pulsatile haematoma)

Results from ongoing arterial bleeding from the puncture site into a haematoma where compressed adjacent tissues form a fibrous sac. False aneurysm is uncommon following diagnostic arteriography. It is most likely to occur when large catheters and sheaths are used, and is particularly likely if the superficial femoral artery has been punctured. Ultrasound shows a typical 'to and fro' flow pattern and confirms the diagnosis.

Management: false aneurysms are likely to rupture if left untreated. If the patient has a normal clotting screen, duplex-directed compression and/or thrombin injection usually thrombose the false aneurysm. Surgery is indicated in patients with compression symptoms. The haematoma needs to be evacuated and the arterial defect repaired.

Arterial dissection

Flow-limiting dissection is commoner with antegrade puncture, particularly when catheterizing calcified atheromatous vessels.

Management: if the dissection is not flow-limiting it is not clinically important. Flow-limiting dissections must be rectified either by low-pressure angioplasty, stenting, or surgery.

Local thrombosis

Puncture-site thrombosis rarely occurs in the absence of significant plaque at the point of puncture. Plaque damage activates the coagulation cascade and platelet aggregation, resulting in vessel occlusion.

Management: the patient should be reviewed by an experienced vascular surgeon. Immediate intervention is necessary if the limb becomes acutely ischaemic. If the limb remains well perfused the patient can be observed pending definitive management of the initial problem.

Arteriovenous (AV) fistula formation

Iatrogenic AV fistula is a very rare complication of percutaneous endovascular techniques. It occurs in the presence of simultaneous injury to both the artery and the vein. There is often an arterial bruit and a 'buzzing' pulse, the diagnosis is confirmed on ultrasound.

Management: symptomatic or enlarging fistulas require intervention. Treatment options include stent grafting and surgical exploration and repair.

Vasospasm

This can occur at the puncture site or in the adjacent artery. Small- and medium-size muscular arteries are most often affected, so it occurs most commonly in the arm vessels and the crural circulation.

Management: prophylactic vasodilators (glyceryl trinitrate (GTN) and papaverine) are used to prevent spasm. Vasodilators also help if there is significant ischaemia. If there is refractory spasm the patient should be heparinized to prevent thrombosis.

Femoral nerve injury

This can be caused by the administration of local anaesthetic and by haematoma. The former is very uncommon, but the latter is a cause of significant morbidity and can lead to causalgia lasting many months.

Complications at the intervention site

Complications here may relate to injudicious catheter and guide-wire manipulations. They may also occur at the angioplasty site, as a result of balloon inflation, or during stent deployment.

Primary success in angioplasty to iliac stenoses is around 95–100%. This is, however, worse when treating occlusive disease and may fall to 80% for 5-cm long occlusions. Primary stenting is reserved for iliac occlusions over 6 cm. In the femoropopliteal segment primary success is around 90% for short stenoses, but it is worse for occlusions and diffuse disease. Lesions measuring more than 10 cm require surgical intervention. Complications resulting in an acute deterioration in lower limb ischaemia occur in up to 5% of patients undergoing femoropopliteal segment angioplasty. In the infrapopliteal segment the incidence of complications exceeds 5% and it is therefore reserved for critically ischaemic patients.

Primary success is achieved in around 90% of iliac stents deployed for short iliac occlusions.

Subintimal dissection

The passage of the guide-wire subintimally can raise an intimal flap which may be flow-limiting or that may precipitate thrombosis. Subintimal dissection may also damage collaterals in the femoropopliteal segment which can convert a claudicant into critical ischaemia. Subintimal angioplasty (SIA) is based upon this principle with the guide-wire being passed subintimally and a new lumen being created within the vessel wall. It is often used for infrapopliteal angioplasty.

Treatment: In the absence of symptoms this may be observed, but in those patients with a significant residual pressure gradient re-angioplasty may be attempted or a stent inserted. When these measures fail, and in the presence of critical ischaemia, a vascular opinion should be sought for surgical repair.

Thrombosis and/or macroembolization

Affects 3–5% of patients. Pericatheter thrombosis may occur and distal embolization can involve a thrombus or friable atheromatous plaque. All stents are thrombogenic and thrombosis may occur during deployment, although it is very rare. Thrombosis or distal macroembolization can result in occlusion with consequent acute ischaemia. In these circumstances percutaneous suction thrombectomy or thrombolysis can be undertaken. Failure merits surgical intervention (i.e. thromboembolectomy) if ischaemic symptoms persist.

Vasospasm

Small vessels are prone to vasospasm and thrombosis. This contributes to the high incidence of PTA complications in the crural vessels. In these cases the radiologist can inject a vasodilator at the time of arteriography (e.g. papaverine, GTN) and thrombolysis can be used to clear thrombus. On return to the ward, intravenous prostaglandin or heparin may be a useful adjunct for 24 h.

Elastic recoil

This is more common when treating eccentric, heavily calcified plaques. A residual pressure gradient may exist and suboptimal flow can precipitate thrombosis.

Management: options are to observe alone, or stent the affected segment in the presence of a significant pressure gradient.

Guide-wire perforation

Small arterial perforations can occur as a result of guide-wire passage. They often seal if an angioplasty balloon is gently inflated for several minutes at the site of the injury. If this is not successful then stent grafting or embolization often saves the day. Failing this, an angioplasty balloon is inflated in the inflow vessel to control the bleeding until urgent surgical repair is performed.

Vessel rupture

Rare. When this is due to overdistension during balloon angioplasty it is rare, but it can result in catastrophic bleeding and thrombosis with distal ischaemia when it requires urgent surgical intervention.

In this situation the radiologist can inflate a balloon above the site of the puncture to control the haemorrhage and send off an urgent request for cross-match. The patient should be transferred immediately to theatre for surgical exploration and definitive repair (excision of the affected segment and end-to-end anastomosis or an interposition graft).

Remote complications

Cholesterol and platelet embolization

Microemboli detach from the surface of an atheromatous plaque or from a thrombus within an aneurysm wall. Small emboli pass distally and usually present with livedo reticularis and small cutaneous infarcts to the feet ('trash foot'). Widespread visceral embolization is a rare but devastating complication.

Management: peripheral emboli are usually managed conservatively, in some cases a lumbar sympathectomy may be useful to improve skin perfusion and reduce pain. Systemic embolization may be fatal: expert renal management is imperative and signs of bowel ischaemia must not be ignored.

Other remote complications

- Macroembolization—see thrombosis and embolism, above.
- Contrast reactions with iodinated contrast media—up to 2% of patients require treatment for adverse reactions to intravascular contrast agents. Contrast reactions can be due to direct or idiosyncratic reactions.
- Direct cellular effects are secondary to the osmolarity and chemotoxicity of the contrast agent. These commonly cause heat, nausea, and pain. Nephrotoxicity (see below) and cardiac ischaemia and dysrhythmias may also occur.
- Idiosyncratic reactions are rare. Vasoactive agents, including histamine, serotonin, bradykinin and complement have been implicated, although a causal role has not yet been established. Reactions can be classified as:
  - **Mild**—common (1 in 30)—metallic taste, nausea, sneezing—do not require treatment;
  - **Intermediate**—common (1 in 100)—urticaria—respond quickly to treatment;

- **Severe**—rare (1 in 3000)—circulatory collapse, arrhythmias, bronchospasm—require immediate treatment—may be life-threatening;
- **Death**—rare (1 in 40 000)—due to arrhythmias, pulmonary oedema, respiratory arrest or convulsions.

Treatment: the vast majority of severe contrast reactions will occur within 20 minutes of contrast administration and all patients require close monitoring of pulse, blood pressure, oxygen saturation, and ECG. Resuscitation equipment and drugs should be available within the angiography suite:

- Urticaria—give chlorphenamine (chlorpheniramine) 20 mg.
- Vasovagal syncope—give atropine 0.6–1.2 mg for bradycardia and volume expansion for hypotension.
- Bronchospasm—use nebulized salbutamol 2.5–5 mg. 200 mg intravenous hydrocortisone. Monitor. Subcutaneous adrenaline (epinephrine) (0.3–0.5 ml of 1 in 1000 solution) if bronchospasm fails to improve. If shocked, adrenaline can be given intravenously: 1 ml of 1 in 10 000 solution.
- Laryngeal oedema and refractory hypotension—adrenaline, chlorphenamine, and hydrocortisone. An anaesthetist should assess airway, and tracheostomy may be required.
- The definitive treatment of all patients with intermediate or severe contrast reactions is on the intensive care unit, where close monitoring can be undertaken and cardiovascular, respiratory, and renal support utilized if necessary.

Reducing the risk of contrast reaction

Certain patients are known to be at increased risk, including: those with a previous iodine-based contrast reaction or shellfish allergy (10-fold); cardiac disease (5-fold); asthma (5-fold); general allergic responses (3-fold); and β-blockade (2–3-fold). The risks can be reduced by avoiding the use of non-ionic contrast agents and the administration of steroids as a premedication (i.e. hydrocortisone 200 mg).

In the presence of contraindications to conventional iodinated contrast, an alternative contrast agent could be considered. This includes carbon dioxide, which does not cause contrast reactions or nephrotoxicity. CO_2 dissolves in the blood and is excreted from the lungs. Gadolinium can be used for angiography as well as an MRI contrast agent, it has no reported nephrotoxicity.

Acute renal impairment

Nephrotoxicity can occur in patients with pre-existing chronic renal impairment and with a creatinine concentration of >150 mmol/l. This is a particular risk in elderly and diabetic patients. Strategies to reduce the incidence of acute renal impairment include: using other tests when possible; keeping the contrast dose to a minimum; using alternative contrast agents such as CO_2 and gadolinium. Prehydration is essential and theophylline may also be helpful.

• An example of a renal protection protocol for patients over 70 years of age with creatine concentrations of:
  – <120 mmol/l—require no protection;
  – 121–200 mmol/l—require 1 litre of normal saline commenced during the procedure and infused over 4 h;
  – >200 mmol/l—require admission for prophylaxis, and oral theophylline (3 mg/kg) should be given 1 h before the procedure and 12, 24, and 36 h postprocedure. Normal saline should also be given as shown above.
• Renal protection for patients 69 years or below:
  – similar guidelines to the above should be followed, although a creatinine concentration >300 mmol/l merits admission, oral theophylline, and normal saline prophylaxis.

Lactic acidosis and acute renal failure

Has been reported following intravascular iodinated contrast in diabetics taking metformin, and it is extremely rare. Current practice is to stop metformin at the time of examination and for 48 hours postoperatively. It should only be restarted when renal function has been evaluated and found to be normal.

Intermediate and late complications—after 30 days

Re-stenosis

Some 25–30% of angioplasties develop re-stenosis within 12 months. The tearing of intima and plaque stimulates myointimal hyperplasia, which can result in a localized stenosis causing recurrent symptoms and with an inherent risk of *in situ* thrombosis. Long-term patency rates are around 70–80% at 2 years for iliac stenosis angioplasty but are lower for occlusive disease. Patencies of 70–80% at 1 year for femoral segment stenoses can be expected. Myointimal hyperplasia may also affect stents in a manner analogous to bypass graft stenosis. This can result in stent failure as a result of thrombosis. Long-term patency rates are around 70–80% at 2 years for iliac occlusions, which are superior to angioplasty. This is likely to arise from better initial luminal dilatation. Stenting of the femoropopliteal segment confers no benefit in long-term patency to angioplasty. High rates of thrombosis and re-stenosis mean that the use of stents here should be reserved for salvage procedures.

Thrombosis

All metal stents are thrombogenic and thrombosis may occur below the threshold thrombotic velocity (even in the absence of a significant stenosis), resulting in stent failure and a recurrence of symptoms.

Infection

Rare, occurs in less than 1% of cases. Infection is likely to result from bacterial contamination at implantation, although any cause of bacteraemia may potentially infect a stent.

Intra-arterial thrombolysis

The aim of thrombolysis is to re-establish perfusion by the local infusion of a thrombolytic agent (e.g. recombinant tissue plasminogen activator (rtPA), streptokinase, or urokinase), via a transluminal catheter, into the thrombus. This can be administered by a bolus dose, low-dose infusion, or rapid pulse–spray boluses. Removal of thrombus can be enhanced by percutaneous thrombus aspiration. Angiograms are repeated every 4–6 h to ensure successful lysis. Heparin may be administered concurrently and may be continued until definitive treatment to any underlying flow limiting lesion is performed (i.e. angioplasty, stent, or surgery).

Activation of the fibrinolytic cascade can cause serious bleeding complications and therefore thrombolysis is reserved, in the absence of contraindications, for the treatment of limb-threatening acute ischaemia. This can include *in situ* native-vessel thrombosis, graft thrombosis, thromboembolism, and thrombosed popliteal aneurysms. If the degree of ischaemia merits immediate revascularization, then surgery is more appropriate. Successful lysis is achieved in 80% of cases, with limb-salvage rates of 70–80% following adjunctive procedures (e.g. angioplasty to an underlying stenosis).

Early complications from the administration of local lytic agents

+ Mortality—the overall mortality rate is around 2–3% from fatal stroke or uncontrollable haemorrhage. Delivery of the lytic agent locally into the thrombus, rather than systemically, aims to reduce this.
+ Major haemorrhage—occurs in 5–10% of patients. This can be pericatheter, retroperitoneal, or gastrointestinal. Particular vigilance should be paid to occult bleeding in to the retroperitoneal space following transfemoral puncture. The classic signs are tachycardia and hypotension, but with no obvious source of external blood loss. Occasionally these patients may present with signs of femoral nerve irritation, and severe groin pain should not be dismissed lightly. Significant bleeding requires stopping the thrombolytic infusion, checking the clotting, and administering fresh-frozen plasma and packed cells as necessary.
+ Minor haemorrhage—occurs in 10–30% of patients and is usually puncture-site related. For this reason intramuscular injections and venepuncture should be avoided. Haematomas and femoral false aneurysms can result as a consequence.
+ Stroke—occurs in between 2 and 3% patients and is usually haemorrhagic. Cerebral hypoperfusion and ischaemic stroke may result from major haemorrhage.

- **Distal embolization**—occurs in 4% of patients and is usually managed with continued lysis or suction thrombectomy. In those patients who fail to improve, surgical thromboembolectomy may be required to salvage the limb.

- **Pain**—results from distal reperfusion. Most patients require opiate analgesia.

- **Reperfusion damage**—is reported in 2% patients and includes the risk of acute compartment syndrome (see Chapter 2).

- **Anaphylaxis with streptokinase**—rare complication; unreported in rtPA.

Chapter 16
Complications of varicose vein surgery

Introduction

Varicose veins are common, affecting 10–15% of men and 20–25% of women in the Western world. Surgery is undertaken for symptomatic veins or for the complications arising from them. 80% of procedures are undertaken for primary varicose veins arising from saphenofemoral junction (SFJ) incompetence with long saphenous vein (LSV) reflux or saphenopopliteal junction (SPJ) incompetence with short saphenous vein (SSV) reflux. Surgical treatment is performed under general anaesthesia and consists of a high tie, LSV strip, and multiple stab avulsions (MSAs) for the former and SPJ ligation and MSAs for the latter. 20% of operations are for recurrent varicosities requiring revisional or redo surgery. Increased operating times and technically more complex and challenging surgery mean that the complications in this group of patients are higher.

Early complications

Bleeding/haematoma

All patients are invariably bruised following venous surgery and this relates to stripping of the long saphenous vein and the multiple stab avulsion sites. Intraoperative head-down tilt, evacuation of haematoma in the LSV tunnel, and compression dressings are applied immediately postoperatively to minimize this effect. Some advocate the use of a tourniquet to minimize intraoperative blood loss. Dressings are left on for between 24 hours and 1 week. 5% of patients develop a discrete haematoma, which can affect the groin, long saphenous tract, or multiple stab avulsions sites, and is a potential risk for infection. In some cases the bruising can persist as a brown stain that may be permanent. Many patients, particularly those undergoing revisional surgery or surgery for large varicosities, are left with lumpiness around avulsion sites which can take many weeks to resolve and patients may be left with unsightly brown pigmentation as a result of haemosiderin deposition within the subcutaneous tissues.

Deep venous thrombosis

The overall incidence of deep venous thrombosis is around 1% after varicose vein surgery. There is, however, no evidence to suggest that uncomplicated primary varicose vein surgery in an otherwise fit individual, who mobilizes rapidly, is a risk factor for venous thromboembolic disease. The administration of prophylactic low molecular-weight heparin (LMWH) is based on the surgeon's personal preference in these patients. Those patients undergoing revisional surgery, with pre-existing deep venous incompetence and/or delayed postoperative mobility (e.g. elderly, obese) have a higher thromboembolic risk and should receive routine thromboembolic prophylaxis (i.e. Fragmin, Clexane). In the case of a prior DVT or a family history of venous thrombosis, a blood sample should be sent for a thrombophilia screen.

Women on the combined contraceptive pill are also likely to be at increased risk and this should ideally be discontinued 6 weeks prior to surgery. If not, and they wish to proceed with surgery, then they should be given subcutaneous LMWH at home for 1 week postoperatively. In the case of women on HRT there is little evidence-based medicine on which to advise. A 1-week course of an LMWH can be offered.

Wound infection

Wound infection occurs in 2–3% of patients and tends to involve the groin wound. This is particularly so in the obese, diabetics, and where large amounts of bleeding takes place (i.e. revision veins and large-calibre varicosities). The sites of avulsion can remain lumpy for at least 3 months and may persist up to 1 year after surgery.

Nerve injury

Saphenous nerve

The saphenous nerve joins the LSV just over one-hands breadth below the knee. Saphenous neuritis occurs in 5% of patients if the LSV is stripped to below the knee. Nerve injury presents with paraesthesia affecting the medial aspect of the leg down to and including the first toe. This may take many months to settle or be permanent. If the long saphenous vein is stripped to the ankle the incidence of injury rises to around 10%, and for this reason this has largely been abandoned. The LSV may also be injured during below-knee MSAs. A variety of drugs can be used for disabling saphenous nerve paraesthesia, including: carbamazepine, amitriptyline, gabapentine, and capscoid ointment.

Sural nerve

The sural nerve accompanies the short saphenous vein (SSV) in the leg. Stripping of the SSV is associated with a 10–20% incidence of sural nerve injury and is therefore rarely performed. Sural nerve injury presents with paraesthesia over the lateral aspect of the leg.

Femoral nerve

True femoral nerve injury is a rare, but documented, complication of groin dissection. More common is femoral nerve block as a result of infiltration with local anaesthetic to reduce postoperative pain. This results in combined sensory loss to the anterior thigh and quadriceps weakness. Vigilance to this should be maintained postoperatively as the patient may fall and cases of consequent ankle sprains and fractures are documented!

Common peroneal nerve

The common peroneal nerve is vulnerable to injury during dissection of the popliteal fossa and MSAs around the neck of the fibula. Injury results in sensory loss to the lateral aspect of the leg and foot drop. The use of local anaesthetic in the popliteal fossa may block the peroneal nerve and produce a temporary foot drop. Again care should be taken during infiltration of the popliteal fossa with local anaesthetic especially in thin patients.

Superficial cutaneous nerves

These may be damaged at the site of avulsions. This is especially the case at and below the level of the ankle joint. For this reason MSA should be avoided in that region.

Lymphocele

Damage to afferent lymph vessels or saphenous lymph nodes in the groin, particularly after redo surgery, can result in a localized collection of lymph (lymphocele). Lymphatic leaks and lymphoceles may also affect MSA sites. They can be easily aspirated and compressed, although they tend to re-accumulate. Ultimately 90% resolve spontaneously but this may take many months.

Major venous injury

Damage to the common femoral vein (CFV) can occur during groin dissection and particularly during revisional surgery. Bleeding may obscure the operative field and the blind use of clamps and crude attempts at suturing may damage the CFV. Misidentification of the LSV and CFV can lead to inadvertent ligation or even stripping of the CFV, and the saphenofemoral junction should be clearly identified before ligation and division. In those rare cases where the common femoral vein is ligated and/or divided, the long saphenous can be used to create a panel or spiral graft to replace the affected segment of the femoral vein. Following this the patient is heparinized and warfarinized.

The saphenopopliteal junction is less distinct than the SFJ, access more difficult in the popliteal fossa, and the thin-walled popliteal vein easy to tent up and consequently damage.

Arterial injury

Division and even stripping of the common and superficial femoral arteries has been reported.

Overtight bandaging

Ischaemia can result if the compression dressings are applied too tightly, this is a particular risk in patients with pre-existing peripheral vascular disease. Capillary return in the toes should be inspected postbandaging. In the presence of disproportionate postoperative pain all dressings should be removed to allow wound inspection.

Intermediate complication:

Recurrent varicosities

Inadequate surgery

Neovascularization

The development of new sites of reflux

Spider veins

Intermediate complication:

Recurrent varicosities

The incidence of recurrent varicosities after previous surgical intervention stands at 5% within 5–10 years postoperatively. The term 'recurrent varicosities' should be distinguished from those patients with persistent varicose veins (those veins simply missed at the original surgery). Truly recurrent varicose veins can result from the following:

Inadequate surgery

30% of recurrent varicose veins develop as a result of mid-thigh perforator incompetence following failure to strip the LSV. 10% of recurrences are due to developing incompetence through a second saphenous system missed at previous surgery. 50% of recurrences originate from the SFJ in the groin which may be inadequately ligated, or from major tributaries which are not ligated, or a combination of both.

Neovascularization

The formation of small vessels between the ligated SFJ and the remnant of the LSV, often across fibrous scar tissue, is known as 'neovascularization'. This can account for up to half of recurrent saphenofemoral junction incompetence if the LSV is not stripped.

The use of prosthetic patches or autologous materials does not appear to affect the recurrence rate.

The development of new sites of reflux

This complication accounts for 10% of all recurrent varicosities. This usually involves the development of SPJ incompetence, although, in the absence of an initial duplex scan, subclinical SPJ incompetence may have already existed at the time of initial surgery.

Spider veins

Pre-existing spider veins can worsen after superficial venous surgery in around 3% of patients. They tend to develop at the site of stab avulsions.

Complications of sclerotherapy

Venous sclerotherapy can be performed on patients with isolated superficial primary varicose veins, residual veins after surgery, or for spider or thread veins. It involves an intraluminal injection of sclerosant (e.g. 0.5–3% sodium tetradodecylsulphate depending upon the size of the vein, or chrome alum), compression dressings can be applied in the outpatient department. A number of complications exist however:

- Brown pigmentation—postprocedure bruising can occur and the extravasation of blood and subsequent haemosiderin deposition can result in pigmentation in around 3% of patients.
- Thrombophlebitis—injection of sclerosant can cause pain and precipitate thrombophlebitis, especially if inadequate compression is applied allowing thrombus to remain in the vein. Deep venous thrombosis complicates less than 1% of cases, but is a particular risk if pain limits mobility postprocedure.
- Ulceration—extravasation of sclerosant can occur if the vein or venule is not cannulated adequately. This can result in skin necrosis with ulceration and subsequent scarring.
- Inadvertent arterial injection—is a rare but documented complication!
- Anaphylaxis—is a rare but potential side-effect of sclerosant injection.
- Allergic reaction to bandages—this particularly applies to those containing latex.

Chapter 17
Complications of orthopaedic surgery

Complications after specific operations

Total hip replacement

Introduction

Primary total hip replacement arthroplasty is a successful but non-biological solution to painful hip disease in adults, which carries with it the risk of complications. Broadly speaking, hip replacement arthroplasties can be of a cemented or uncemented (bio-ingrowth) type.

Early complications

Dislocation

Dislocation of hip prostheses occurs in 1–5% of patients in the first 3 months following hip replacement performed electively for hip arthritis. The incidence of dislocation is much higher, usually around 10% if this procedure is performed early for a femoral neck fracture. At least 40% of dislocations occur in the first month after surgery. The direction of dislocation is generally determined by the surgical approach used, thus posterior dislocation is more common with the posterior approach.

Causes

Improper orientation and positioning of the components or inadequate soft-tissue tensioning predispose to hip dislocation postoperatively. Improper compliance of the patient with the prescribed postoperative regime usually precipitates the dislocation.

Recognition

Sudden onset of pain (different from the usual postoperative pain) with shortening of the affected leg, which will be either internally or externally rotated, depending on the direction of the dislocation. Diagnosis can be confirmed by a plain X-ray of the hip.

Treatment

The hip dislocation should be reduced under a general anaesthetic by closed manipulation as soon as possible. If successful, check for stability in various positions of the limb. The joint is, usually, most stable in abduction. Following reduction the hip is maintained in the most stable position, determined by image-intensifier screening (usually in abduction). This is accomplished using an abduction brace, which should be continuously worn by the patient for a period of 6–12 weeks. About two-thirds of these cases stabilize with treatment in the brace. If dislocation recurs following removal of the brace, surgical treatment is likely to be essential for either repositioning of the components or re-tensioning of the hip. If closed reduction fails, open reduction of the dislocation should be undertaken and the above regime of bracing followed.

Infection

This is a dreaded complication following hip replacement and with modern techniques, prophylactic antibiotics, and laminar-flow (clean air) theatres, the early postoperative incidence should be 0.5% or less. Overall, it is estimated that the incidence of infection is approximately 1% over the lifetime of the prosthesis.

Recognition

Redness and raised local temperature around the wound or a dusky discoloration around the wound with associated tenderness and pain in this area are the key features. This may be associated with systemic features of pyrexia, tachycardia, malaise, leucocytosis, connected with toxaemia. Early infection is usually obvious clinically and does not require any extensive investigation, but may be covert when it occurs late.

Treatment

Superficial infections usually settle with a course of intravenous followed by oral antibiotics. Treatment should be aggressive, with an anti-staphylococcal agent (flucloxacillin 1 g every 6 h). Superficial wound infection usually settles with this regimen within 2 weeks. If infection is not controlled by this regimen or a deep infection is suspected, re-exploration of the wound, arthrotomy, and thorough debridement with copious irrigation can salvage the prosthesis. This should be undertaken promptly if a deep infection is suspected. If infection fails to settle in spite of this, management (as detailed in the section on delayed/late complications below), should be more radical. Microorganisms include *Staphylococcus aureus* and *Staph. epidermidis* (the latter typical in late infection).

Periprosthetic fractures

These can occur at any time following hip replacement and result from an injury to the area. They may also occur intraoperatively (iatrogenic).

Recognition

Presentation is with pain and an inability to weight-bear and usually follows an episode of injury (e.g. a fall). Diagnosis is confirmed by X-ray and it is important to obtain anteroposterior and lateral X-rays of the femur to determine the extent of the fracture.

Treatment

This depends on the location of the fracture. If located proximal to the intertrochanteric line conservative treatment, with a period of relative rest and partial weight-bearing/toe-touching, will lead to healing of the fracture if the rest of the femoral stem is well anchored. Fractures extending to below the lesser trochanter up to the lower third of the femoral prosthesis can still be treated in the same fashion, provided the distal femoral stem is well anchored in the femur. These fracture are associated with a high rate of late femoral-component loosening. Fractures at the level of and below the distal third of the femoral prosthetic stem have a high incidence of malalignment and malunion with closed treatment and are treated by open reduction and internal fixation with plates, screws, circlage wires, and cables (with or without bone allografts). Postoperative management must follow the principles of standard fracture management, with protective casing or bracing and restricted weight-bearing until there is fracture union. Fractures associated with an existing loose femoral prosthetic component are best treated by revision hip replacement to provide stable fixation and early mobilization of the patient.

Other complications

Persistent pain following the hip replacement should prompt consideration of aetiologies that are extrinsic to the hip, e.g. a spinal pathology or vascular claudication. Intrinsic hip pain from any stress fracture, infection, or bursitis should also be considered. Sciatic nerve neuropraxia from traction is rare, but usually recovers within 6–12 weeks. Inadvertent division of the sciatic nerve whilst performing the posterior hip approach has been reported and should be promptly repaired surgically. This has a poor prognosis for recovery of function below the knee.

Delayed/late complications

Deep infection

This occurs through haematogenous spread and is somewhat more common if there has been a superficial wound infection in the earlier postoperative period.

Recognition

Onset of pain in the hip after a pain-free period should raise suspicion of sepsis. X-rays of the hip show osteolytic lesions around the prosthesis, eventually the prosthesis becomes loose and may cause dislocation of the hip or a prosthetic fracture. In doubtful cases, isotope bone scan, using ^{99}Tcm- or ^{111}In-labelled leucocyte scintigraphy may be helpful. Hip-joint aspiration is diagnostic in up to 70% of cases when there is a leucocytosis >10 000/mm^3 or when the offending organism is cultured.

Treatment

Once the diagnosis is confirmed, surgical treatment is indicated. The existing implants should be removed and revised to a new set of prostheses; this is usually done in two stages, where the old prosthesis is removed with the first operation and systemic antibiotic therapy instituted. Gentamicin-impregnated beads can be used locally in the wound for delivery of antibiotics. The leg is maintained in Hamilton Russell traction and a second-stage procedure for implanting a fresh hip prosthesis is done, usually 4–6 weeks later, once all evidence of infection has gone.

Aseptic loosening

This is the mechanism by which hip replacements usually fail over a period of time. Some 5–10% of prostheses become loose in this fashion over a period of 10 years from the time of surgery.

Mechanism

Over time, small particles of polyethylene from the acetabular cup incite a foreign-body type reaction and granuloma formation. Once these are ingested by local macrophages there is a release of osteolytic enzymes which leads to loosening of the prosthetic components.

Recognition

Serial plain X-rays of the hip. Progressive radiolucent lines occur around the bone/cement or bone/prosthesis interface (with cemented or uncemented components, respectively) and may show a change in orientation of the components with time (e.g. the acetabular cup may become more vertical compared to previous radiographs). Clinically, this presents with pain in the hip, with or without associated 'clunking' or late dislocation. The leg may become shorter and the 'telescoping' sign may be positive.

Treatment

The standard treatment for aseptic loosening of a total hip prosthesis is surgical one-stage revision hip replacement.

Implant failure where there is a fracture of the prosthesis may occur following loosening or be due to true fatigue fracture of a well-fixed component (e.g. fracture of the modular head/neck of a well-fixed, uncemented, femoral component). This is usually treated by a revision hip replacement.

Total knee-replacement arthroplasty

Infection

The incidence of infection is low, generally around 0.5%, with risk factors including malnutrition, immunocompromise, diabetes, psoriatic arthropathy, and previous periarticular infection, which are all more likely to relate to a deep infection following a knee replacement. The presence of persistent erythema, poor wound healing, fever, or more than expected pain during rehabilitation should raise the suspicion of an early infection. Elevated white cell count, erythrocyte sedimentation rate (ESR) or C-reactive protein (CRP) are also suggestive of an infection. Aspiration of the joint and evaluation of the Gram stain and culture is diagnostic in 75% of cases.

Treatment

Early infection, i.e. 2–4 weeks following surgery, should be treated by re-exploration of the wound, arthrotomy, thorough debridement and copious lavage, followed by appropriate parenteral antibiotics. If the knee components are well fixed they may be left in place, and this strategy has the best chance of salvaging the prosthesis. If, in spite of this, infection persists or if subsequent late infection occurs by haematogenous spread at continued follow-up, a two-stage revision knee replacement is indicated.

Thromboembolism

Without prophylaxis, the rate of venous thrombosis following a total knee arthroplasty is as high as 84%, but it is debatable whether prophylaxis reduces the incidence of fatal pulmonary embolism. Various mechanical and pharmacological modes of prophylaxis are available (e.g. compression stockings, sequential compression devices, pedoplexus compression devices, aspirin, low molecular-weight heparin (LMWH), warfarin). There is no consensus about the ideal method of prophylaxis at present, although low molecular weight heparin is the most favoured.

Periprosthetic fractures

These are defined as fractures occurring within 15 cm of the joint line and occur in 0.6–1.6% of patients, usually on the femoral side. These occur in association with minimal trauma and osteoporosis. Most of these injuries are of low-energy type and heal rapidly with immobilization and closed treatment if reduction can be maintained. However, proper alignment is difficult to maintain by closed methods in some of these fractures and, in these, open reduction and internal fixation with either an extramedullary plate and screws or an intramedullary locked nail is indicated.

Arthrofibrosis

This is a rare complication that presents with a painful knee which has a poor range of motion following knee replacement. These patients may never gain a functional range of motion following surgery, or they may lose motion after initially doing well. This condition has to be differentiated from reflex sympathetic dystrophy and, after ruling out infection, can be successfully treated by manipulation and physiotherapy. Rarely, an arthrotomy with removal of intra-articular adhesions and scar tissue may be necessary.

Extensor mechanism problems

Fractures of the patella around the patellar component of the prosthesis may occur and, if undisplaced, are usually managed conservatively. Immobilization for 4–6 weeks with external cast/splintage, followed by guided active exercises usually lead to full recovery. Displaced fractures may need to be treated by internal fixation, with or without revision of the patellar component.

Progressive patellar maltracking with lateral subluxation of the patella may occur with continued follow-up. Patellar tendon avulsion is a serious complication for which treatment is frequently unsuccessful. Primary repair, if unsuccessful, leads to a lack of extensor mechanism for the knee, which will have to be treated by a locked knee brace or surgical arthrodesis.

Aseptic loosening

Particulate polyethylene debris incites a granulomatous foreign-body type reaction that leads to bone osteolysis, synovitis, and swelling in the knee. Radiological examination reveals progressive radiolucent lines with loosening of the prosthetic components. Once infection is excluded, treatment is by a single-stage revision knee replacement.

Complications following surgical treatment of fractures

The following complications can occur with any of the various types of internal fixation or external fixation of fractures.

Infection

Superficial wound infection or deep infection (osteomyelitis) can both occur after surgical treatment of fractures, and present with local pain, redness, swelling, warmth, and, in the later stages, wound gaping and discharge. Systemic features of toxaemia with pyrexia and leucocytosis may be present. X-rays of the involved part show soft-tissue swelling only in the first 2 weeks, but later show osteolysis around the implants. In the case of external fixators, the pins may become loose due to a surrounding osteolysis.

Treatment

A wound swab and blood for culture should be taken. Intravenous antibiotics should be given with activity against *Staphylococcus aureus*. If there is any suspicion of deep infection or suppuration, the wound needs to be surgically re-opened with thorough debridement. Anaerobic and bowel flora organisms are a serious problem, particularly in lower limb fractures with severe contamination *or* associated vascular injury. If implants are well fixed they can be left alone after thorough lavage of the wound. If internal fixation implants are loose, they have to be removed and fixation revised or alternative methods of fixation used, such as an external fixator. In the case of pin-site infection in an external fixator, treatment with antibiotics is required with local pin-site dressings and care. If pins become loose, the pins need resiting with reapplication of an external fixator and a course of antibiotics.

Non-union

This is failure of the fractured bone ends to unite by bony union.

Causes

Local infection, abnormal movement at the fracture site with inadequate fixation of the bony fragments, and poor blood supply to the bone ends at the fracture site are the causes. Also, distraction with a gap at the fracture site predisposes to non-union.

Types

+ **Atrophic types**—the bone ends are thin and look rounded-off with sclerosis, usually due to inadequate blood supply and revascularization.

- **Hypertrophic non-union**—this is where the bone ends are expanded and are attempting to heal but there are other factors preventing them healing, e.g. infection, local fracture site movement. X-ray appearances of the bone ends are usually described as a 'horse's hoof' or an 'elephant's foot'.
- **Pseudoarthrosis**—this is when there is established non-union with rounding of bone ends, and there may be an artificial synovial-type cavity formed around these.

Treatment

This is usually surgical, requiring rigid internal fixation to eliminate movement at the non-union site. Freshening of the bone ends and bone grafting of the defect is the standard treatment for an established non-union. Other methods used are a vascularized bone graft (e.g. fibular graft) for segmental bone loss, or bone transport with a three-dimensional fixator (Ilizarov frame) which is being used more frequently for treating segmental bone loss. Other methods, like electrical stimulation and pulsatile electromagnetic fields, have been tried with variable success. If there is a small fracture gap, a percutaneous bone-marrow injection may be used. It is important to eradicate any infection at the non-union site before attempting definitive surgical treatment.

Malunion

This is where the fractured bone unites in a non-anatomical alignment.

Causes

Inadequate initial reduction of fracture, inadequate internal or external fixation/splintage, or failure of fixation (implant failure or infection and loosening).

Treatment

This depends on the site and degree of malunion. If correction is indicated, planned corrective osteotomy with further internal fixation should be carried out. Alternatively, osteotomy with external fixation (Ilizarov frame) can be used.

Avascular necrosis (aseptic necrosis)

This is death of bone from a deficient blood supply. It may cause local pain, non-union of fractures, and may lead to disabling arthritis or disorganization of a joint. Avascular necrosis is important clinically only when it involves the articular end of the bone.

Sites

Common sites are: the femoral head after a femoral neck fracture or after dislocation of the hip; the proximal part of the scaphoid bone after fracture through its waist or more proximally; and the body of the talus after a fracture through the neck of the talus. This can also occur spontaneously in patients on steroid therapy, in sickle-cell disease, and as part of decompression sickness (e.g. deep-sea diving).

Pathology

Loss of blood supply makes the bone lose its rigid trabecular structure and become more granular or 'gritty'. This makes the bone crumble more easily with stresses imposed by a muscular tone or body weight, and it may collapse into an amorphous mass as a result of these stresses. These changes usually occur within a year of injury but, sometimes, take up to 2–3 years to develop. Radiologically, this develops as increased density of the avascular fragment with some relative osteopenia of the surrounding bones from the reactive hyperaemia and disuse of the surrounding area.

Diagnosis

Usually evident with follow-up radiographs. ^{99}Tcm-radioisotope bone scanning with high resolution may show the area as a cold spot. A magnetic resonance imaging (MRI) scan can reliably pick up areas of avascular necrosis as early as 2 weeks following the injury.

Treatment

Attempts to revascularize the area have been tried with vascularized bone grafts or muscle pedicle grafts, but success is variable.

Septic arthritis

This is used to describe an infected joint. Prompt treatment of this is imperative, otherwise major joint destruction and systemic complications are likely to ensue.

Causes

Any surgical procedure in a joint, e.g. arthroscopic surgery or fixation of articular fractures, reconstruction of the knee, or synovectomy. This can also occur after penetrating injuries in the joint in spite of wound exploration and debridement. Intra-articular injections, in particular steroid injections, can cause this condition. Haematogenous spread can also cause a joint infection, a particularly common event in intravenous drug abusers and immunocompromised individuals.

Clinical features

Pain and swelling in the joint with stiffness of the joint with pain on movement are the usual symptoms. Usually, synovial tenderness and joint-line tenderness with an effusion in the affected joint are seen. There is increased local warmth and movements of the joint are restricted and painful. There may be features of toxaemia, like pyrexia, tachycardia, sweating, and rigors.

Investigation

Blood investigations reveal leucocytosis, predominantly increased neutrophils, and blood culture may be positive, particularly if the sample is obtained in association with pyrexia and rigors. X-ray of the affected joint shows soft-tissue swelling in the initial stages and periarticular osteoporosis with joint destruction in the later stages. Confirmation of the diagnosis is by obtaining a joint aspirate for Gram stain microscopy and culture. Synovial biopsies may also be obtained for culture.

Microorganisms

Most commonly *Staph. aureus*. May also be caused by *Haemophilus influenzae*, *Streptococcus pneumoniae*, *Gonococcus* and *Pseudomonas* spp., and other Gram-negative bacteria. *Salmonella* and *Mycobacterium* spp. are also other important but less common microorganisms.

Treatment

This is a surgical emergency. Radical treatment by arthrotomy, copious irrigation of the joint, and synovectomy with systemic intravenous antibiotics (initially flucloxacillin and modified as necessary depending on the results of culture and sensitivity) stands the best chance of eradicating the infection.

Complications following hand surgery

Reflex sympathetic dystrophy (RSD)

This complication can arise after any hand surgery or injury, and is fully described later in this chapter.

Infection

Infection in the hand occurs in one or more of the following palmar spaces:

+ **Hypothenar space**—this encloses the hypothenar muscles but not the long flexor tendons or their sheaths. If infection is confined to this space, it is less problematic than the other areas in the hand.
+ **Mid-palmar space**—this is a space that lies deep to the flexor tendons and the common synovial sheath; it contains the lumbricals and dorsally is bounded by the interossei.
+ **Common flexor sheath**—this is the area that contains the long flexor tendons to the fingers, particularly the little, ring, middle, and, sometimes, the index. Infection here can lead to serious involvement of function of these fingers.
+ **Thenar space**—this space encloses the thenar muscles, the flexor tendon of the thumb, and, sometimes, the flexor tendon of the index finger. Infection here causes abnormal function of these fingers.

Infection in the above spaces generally presents with pain in the hand with swelling, which is most marked over the **dorsal** aspect of the hand. If the flexor tendons are involved this can lead to some local tenderness over the area of the common flexor sheath (Kanavel's sign), which is detected by pressure on the ulnar side of the palm. There is pain on passive or active movements of the involved fingers, and the finger assumes a flexed posture with any passive stretching/straightening leading to severe pain along the flexor sheath. With an extension of the infection, tenderness and swelling can be noted in Parona's space, just proximal to the carpal tunnel on the volar aspect of the wrist.

Treatment

In the acute stage, intravenous antibiotics are needed with hand elevation and gentle physiotherapy to prevent contractures. If infection does not respond to these measures or if the patient presents late (after 48 hours of onset) there may be local suppuration. This requires urgent investigation using ultrasound or MRI to localize the collection. Surgical drainage is needed as an emergency procedure, with the exception that in the hand the skin is closed primarily following the drainage. Hand elevation and intravenous antibiotics should be continued. If a flexor sheath is involved, a window is made proximally and distally in the sheath and the sheath is irrigated copiously with warm Ringer's lactate or saline, in addition to draining any other collection. Physiotherapy is continued postoperatively to maintain hand and finger function.

Tendon adherence

This occurs following any tendon repair or a surgical procedure or injury in the proximity of a tendon. Adherence is most common following flexor-tendon repair in zone 2, and presents with a reduced active range of movements in spite of continued physiotherapy. Diagnosis should always be considered when the passive range of movement exceeds the active range of movements in a finger.

Treatment

This is treated by surgical tenolysis (freeing of the tendon adhesions) but should not be undertaken for several weeks following the repair, until the tendon strengthens up, as there is a risk of re-rupture of the tendon following tenolysis. A further course of active rigorous physiotherapy following the tenolysis restores active finger movements.

Scar contracture

This is another complication which can reduce the range of finger movements. Longitudinal incisions forming scars across flexion creases in the fingers usually lead to this complication, such incisions should therefore be avoided. Contractures present with tightness of the scar with an inability to extend the fingers fully. This is treated in the initial stages by scar massage and gentle stretching and, once the scar matures, if there is a significant residual contracture, a surgical release by Z plasty cures the condition.

Inadvertent neurovascular injury

This complication may occur with injury to digital neurovascular bundles, particularly whilst doing a fasciotomy for Dupuytren's disease. If recognized at the time of surgery, the digital nerve should be repaired by epineural sutures under magnification. If recognized following surgery, there is the risk of neuroma formation and loss of protective sensation in the finger and re-exploration with surgical repair of the nerve should be carried out. The aim of surgery is to restore the protective sensation in the finger and to prevent neuroma formation.

Complications after spinal surgery

The following complications may occur following any form of spinal surgery.

Paralytic ileus

This complication may occur due to reflex inhibition of bowel function. It is more common with anterior approaches to the lumbar spine and is treated in the usual way, as detailed elsewhere in this book. This complication is temporary and bowel function returns within a day or two following surgery. If not, a more organic cause should be suspected and investigated (e.g. inadvertent bowel injury).

Infection

Vertebral osteomyelitis and/or an epidural abscess may occur and presents with increasing local pain. There may be systemic features and if an epidural abscess or a granulomatous lesion develops in association with this, a corresponding neurological abnormality might develop. It is important to chart neurological signs regularly after any spinal surgery.

Treatment

Treatment is along the usual lines with intravenous antibiotics and close observation. If there is suspicion of an abscess formation, this will need surgical drainage.

Neurological deficit

Usually, there is some neurological dysfunction preoperatively in most of these cases and it is important to document this carefully. If any fresh neurological abnormality occurs postsurgery or if there is progressive neurological involvement then prompt investigation and action are indicated. Carefully watch for these events, particularly any postoperative sphincter disturbances.

Causes

Haematomas can cause neurological compression. Residual intervertebral disc fragments/sequestration/prolapse at another level may not be recognized at the time of surgery, thereby leading to abscess formation. Inadvertent neurological injury, particularly with instrumented spinal surgery, using pedicle screws and distraction, is another cause.

Management

Determine the level of possible neurological involvement, obtain urgent local imaging (e.g. CT or MRI scanning), and treat the pathology detected. Neurological injury may cause causaulgic type nerve pain and may need the involvement of a chronic pain-management team.

Other complications

Failure of fusion and persistent pain with attempted intervertebral fusions (particularly multiple levels), instability following extensive laminectomy, and undue stresses adjacent to fused vertebral segments cause persistent low back pain (the Failed Back syndrome). Empyema, persistent pneumothorax, or excessive blood loss from a large haemothorax may occur following a thoracotomy for anterior thoracic spinal operations. It is important to learn to anticipate these complications and institute prompt treatment.

Arthroscopic surgery

The following specific complications can occur following arthroscopic surgery of any joint.

Infection

Septic arthritis of the joint may occur and needs to be treated promptly, as described earlier.

Synovial fistula

Persistent discharge of synovial fluid occurs from a fistula opening out to the skin surface through an arthroscopy port. This is a rare complication, and is treated by splintage of the joint and occlusive dressings with non-steroidal anti-inflammatory agents in the early stages. If drainage fails to cease by 8 weeks, surgical excision of the fistula needs consideration with or without a synovectomy of the involved joint.

Compartment syndrome

This is a rare complication, particularly after a knee arthroscopy, and may occur if the irrigation fluid extravasates into the calf through a capsular tear, causing abnormal tension in the muscle compartment of the leg. If suspected, treat by a prompt fasciotomy.

Neurovascular injury

This should not occur with safe arthroscopic practice. Injury to nerves may cause painful neuromas (usually related to subcutaneous nerves) or may cause a patch of numbness in the distribution of the cutaneous nerve. If a troublesome neuroma occurs, surgical resection and nerve repair are indicated.

Other complications

Quadriceps inhibition may occur after knee arthroscopy, but this is temporary and can be treated by active physiotherapy. Joint stiffness and florid RSD may occur, particularly in the hand following a wrist arthroscopy. This is managed in the usual fashion. Haemarthrosis is rare, but it can occur after an arthroscopic synovectomy. If bleeding is not controllable arthroscopically, an arthrotomy with drainage of the arthrosis and diathermy haemostasis might be necessary. Treatment is indicated if there is symptomatic joint involvement.

Treatment usually involves surgical removal of the avascular part followed by the salvage procedure for the joint (e.g. arthrodesis or joint replacement arthroplasty).

Non-specific orthopaedic complications

Post-traumatic ossification (myositis ossificans)

This complication is encountered most commonly around the elbow, but it can occur around any joint following a severe injury, especially a fracture dislocation.

Mechanism

With severe injury there is stripping of capsule and periosteum from the bones and displacement of the fracture fragments. Blood collects under the stripped periosteum forming the haematoma around the joint. Osteoblasts are activated by the periosteal stripping and, instead of the haematoma being reabsorbed, it becomes calcified and forms a mass of bone.

Recognition

Myositis ossificans presents with subjective stiffness and a reduced range of movement which fails to improve with continued follow-up and physiotherapy. It should be suspected in patients in whom joint movement does not recover within the anticipated period. X-rays of the involved part show 'fluffy' calcification around the joint which looks similar to immature callus. Serum alkaline phosphatase is raised and an isotope bone scan demonstrates a hot spot in this area in the active stages of bone formation.

Treatment

Gentle active exercises in the initial phases, but passive stretching should be avoided altogether. It is necessary to wait for the heterotopic bone to mature (indicated by maturation of the bone with serial radiographs), return to normal of the serum alkaline phosphatase level and the isotope bone scan (which then indicates that the process has reached an inactive stage). The heterotopic bone can be removed at this stage with improvement of joint function. There is a risk of recurrence of heterotopic ossification with surgical excision.

Post-traumatic arthritis

This occurs due to damage of a joint surface from a displaced intra-articular fracture. Surgical reconstruction aims to restore normal joint congruity. Accurate reconstruction of the joint surface minimizes, but does not eliminate, the risk of post-traumatic arthritis. Treatment of this complication should follow the general principles of managing painful arthritis in a joint.

Fat embolism syndrome (FES)

This is a condition characterized by unanticipated respiratory compromise following long-bone fractures.

Pathomechanics

The syndrome follows small-vessel occlusion by fat globules. There are two current theories to explain this phenomenon: the fat emboli are thought to originate directly from the bone marrow of the fractured bone; or through aggregation of fat from soft-tissue stores in the bloodstream during post-traumatic shock.

Clinical features

These usually follow long bone fractures in the lower limb (femur, tibia/fibula). The syndrome presents with dyspnoea, tachycardia, anxiety, tachypnoea (sustained respiratory rate >35/min), a petechial rash above the level of nipples, fever, retinal changes, and, sometimes, jaundice. There is a 'lucid' symptom-free period of 1–2 days after the fracture before the onset of these symptoms. Gurd and Wilson's criteria for diagnosis are shown below:

- **Major signs:** Respiratory insufficiency, cerebral involvement, and petechial rash
- **Minor signs:** Fever, tachycardia, retinal changes, jaundice, and renal changes

FES can be diagnosed when one major and four minor signs are present.

Investigations

- Arterial blood gases—PO_2 <9 kPa, PCO_2 >8 kPa, pH <7.3 breathing room air
- Fat globules in blood (macroglobulinaemia), urine, and sputum
- ST segment changes on ECG and $S_1Q_3T_3$ suggesting right ventricular strain

Treatment

Supportive, maintaining respiratory function with appropriate supportive measures whilst awaiting spontaneous resolution. Early surgical stabilization of fractured long bones, especially in polytrauma, within 24 hours of injury. O_2 administration in the postinjury period reduces the incidence of FES. Corticosteroids in high doses have been shown to reduce the incidence of FES, but their routine use is not recommended and steroid therapy remains controversial.

Multiple system organ failure (MSOF)

This is defined as the sequential failure of two or more organ systems following injury, operation, systemic inflammatory response syndrome (SIRS), or multiorgan dysfunction syndrome (MODS). It is important to take extra care to prevent this complication, as the mortality rate following failure of two or more organ systems after trauma is 75% and if one of these is the renal system then mortality may approach 100%.

Mechanism

Patients with polytrauma, uncontrolled sepsis, or the presence of gangrenous tissue or a limb are at risk. These trigger SIRS followed by the cascades that lead to MODS and decompensation of organ systems.

Recognition after multiple trauma

Beware of the polytraumatized patient and one with a focus of infective, necrotic, or inflammatory tissue (e.g. extensive burns). A high index of suspicion should be maintained in these patients. Lung involvement usually occurs first (acute respiratory distress syndrome, ARDS) with the ensuing reduction in PO_2 contributing to the failure of other systems, i.e. renal, ileus and gastritis, liver, and derangement of coagulation.

Treatment

Early recognition is important. Usual methods to control and treat pneumonia, GI bleeding, and renal failure appear to be ineffective and an aggressive multidisciplinary approach to management is essential. Surgical stabilization of any long-bone, pelvic, or spinal fractures as indicated, should be performed urgently, if not already done, and all necrotic tissue radically excised. The patient usually needs blood, fluid and electrolyte balance, effective antibiotics, calories, and nutrition. Controlled ventilation and renal dialysis may be necessary. All of these must be continuously monitored in an intensive care setting.

Prevention

Prompt surgical treatment, e.g. stabilization of fractures within 24 h of injury in the polytraumatized patient is mandatory. Pulmonary failure should be anticipated and early mechanical ventilation for respiratory failure may be necessary. Nutrition must be monitored.

Osteomyelitis

This is the term applied to an infective process in bone and is a potential local complication of any elective surgical procedure on the skeleton or fracture treatment. It may occur without surgery or trauma in the paediatric age groups or in immunocompromised individuals by haematogenous spread.

Types

Osteomyelitis may be acute, subacute, or chronic depending on the clinical presentation, including the time-scale. Four types have been described based on the extent of bone involvement—medullary (in haematogenous type), superficial, focal, and diffuse.

Bacteriology

Staph. aureus is the commonest pathogen. *Strep. pneumoniae, Haemophilus influenzae, Brucella abortus, Salmonella* spp., *Mycobacterium* spp., spirochaetes, and fungi may also cause osteomyelitis.

Pathology

The presence of bacteria within the musculoskeletal system is abnormal. It is important to recognize the difference between 'colonization' and 'infection'. Bacteria can be cultured from pin-sites of an external fixator, or an open wound associated with a fracture—this is colonization. Osteomyelitis is the presence of bacteria with an inflammatory response that leads to progressive destruction of bone. Once a critical bacterial load that overwhelms local defences is introduced (usually $>10^5$ colony-forming units/g of tissue) into bony tissue, this sets up a local hyperaemia and inflammatory response. There is bone necrosis with formation of infective thrombi. Reactive periosteal bone (involucrum) may form around the infective focus (sequestrum), and, if suppuration evolves further, the pus tracks through holes in the involucrum (cloacae) to the skin, forming discharging sinuses. This heralds the transition to a chronic phase subsequent to uncontrolled acute osteomyelitis.

Clinical features

Manifestation is usually at least a week after fracture treatment or a surgical procedure on bone. In acute osteomyelitis there is local warmth, swelling, skin oedema, and erythema. These signs may be absent if infection occurs deep to the deep fascia, particularly in the femur. The patient is usually febrile with a leucocytosis. Subacute osteomyelitis presents with pain, but local and systemic features are remarkably absent. There may be percussion tenderness on the affected part of the bone.

Chronic osteomyelitis presents a few months after the inciting event or after an acute osteomyelitis that has been modified in its course by inadequate treatment. There may be some local pain, swelling, and erythema but these are usually not severe. One or more sinuses on the skin may be discharging purulent material, sometimes containing pieces of white necrotic bone. Systemic features are typically absent.

Investigations

Acute osteomyelitis is a clinical diagnosis and treatment should not be delayed. Blood culture and local wound swab is appropriate for culture and sensitivity to confirm the empirical choice of therapy. Blood cultures are positive in only about 50% of cases. Leucocytosis and periosteal reaction on local X-rays may be present. Chronic and subacute osteomyelitis may be more difficult to diagnose clinically, and may need further investigation.

Plain radiographs of the involved part are mandatory and remain the single most useful investigation. They may demonstrate osteolysis and a periosteal reaction. Haematological investigations are usually normal. Isotope bone scan, using technetium-99m, shows the infective focus as a hot spot, but occasionally can give false-positive and false-negative results. The ^{111}In-labelled leucocyte scan is more specific. Bone biopsy is the definitive confirmatory investigation in doubtful cases. This also helps in identifying the offending organisms and its antibiotic sensitivity.

Treatment

Acute osteomyelitis

Splint the affected limb for pain relief. Start intravenous antibiotics after obtaining a blood sample for culture and any local sample from the affected part, if feasible. Use an antibiotic with activity against *Staph. aureus*, e.g. flucloxacillin. Clinical signs should be monitored: leucocyte count, CRP, ESR (or plasma viscosity) to determine response to treatment. Continue IV antibiotics until CRP returns to normal, and switch to oral antibiotics for a further 4 weeks. Usually a 6-week course of antibiotics (at least) is needed for eradication of infection.

Subacute and chronic osteomyelitis

Treatment usually requires surgical sequestrectomy and drainage of any abscesses, augmented by local or systemic antibiotics. Multiple surgical procedures may be necessary.

Complications

Local deformity, scarring, and growth disturbance may occur. Sinuses may rarely turn malignant (Marjolin's ulcer) and chronic infection may lead to systemic amyloidosis.

Reflex sympathetic dystrophy

This is a clinical condition that can occur after any limb injury or surgery, application of plaster casts, accidental insertion of needles into nerves, or extravasation of thiopental during induction of anaesthesia.

Causes

It is trigged by injury to peripheral nerves or following any type of surgery. It is more common in the upper limb (sometimes referred to as the 'shoulder hand syndrome') but has been recognized around the knee following any injury or surgery in this region.

Mechanism

This is unclear. A widely accepted hypothesis is that the condition is mediated and maintained by the autonomic nervous system, and is thought to be a prolongation of the normal sympathetic response to injury.

Clinical features

Three phases are recognized:

1. **Acute (hyperaemic) phase**—pain, hyperaesthesia, increased local warmth, and oedema, also the skin looks stretched and shiny with loss of normal wrinkles and creases.

2. **Dystrophic (ischaemic) phase**—the oedema spreads further, joints become stiff, and muscle wasting develops. Pain remains the main symptom and is usually burning in nature. The skin becomes moist, cyanotic, and cold. The hair is coarse, the nails show ridges and are brittle.

3. **Atrophic phase**—trophic changes become irreversible. Skin becomes pale, smooth, glossy, and tight. Temperature is lowered. The thickened hair falls out. There is extreme weakness and limitation of movement of all involved joints (e.g. fingers and wrist). Pain, although less prominent, persists.

Diagnosis

This is usually clinically obvious. X-rays of the involved part (e.g. hand) show patchy osteoporosis (known as Sudeck's atrophy). Three-phase isotopic bone scans show increased uptake in early and delayed phases with increased activity in a periarticular distribution.

Differential diagnosis

Tenosynovitis, bursitis, myofascial pain, Raynaud's phenomenon, and, sometimes, peripheral nerve injury without a sympathetic nervous system component.

Treatment

This is difficult. Different modalities may have to be tried simultaneously or sequentially. These are: physiotherapy; nerve blocks, especially regional block using guanethidine; surgical or chemical sympathectomy; and psychotherapy. It is important to maintain function of the involved part and alleviate the stresses produced by the syndrome on the central nervous system.

Compartment syndrome

This is a very important condition, characterized by raised pressure within a closed space with the potential to cause **irreversible** damage to the contents of the closed space. It is usually seen in muscle compartments in the limbs and occurs most commonly in the leg, but can also occur in the forearm, thigh, foot, and hand. Abdominal compartment syndrome is a similar condition, this can occur after laparotomy or ileus.

Causes

Closed or open fractures, direct blow blunt injuries, and crush injuries are usually responsible. The syndrome can occur when compartments are reperfused after arterial repair (ischaemia-reperfusion injury).

Recognition

Persistent pain in a compartment(s) after surgical stabilization of fractures or splintage is the key symptom. Pain on active and passive movements of the muscles in the involved compartment is the earliest sign. The compartment may feel tense to palpation. Other signs (anaesthesia of skin, impaired circulation) appear later but treatment should be instituted before most of these are manifested.

Investigation

This is unnecessary in an alert and lucid patient and treatment is based on clinical findings. Investigation is only needed if diagnosis is unclear clinically, or in cases of head injury or drug overdose causing altered level of consciousness, or after polytrauma. Compartment pressures are usually measured with a needle manometer. Fasciotomy is indicated if the compartment pressure rises to within 30 mmHg of the diastolic pressure.

Treatment

Urgent fasciotomy where the skin and enveloping fascia of the involved compartment(s) are incised in their **entire** length and left open. In the leg, all four compartments (anterior, lateral, superficial posterior, and deep posterior) should be decompressed.

Chapter 18
Complications of amputation

Introduction

The major indications for lower limb amputation in vascular surgery are for non-reconstructable critical limb ischaemia, non-viable acute limb ischaemia, trauma, and for the diabetic foot. Amputation is therefore needed to preserve life, prevent the spread of infection, alleviate pain, and promote mobility. Common amputations performed are digital, ray (digit plus metatarsal), transmetatarsal, below knee (BKA), and above knee (AKA).

Early complications (within 30 days)

Wound breakdown

The primary aim of any major lower limb amputation is to achieve primary wound healing and permit postoperative rehabilitation. It is well established that following AKA only 40% of patients achieve grade III–V mobility (i.e. unlimited household mobility or better) compared to 80% of those with BKA (note: grade 0 is bedridden and grade V has unlimited mobility). The risk of wound breakdown must consequently be balanced against the enhanced mobility associated with BKA when choosing the amputation level. Certain techniques have been investigated to predict wound healing in BKA (e.g. angiography, ankle systolic pressures, transcutaneous oxygen partial pressures, isotope blood studies, thermography, and laser Doppler flowmetry), but none have been shown to be sensitive enough. In practice, if the skin of the calf is warm, free from trophic change and infection, and tissue bleeding is adequate intraoperatively then primary healing with BKA is likely to take place. Wound breakdown occurs in around 20% of all BKAs and requires conversion to an above knee level. It usually results from ischaemia (due to peripheral vascular disease, excess suture tension and haematoma formation may exacerbate), infection, or a combination of the two.

Infection

Operating on dirty and devitalized tissues means that wound infection is always a risk. Broad-spectrum antibiotics (e.g. intravenous cefuroxime and metronidazole—unless preoperative sensitivities dictate otherwise) are thus given prophylactically; in the presence of preoperative infection a full treatment course should be given. Infection can result in oedema with resultant increased tissue tension, and ischaemia can result in wound breakdown or skin flap necrosis. Consideration should be given to leaving the skin flaps open in the presence of gross infection or contamination. Osteomyelitis is another potential consequence and invariably requires conversion to a higher level. Bacteraemia may follow and can result in a systemic inflammatory response or multiorgan failure and death. Common pathogenic organisms include *Staph. aureus*, streptococci, coliforms (pseudomonads, *Proteus* spp.), and *Bacteroides* spp. Vigilance should be paid to an increasing prevalence of MRSA-related wound colonization, with the potential risk of postoperative wound infection and systemic disturbance. All patients with an open wound should be screened on admission to hospital. Clostridial fasciitis and myonecrosis (gas gangrene) is a rare cause of infection, particularly following trauma. It should be distinguished from anaerobic cellulitis (necrotizing fasciitis) which may be caused by anaerobic streptococci or a synergistic infection. Both are gas-producing infections and cause profound systemic disturbance with high mortality. Some advocate the use of penicillin as prophylaxis for all patients, particularly diabetics or patients who are immunosuppressed.

Bleeding and haematoma

Many surgeons place a small-calibre suction drain to avoid this complication. Haematoma formation carries the risk of infection and wound breakdown. Intraoperatively, care should be taken to individually ligate all bleeding points.

Stump pain

Postoperative pain is a common occurrence and is usually managed in the immediate postoperative period with a patient-controlled analgesia system (PCAS) pump or epidural anaesthetic. In those cases where an epidural cannot be used, an epidural catheter can be inserted into either the tibial or sciatic nerve sheath depending upon the level of the amputation. The same local anaesthetic infusion regimen can be used. Excessive pain can result in joint contractures and limit ambulation. The preoperative siting of an epidural anaesthetic has been shown to reduce the incidence of post-operative stump pain and the development of phantom limb pain.

Joint contractures and muscle wasting

Adequate pain control and intensive physiotherapy are required to prevent joint contractures and muscle wasting. In the knee, a fixed flexion deformity above 20 degrees results in increased hip flexion and lumbar spine extension which makes mobilization difficult. An angle over 35 degrees makes it impossible to fit even a kneeling prosthesis. To achieve a good functional result for mobility, patients require a minimal fixed-flexion deformity at the knee and certainly less than 20 degrees. All patients should have access to tricep springs, monkey bars, and rope ladders. These are essential for early mobilization in bed and promote the development of upper body strength, which is essential for early mobilization. Patients should have access to their own wheelchair and be referred on to the regional limb-fitting service. Finally, an early comprehensive assessment is essential to facilitate an early discharge from hospital. A full nutritional assessment, with support if intake is inadequate, should be made in the elderly and debilitated (i.e. chronic sepsis) to enhance rehabilitation.

The complications of recumbency

Prolonged recumbency particularly affects elderly patients undergoing AKA. It carries the risk of thromboembolic events and chest infections.

Late complications (after 30 days)

Stump neuritis

Stump neuromas tend to affect the sciatic nerve following AKA. The bulbous nerve end can cause severe pain when compressed against a prosthesis, and for this reason the sciatic nerve is always divided as high as possible. They may require excision if they are persistently problematic after injection with local anaesthetic and steroids.

Phantom limb pain

This describes the painful sensation derived from the non-existent limb and affects many amputees. The cause of phantom limb pain is not fully understood but may be due to the persistence of the sensory cortex. Pain is often more severe in the distal extremities which have the largest cortical representation. Treatment can involve antiepileptics (e.g. carbamazepine, sodium valproate), antidepressants (e.g. amitriptyline), regional nerve blocks, or transcutaneous electrical nerve stimulation.

Causalgia

Causalgia is a form of sympathetic dystrophy that follows nerve injury incurred during amputation. It may arise from sympathetic fibres growing down peripheral nerves. It presents with intractable burning pain in the amputation stump which may be accompanied by trophic change to the skin or vasomotor disturbance. Treatment is similar to phantom limb pain and may include sympathectomy.

Poorly fitting prosthesis

Having achieved primary healing the ideal amputation stump should be conical, have adequate muscle coverage without redundant tissue, and have minimal pressure through the suture line. If these criteria are not met due to a technically poor operation the fitting of limb prostheses is difficult, with an adverse effect on mobilization and the risk of ulceration.

Bone spikes or spurs

These arise if the bone ends are not adequately rasped. They can cause pain and ulceration. If the amputation stump is required for mobility then revision of the stump should be considered.

Stump ulceration

Ulceration can occur as a result of bone spikes, inadequate muscle coverage of the bone ends (in the wasted or debilitated patient), infection, ischaemia, and an ill-fitting prosthetic device causing pressure or friction. Ulceration can also allow recurrent infection and the development of osteomyelitis. This invariably requires revision of the stump.

False aneurysms and arteriovenous fistulas

Although these are rare, they can involve the superficial femoral or crural vessels.

Chapter 19
Postoperative complications in urology

Kidney

Radical nephrectomy

Radical nephrectomy is considered the optimal treatment for patients with non-metastatic, renal-cell carcinoma and is usually performed through a transabdominal–transperitoneal or a thoracoabdominal approach.

Postoperative complications

- Pulmonary complications of atelectasis and lobar collapse can be prevented by assiduous anaesthetic attention to ventilation and suctioning during the operation. Remember that pulmonary vital capacity is reduced by thoracoabdominal incisions. Adequate pain relief and physiotherapy must be ensured postoperatively.
- For a collapsed lung that fails to expand, arrange for bronchoscopy.
- A tension pneumothorax can occur if the lung is inadvertently injured. In an emergency, put a needle into the second intercostal space; then insert a pleural drain.
- Pleural effusions should be aspirated.
- Pancreatic injury may not be recognized intraoperatively. After operation an increase in serum amylase levels, an alkaline pH drainage from the wound, or a retroperitoneal collection of fluid is highly suggestive. Drain the collection under ultrasound or computed tomography (CT) guidance if needed. Expect spontaneous closure of the fistula, but hyperalimentation via a fine-bore enteral tube may be required.
- If splenic injury occurs consider splenorrhaphy and try to avoid splenectomy, which increases the susceptibility to pulmonary infections and septicaemia. Pneumococcal vaccine should be given routinely to patients over the age of 65 undergoing left transperitoneal nephrectomy.
- Bleeding from the wound is usually from an unsecured vessel in the muscle or superficial layers. A pressure dressing on the area often arrests the bleeding.
- 'Sagging of the flank' resembling a hernia may result from division of more than the XIIth intercostal nerve.

Vena caval thrombectomy

Propagation of neoplastic cells along the renal vein and into the inferior vena cava (IVC) requires removal, but this may result in a vena caval thrombus which is managed in conjunction with radical nephrectomy.

Postoperative complications

- Pulmonary embolism may occur.
- Duodenal obstruction has been reported.

+ Low urinary output may respond to furosemide (frusemide), providing the fluid balance is optimal.
+ Acute renal failure may require haemodialysis.
+ Excessive bleeding after cardiopulmonary bypass can be avoided by transfusing platelets and fresh-frozen plasma plus desmopressin acetate, aminocaproic acid, or a combination of these during the immediate postoperative period. Re-operation for massive bleeding may be required for a minority of patients.

Simple nephrectomy

Simple nephrectomy is performed when the function of the kidney has been irreparably destroyed due to disease processes including calculi, obstruction, infection, trauma, uncontrolled renal vascular hypertension, and haemorrhage.

Postoperative complications

+ Haemorrhage can arise from the renal artery, aorta, or inferior vena cava. A vessel in spasm may be overlooked during closure leading to reactive haemorrhage. Carefully monitor vital signs and restore blood volume. Re-operation may be needed.
+ Ileus can be a problem secondary to retroperitoneal dissection around the coeliac axis. Because of this reaction, even after a flank approach, the patient should not resume oral intake until peristalsis returns or nausea is resolved, there is absence of abdominal distension, and there is passage of flatus per rectum.

Partial nephrectomy

Partial nephrectomy is indicated for patients with bilateral tumours or a tumour in a solitary kidney. Removal of a lower non-functioning renal pole for stone disease is an appropriate objective for partial nephrectomy.

Postoperative complications

+ Urinary leakage; look for a distal obstruction if it is persistent.
+ Fistulas are not common but occur with central and large tumours or following collecting system reconstruction. They usually resolve spontaneously, or after ureteral stent placement (or removal).
+ Urinomas are secondary to poor drainage. Placement of a ureteral catheter or stent is rarely necessary.
+ Wound infections can occur and often follow operations for infected stones.
+ Renal artery thrombosis is rare.
+ Acute renal failure may follow partial nephrectomy of a solitary kidney, related to the large size of a tumour, excessive removal of parenchyma, and/or prolonged ischaemia time.

Nephroureterectomy

The purpose of nephroureterectomy is removal of the kidney, ureter, and bladder cuff in continuity, to treat an upper urinary-tract, transitional-cell carcinoma.

Postoperative complications

+ These are the same as after radical nephrectomy.
+ Urinary leakage through the bladder incision is rare, but settles spontaneously with the insertion of a urethral catheter.

Pyelolithotomy and nephrolithotomy

Nowadays, open renal stone surgery is rarely indicated due to the advent of percutaneous and shock-wave modalities.

Postoperative complications

+ Pain is a common problem due to the large incision that is required.
+ Pulmonary atelectasis is common. Encourage coughing, deep breathing, and early ambulation.
+ Pneumothorax is a possible complication. Do not wait for portable chest radiography if pneumothorax is clinically obvious, but insert a chest tube.
+ Bleeding may occur postoperatively. It usually stops spontaneously. Treat haemorrhage expectantly with fluids and blood transfusions. If haemorrhage continues, re-operation is needed to open the kidney and place sutures appropriately.
+ Suspect the development of an arteriovenous fistula or a false aneurysm. Consider arteriography to define the site and try to embolize it. Re-operation is the next step to suture-ligate the offending vessel.
+ Prolonged urinary drainage should be prevented by ureteral stent insertion intraoperatively.
+ Exclude residual calculi causing obstruction. If it is a problem postoperatively insert a stent or a percutaneous nephrostomy and remove the stone.
+ Renal damage from prolonged ischaemia during nephrolithotomy is uncommon.

Pyeloureteroplasty

Main indications for pyeloureteric junction obstruction repair are renal impairment, pain, and/or infection. Among open procedures, the Anderson–Hynes pyeloplasty is the most commonly used technique because it allows removal of diseased portions of the pelvis and ureter. Endoscopic incision and laparoscopic procedure are alternatives to open pyeloplasty.

Postoperative complications

+ Bleeding and formation of clots can obstruct the outlet and jeopardize the repair. The source of bleeding is usually the nephrostomy tract. Tamponade the tract by temporarily closing the nephrostomy, but re-exploration may be required if bleeding persists. Do not irrigate through the nephrostomy tube because this increases the infection rate and can disrupt the suture line.

+ Acute pyelonephritis indicates infection above an obstruction. If a nephrostomy tube was not inserted at operation, one can be placed percutaneously.

+ Urinary leakage can be expected in the early postoperative period. It should be investigated if it persists for more than a week. A bladder catheter should be inserted if the patient does not have one. Be sure that the drain is not in contact with the anastomosis. Shorten it and subsequently remove it if the leakage stops. It is usually necessary to insert a double-J stent from below or to place a nephrostomy tube and a stent from above as soon as an obstructed system is suspected.

+ A urinoma may form if the drain is removed too soon. The collection and the pelvicalyceal system should be drained percutaneously. Before removing a stent, fill the system with contrast medium to test for leakage, removing the drain only after making sure the ureter is intact.

+ Obstruction at the pelviureteric junction (PUJ) after the stent is removed can be managed by leaving the nephrostomy tube in place, by placing one percutaneously until nephrostography shows an open tract, or by passing a double-J stent from below. For persistent obstruction, balloon dilatation or endopyelotomy by either a retrograde, or more often, a percutaneous route can solve the problem.

Open renal biopsy

Open renal biopsy is preferable to percutaneous biopsy in adults who have solitary or small contracted kidneys and very poor renal function, who are obese, or who have some bleeding disorders.

Postoperative complications

Bleeding occurs in hypertensive patients or those with major coagulation problems in particular. Gross haematuria usually stops after 24 hours of bed rest. A retroperitoneal haematoma may form, but wound infection is uncommon.

Repair of renal injuries

Most penetrating renal wounds, particularly gunshot wounds, and occasionally closed renal injuries, need surgical repair.

Postoperative complications
Early complications

+ Delayed renal bleeding and infection with possible perirenal abscess formation. Open urinary drainage may continue, or closed urinary leakage may lead to the formation of a urinoma or abscess. This should be suspected when there is a prolonged ileus. Percutaneous drainage techniques may be effective and prevent the need for re-operation.

Delayed complications

+ Hypertension, hydronephrosis, or arteriovenous fistula may occur. Hypertension should be treated conservatively and if this fails, or if the cause of hypertension is renal artery stenosis, nephrectomy is usually required.

+ Hydronephrosis is usually due to ureteral obstruction. Endoscopic dilatation of the ureteral stricture or open ureterolysis is the treatment of choice, but nephrectomy is often needed.

+ Arteriovenous fistula is a troublesome problem and haematuria is the most common presenting symptom. Management is controversial. Embolization could lead to material shunting into the venous system. Partial or complete nephrectomy is the alternative.

Bladder

Radical cystectomy

Radical, and occasionally partial cystectomy, is the treatment of choice for the majority of invasive bladder cancers. Pelvic lymphadenectomy is performed at the same time. Radical cystectomy is usually accompanied by urinary diversion in the form of non-continent diversion, heterotopic continent diversion, or orthotopic continent-bladder substitution.

Non-continent urinary diversion is created using a bowel segment (usually small bowel) to form a conduit. The ureters are anastomosed to the proximal end of the segment, while the distal end forms a cutaneous stoma. Urostomy bags are needed permanently thereafter.

Continent heterotopic (not to native urethra) urinary diversion uses various bowel segments to create a reservoir with a continence mechanism, again with the formation of a cutaneous stoma. Patients have to catheterize themselves but no urinary bags are needed.

Continent orthotopic (to native urethra) bladder substitution implies the use of a bowel segment to create a 'neobladder', which is anastomosed to native urethra thereby preserving urinary continence.

Postoperative complications
Complications of cystectomy

- Bleeding can arise from several sources and must be controlled intra-operatively. Careful measurement of drain output and patient vital signs are needed postoperatively. If bleeding persists the patient needs to go back to theatre.
- Pulmonary problems are common and can be prevented with aggressive chest physiotherapy, early mobilization, and adequate pain relief. Treat atelectasis with early bronchoscopy if needed. Treat pneumonia with specific antibiotic therapy.
- Cardiac problems are usually the result of fluid overload. Monitoring central venous pressure (CVP) and fluid balance should avoid this.
- Deep vein thrombosis can be prevented by the use of intermittent-pressure stockings, low molecular-weight heparin, and early mobilization. Cystectomy is a high-risk procedure.
- Ileus is reduced if nasogastic suction is maintained for several days. Intestinal obstruction must be considered if it persists. Investigate accordingly, but nutrition must be addressed early on.
- Wound infection and dehiscence may occur.
- The incidence of gastric stress ulcers and bleeding postoperatively can be reduced by the use of H_2-antagonists (e.g. ranitidine) or cytoprotective agents (e.g. sucralfate).

- Rectal injury, although rare, requires primary repair or temporary colostomy and a later repair. It is a serious complication because of ensuing sepsis.
- A faecal fistula or pelvic abscess may develop, which needs a defunctioning colostomy or ileostomy, drainage of the abscess, and parenteral nutrition. The fistula will usually close spontaneously.
- Sexual dysfunction in males is common following cystectomy, although function may be preserved by a nerve-sparing procedure.

Complications of pelvic lymphadenectomy

- Persisting lymphatic drainage from the wound is rarely a problem and responds to tetracycline instillation into the draining tract.
- Lymphocele is rare. It is usually small but may become symptomatic. Locate, aspirate, and inject tetracycline under ultrasound guidance. Laparoscopic or open surgical drainage is seldom needed.
- Obturator nerve injury may occur leading to significant weakness of the adductor thigh muscle. Prescribe physiotherapy. Usually, other muscle groups take over if appropriate physiotherapy is instituted
- Paraesthesiae in the groin, labia, and anterior thigh may present if the lateral femoral cutaneous and genitofemoral nerves are injured.

Complications of urinary diversion

- Urinary leakage can be managed conservatively with adequate drainage. Silastic ureteral stents placed intraoperatively reduce the incidence of leakage. The urine can be diverted by percutaneous nephrostomy to allow healing of the defect. A catheter should be inserted into the conduit or the reservoir even if the ureters have been stented. Be certain that mucus is not blocking the outlet. Should dehiscence of the ureteral anastomosis occur re-operation is needed.
- Early obstruction of the ureteral anastomosis is due to oedema or haematoma. A percutaneous nephrostomy should be placed. Late obstruction of the ureteral anastomosis is more common—increasing with time—usually due to fibrosis, stone formation, or recurrent cancer. Endoscopic dilatation or open re-anastomosis is needed depending on the causes.
- Leakage at the intestinal re-anastomosis is rare but usually leads to peritonitis and needs open surgical correction. Obstruction at the intestinal re-anastomosis is also rare and requires surgical exploration if conservative treatment fails. Intestinal fistulas can occur from the site of the bowel anastomosis and are indicative of local mesenteric ischaemia. They need surgical correction.
- Stenosis at the site of bowel anastomosis to urethra in orthotopic bladder reconstruction is usually treated with dilatation. Urinary retention is likely in these patients for different reasons and requires lifelong self-catheterization.
- Pyelonephritis is common. Ureteral obstruction and stone disease need to be excluded.

- Short-bowel syndrome presents with diarrhoea, malabsorption of bile salts, and vitamin B_{12} deficiency.

- Hyperchloraemic acidosis may infrequently occur. It is usually associated with obstruction of the stoma. Catheterization of the conduit is needed, but revision of the stoma may be required in long term.

- Renal calculi secondary to urinary tract infections are not rare. Treat infection, correct any obstruction, and remove the stones endoscopically or with the use of extracorporeal shock-wave lithotripsy (ESWL).

- Secondary malignancy can occur in some forms of urinary diversion many years following the operation.

Complications of stoma creation

- Fungal infections (*Candida albicans*) are caused when urine accumulates under the barrier and are more frequently seen in diabetics. Dry the skin thoroughly and apply nystatin powder for resolution.

- Allergic contact dermatitis. Sensitivity to solvents, adhesives or detergents is not uncommon. Identify and discontinue the irritant. Apply hydrocortisone cream and avoid solvents and soaps.

- Mechanical trauma. This can be minimized by reducing the number of pouch changes, encouragement of gentle skin care, and less use of sealant and adhesives.

- Stoma stenosis increases with time. It is easily recognized by catheterizing the stoma and measuring the residual urine volume. It is corrected by revision of the stoma.

- Parastomal hernia formation is easily diagnosed on physical examination and needs surgical correction.

The services and advice of an expert stoma nurse are particularly important in the satisfactory resolution of the above.

Bladder augmentation

Augmentation cystoplasty is usually undertaken for reduced bladder capacity due to several causes. The ileum, colon, stomach, or dilatated ureter can be used.

Postoperative complications

- These are similar to radical cystectomy and urinary diversion.

- Ischaemia and necrosis of the segment usually requires surgical exploration and correction.

- Rupture of the augmented bladder occurs with overfilling.

- Malignancy is not uncommon and cystoscopy on a regular basis is needed.

Repair of bladder injuries

Surgical exploration is required for all the intraperitoneal and some of the extraperitoneal ruptures of the bladder.

Postoperative complications

- Persistent pelvic bleeding usually occurs secondary to major traumatic injuries of the bony pelvis and pelvic vessels. Surgical therapy is the primary treatment, although pelvic angiography and embolization may be successful.
- Pelvic abscess. Percutaneous or surgical drainage is required.
- Incontinence needs thorough urodynamic investigation and appropriate treatment.
- Vesicocutaneous or vesicovaginal fistulas require surgical correction.

Surgery for female stress incontinence

Many forms of bladder reconstruction for urinary incontinence exist, including: elevation of the bladder neck; constriction of the urethra; and formation of a new outlet. Postoperative complications are reduced by careful preoperative patient selection.

Postoperative complications

- Urinary infection is rare but can lead to sepsis; treat with appropriate antibiotics.
- Osteitis pubis is rare and usually responds to bed rest and non-steroidal anti-inflammatory agents.
- Pelvic haematoma is treated conservatively unless the patient becomes haemodynamically unstable, in which case surgical exploration is required.
- Urinary retention is the most common complication. Insertion of a suprapubic catheter or self-catheterization for a few days is required. Rarely, urethrolysis is needed.
- Bladder instability can occur following incontinence surgery but usually responds to anticholinergic medications.
- Persistent incontinence needs urodynamic investigation to decide which appropriate treatment is indicated.

Prostate

Suprabubic and retropubic prostatectomy

Prostate excision, with or without incising the bladder, still remains an alternative to transurethral prostatectomy for large adenomas.

Postoperative complications

- Bleeding may persist after the operation and may be controlled by traction on the balloon of the Foley catheter. If this fails, take the patient to theatre and, with the use of endoscopic instruments, evacuate the clots and fulgurate any bleeding points. If severe bleeding continues, the wound needs to be re-opened with packing of the prostatic fossa with gauze and traction to the balloon.

- Inadvertent loss of the catheter during the early postoperative period is rarely a problem. Try to insert a catheter following instrumental dilatation of the bladder neck. If this fails, take the patient to theatre and insert the catheter transurethrally under direct vision.

- Prolonged suprapubic leakage usually stops with urethral catheter drainage. If leakage does not stop or a suprapubic fistula develops then the catheter must be left in place. Think of residual adenoma which is causing obstruction and needs transurethral resection.

- Ureteral obstruction may result from placing haemostatic sutures too high at the bladder neck. Flank pain postoperatively is an indication for either intravenous urography (IVU) or ultrasound, and insertion of a percutaneous nephrostomy tube.

- Bladder neck contracture usually responds to dilatations, but it may need transurethral incision or resection.

- Urinary incontinence is rare. If it is mild it may respond to pelvic exercises and anticholinergic medication. If it persists, implantation of an artificial sphincter or reconstruction of the vesical neck is needed.

- Retention is usually due to local spasm and relaxation of the bladder detrusor. The catheter should be replaced for 2 days, but think of residual prostatic tissue if it persists.

- Retrograde ejaculation is common and the patient must always be forewarned.

- Wound infection is not common, and even more rare is epididymitis. They usually respond to antibiotic therapy.

Radical prostatectomy

Radical prostatectomy is performed for localized prostatic carcinoma and involves removal of the whole gland together with the seminal vesicles.

Postoperative complications

+ Inadvertent loss of the catheter is rare. Catheter replacement is mandatory, but hazardous. Gradually dilate the urethral anastomosis and try to insert a new catheter; or take the patient to theatre and, under direct vision, place a guide-wire to the bladder and insert the catheter over it.

+ Postoperative haemorrhage requires close monitoring of the patient, blood transfusion, and clotting tests to be performed. Re-operation to control the bleeding or to evacuate a pelvic haematoma is rarely needed.

+ Persistent drainage in the early postoperative period is either of lymph or urine. Send a sample for urea and creatinine to determine which it is. If it is lymph, stop suction and gradually advance the drains. Urine leakage from the urethrovesical anastomosis usually ceases in 3–4 weeks. Suction should be stopped and the drain advanced away from the anastomosis.

+ Deep venous thrombosis and pulmonary embolism are relatively common. Intermittent-compression stockings, low molecular-weight heparin prophylaxis, and early ambulation can prevent them.

+ Ureteral injury can occur during the operation. It can be recognized when it causes colicky pain or fever postoperatively. Percutaneous nephrostomy tubes must be inserted followed by antegrade ureteral stenting.

+ Postoperative complications due to pelvic lymph node dissection (see radical cystectomy above) may occur.

+ Faecal fistulas may appear early or late in the recovery period. They are due either to direct rectal injury at the time of operation or to ischaemia and subsequent necrosis of the rectal wall. They are unlikely to close spontaneously and require surgical repair.

+ Urinary stress incontinence is seen in the majority of early postoperative patients. Perineal exercises and the occasional use of pharmacological agents help resolve this problem within 3–6 months. Total urinary incontinence is fortunately rare. Injection of bulking agents may be helpful. Artificial sphincters should be considered when the degree of incontinence is socially crippling.

+ Pelvic plexus or neurovascular bundle injury during the operation leads to impotence. The patient must be warned of the possibility. Wait 6–12 months for potency to return. If potency does not return in that period consider oral or intracorporal vasodilators, vacuum erection devices, or implantation of a penile prosthesis.

+ Contracture at the vesicourethral anastomosis is caused by a non mucosa-to-mucosa anastomosis of the bladder to the urethra. Prolonged urinary leakage, prior prostatic resection, or disruption of the anastomosis are other causes. Dilate the stricture and teach the patient how to perform self-catheterization. Transurethral incision of the vesical neck may be needed.

Penis and urethra

Circumcision

Circumcision is not a difficult procedure, but is one of great social and psychological importance to the patient. The cosmetic result of this operation is extremely important.

Postoperative complications

* External urethral meatus stenosis. Do not perform circumcision in the presence of inflammation.
* Bleeding. May stop with pressure but often requires a return to theatre and re-suturing.
* Infection. Usually superficial and controlled using topical antiseptics.
* Skin necrosis. Avoid using adrenaline (epinephrine) in the local anaesthetic. For inadvertent excessive removal of skin during circumcision there are several treatment options. If the defect is small it usually granulates without complications. Larger defects should be treated by applying a delayed split-thickness skin graft to the shaft.
* Adhesions from inadequate circumcision may require surgical division.
* Inclusion cysts from inversion of the skin require surgical removal.
* Urethral injury or a urethrocutaneous fistula is rare but needs delay repair with urethroplasty.
* Glandular or penile shaft necrosis is rare but is a difficult problem to solve and requires complicated penile surgical reconstruction.

Penile trauma

Skin avulsion

Avulsion injuries should be carefully cleansed and all necrotic tissue debrided. If primary closure is not feasible, skin grafts can be used to cover the defect.

Postoperative complications

* Infection must be treated with antibiotics.
* Penile contracture must be corrected with the use of thick split-thickness skin grafts.

Penile amputation

Penile amputation is treated either by primary microsurgical re-implantation or by secondary penile reconstruction with the use of a penile prosthesis.

Postoperative complications

+ The major complication of penile re-implantation is skin and soft tissue necrosis. Early debridement and subsequent penile reconstruction is advisable.

Partial and total penectomy

Partial and total penectomy are treatment options in penile cancer. Ilioinguinal lymphadenectomy is important.

Postoperative complications
Penectomy

+ Bleeding is rarely a problem. Pressure or suturing under penile block anaesthesia is adequate.
+ Urethral meatal stenosis is not uncommon. Teach the patient to perform self-dilatations or perform a meatoplasty.
+ Inadequate penile length needs penile reconstruction.

Ilioinguinal lymph node dissection

Complications are:

+ Necrosis of the skin flaps, which needs debridement only if the defect is small. A split-thickness skin graft may be needed for larger defects.
+ Wound infection responds to antibiotic therapy and debridement.
+ Seromas are not uncommon.
+ Lymphoceles need either intermittent aspiration or continuous closed percutaneous drainage.

Hypospadias repair

Hypospadias is a congenital disorder in which the urethral meatus opens not at the tip of the glans penis but more proximally, between the ventral glans and the perineum. The goals of reconstructive surgery for this condition are to produce a penis that is straight when erect, has a urethral opening at the tip of the glans, and is cosmetically acceptable.

Postoperative complications
Early complications

+ Bleeding is not a common problem and usually stops with compression, but it may require re-opening of the wound.
+ Oedema is very common and is reduced by a compressive dressing left in place for 2 days.
+ Wound infection is treated with antibiotics. Clean the wound with topical antiseptics. Incision and drainage to allow healing by secondary intention may be needed to manage a suspected abscess or infected haematoma.

- If wound disruption becomes evident with the removal of the dressing, the skin edges can be approximated with steristrips or stitches.
- Ischaemia and necrosis of the skin flaps usually necessitates new surgical reconstruction.
- Catheter obstruction is uncommon and can usually be relieved by irrigation. Inadvertent loss of a urethral catheter should be managed with insertion of a suprapubic catheter, if one is not already in place.

Late complications

- Urethrocutaneous fistula is a common complication following hypospadias repair. Check for a distal obstruction-stricture and correct it. Patients who have a suprapubic catheter can have their urinary diversion period extended for several days in an attempt to encourage closure of the fistula. Precise application of silver nitrate to a small fistula may cause it to granulate and close. Older children with small fistulas are instructed to void while occluding the fistula with a finger. If the fistula has not healed by 2 months it needs surgical correction.
- Stricture. If it develops at the level of the external meatus perform periodical dilatations. Optical urethrotomy or a second reconstructive procedure may be needed.
- Diverticula if formed need surgical repair. Rule out distal stricture.
- Residual chordee needs surgical reconstruction.
- Persisting or recurrent urinary tract infections after hypospadias repair usually imply a urethral stricture. After treatment, uroflowmetry, retrograde urethrography, and/or cystoscopy make the diagnosis. Surgical repair is needed.

Urethral strictures—urethral trauma

A urethral stricture is a narrowing of the calibre of the urethra caused by the presence of a scar consequent on infection or injury. Treatment options include urethral dilatation, internal urethrotomy, and several forms of urethroplasties.

Postoperative complications

- Bleeding from the corpus spongiosum can usually be controlled by digital pressure over sponges.
- Haematomas can be a problem but rarely do they need open evacuation.
- Re-stenosis and stricture formation needs surgical repair in 4–6 months.
- Fistulas are rare but usually require surgical repair.
- Hairballs become a problem when hair-bearing skin is used for the reconstruction. They are rare.
- Necrosis of the flap is usually secondary to poor technique or infection. Remove the dead tissue, allow healing, and reconstruct the urethra.
- Incontinence, especially after posterior urethral stricture repair, is a major complication. It is usually balanced by an intact bladder neck mechanism.

Before considering surgical intervention exclude uninhibited bladder contractions. Treat them with anticholinergics.

- Impotence is usually secondary to the cause of the stricture (urethral trauma) and rarely to the reconstruction itself. Oral or intracavernosal vasodilators and a penile prosthesis may be needed.

Scrotum

Bleeding

Because the scrotum is distensible the amount of bleeding following scrotal operations can be considerable and quite alarming to the patient expecting a minor operation. In general, make transverse incisions in the scrotum since most of the blood vessels course horizontally. All bleeding points should be cauterized. Scrotal support for 24–48 hours' postoperatively may reduce swelling.

The management of postoperative scrotal haematoma or bleeding requires careful observation. Keep the patient on bed rest with scrotal elevation and observe him. Surgical exploration, although rare, is needed for expanding haematomas and abscess formation.

Vasectomy

- Re-canalization of the vas deferens is fortunately rare. Vasectomy must be repeated.
- Sperm granulomas result from extravasation of seminal fluid into the perivasal tissues. Most cause only mild discomfort and usually resolve spontaneously. Occasionally, it may be necessary to excise a persistent painful granuloma.
- Non-specific epididymitis usually results from epididymis engorgement and can be treated with anti-inflammatory drugs.
- Cystic changes in the epididymis may cause discomfort, but rarely need excision (epididymectomy).

Varicocele ligation

- Damage to the artery leads to testicular atrophy.
- Persistent prominence of the veins is not unusual following correction of a large varicocele. Perform colour-Doppler ultrasonography to exclude recurrence or persistence of the varicocele, which needs re-operation.
- Hydroceles develop because of lymphatic obstruction. They may need surgical correction.
- Dull testicular ache is rare but usually resolves without treatment.

Hydrocelectomy

- Haematoma. This should not happen if haemostasis has been complete—it is significantly less likely with the Lord's procedure.
- Infection. Unfortunately, this may occur and is usually treated with a broad-spectrum cephalosporin. Pus needs incision and drainage.

- Recurrence. When this happens re-operation is necessary. The usual finding is of a pseudocyst, which should be excised, taking as much of the cyst wall as possible.

Testicular biopsy

- In the azoospermic male with normal gonadotrophin levels, testicular biopsy is used primarily as a diagnostic tool to differentiate between testicular failure and obstructive causes of infertility.
- Bleeding and haematocele are rare.
- Inadvertent biopsy of the epididymis is a serious complication and should be avoided—it leads to sterility on the affected side.

Orchidopexy

This means bringing the testis down into the scrotum and is indicated for an undescended or ectopic testicle—it should be performed before the age of 5 years. Scrotal orchidopexy is indicated for torsion—the contralateral testis **must** be fixed at the original operation.

- Inadequate testis position or retraction of the testis is usually corrected with a second operation.
- Ischaemia and testicular atrophy is a major complication and may lead to orchidectomy and the need for insertion of a testicular prosthesis.
- Epididymo-orchitis is treated with antibiotics.
- A hydrocele, if large or symptomatic, requires surgical correction.
- Scrotal bleeding usually stops spontaneously.

Insertion of a testicular prosthesis

- Infection requires removal of the prosthesis.
- Necrosis of the overlying skin is usually secondary to insertion of too-large a prosthesis and requires removal of the prosthesis.
- Scrotal haematoma formation is rare.

Testicular torsion

Testicular torsion is a real emergency that requires prompt diagnosis and surgical treatment.

- Haematoma is rare.
- Re-torsion can occur and is usually due to incorrect fixation of the testicle or to the use of absorbable sutures. It requires re-exploration.
- Fertility can be affected if an ischaemic testicle is left in place.

Orchidectomy

Simple trans-scrotal orchidectomy is usually performed for removal of a non-viable testis following torsion. Intracapsular orchidectomy is a treatment alternative to hormone manipulation in prostate cancer.

Radical inguinal orchiectomy is indicated for testicular tumours. Inguinal orchidectomy may be the only option in boys after the age of 7 when the testis cannot be brought down into scrotum. Microvascular surgery should be considered in young boys.

- Haemorrhage is the major risk after orchidectomy.
- A rapidly expanding scrotal haematoma or evidence of retroperitoneal bleeding signifies haemorrhage from the spermatic cord. Re-operation and control of the spermatic vessels is needed.

Retroperitoneal lymph node dissection

Retroperitoneal lymph node dissection is indicated in stage I and low-volume stage II NSGC testicular tumours. Salvage surgery is indicated whenever possible for masses residual or refractory to salvage chemotherapy.

Postoperative complications

- Pulmonary complications are serious following bleomycin therapy. Enforce pulmonary physiotherapy and cover the patient with a broad-spectrum antibiotic. Judicious fluid replacement is crucial.
- Wound infection and dehiscence is rare.
- Bleeding from major vessel injury requires immediate repair.
- Pancreatitis is usually treated conservatively.
- Ileus is common. If it persists suspect retroperitoneal haematoma, urinary extravasation, or pancreatitis. Mechanical bowel obstruction is rare but requires surgical correction.
- Ureteral injury is usually avoided by freeing the ureter prior to dissection.
- A lymphocele may develop. Aspirate it under CT guidance.
- Chylous ascites is uncommon. Abdominal ultrasonography and paracentesis help establish the diagnosis. Treat with low-fat diet, medium-chain triglycerides, diuretics, and, if necessary, hyperalimentation. Ligation of the open vessel or peritoneovenous shunt may be required.
- Infertility is a major neural complication because removal of the sympathetic nerves causes loss of emission. Retrograde ejaculation or anejaculation can be avoided by preserving the sympathetic nerves when possible. If sperm were not banked, consider sperm aspiration from testis or epididymis.

Ureter

Intraoperative injury of the ureter

- Stent the ureter at the beginning of a difficult abdominal operation.
- When the ureter is cross-clamped or inadvertently ligated insert a double-J stent for at least 10 days.
- If the involved ureteric segment is obviously ischaemic it is better to excise and anastomose it.
- If the ureter is cauterized, inspect it for damage to the adventitial vessels. Ischaemic tissue must be excised.
- When the ureter is severed, spatulation and anastomosis over a stent is necessary.
- Avulsion or extensive damage of the ureter makes the use of a psoas hitch or bladder flap necessary.
- Postoperatively, suspect ureteral injury in the presence of flank pain, low-grade fever, and ileus. Insert a double-J stent retrogradely or antegradely. Percutaneous nephrostomy is an alternative. Wait for the resolution of obstructing absorbable sutures or correct the lesion surgically.

Ureteroneocystostomy

Ureteroneocystostomy is indicated for the correction of vesicoureteral reflux. Several surgical techniques exist, each of which have advantages and disadvantages.

Postoperative complications

- Postoperative ipsilateral persistent reflux or new contralateral reflux is usually of low grade and resolves spontaneously. Previously unrecognized bladder dysfunction, perivesical dissection, or technical failure are the major causes.
- Postoperative ureteral obstruction may occur. In the early postoperative period it is due to oedema. Treat it conservatively. A ureteric stent is rarely needed. Persistent ureteral obstruction is the result of ischaemia, angulation, or a narrow tunnel. Exclude bladder dysfunction. Reimplantation of the ureter may be needed.
- Urinary extravasation indicates obstruction and needs prolonged ureteral stenting.
- Infection and sepsis are rare. Treat with broad-spectrum antibiotics. Rule out obstruction.

Endourology

Percutaneous stone removal (percutaneous nephrostolithotomy, PCNL)

The three essential steps in percutaneous stone removal are nephrostomy tube insertion, tract dilatation, and removal of the stone.

Postoperative complications
Complications related to access

♦ Trauma to intraperitoneal and extraperitoneal organs. Trauma to the spleen will certainly result in severe blood loss. Urgent splenectomy is usually required. Treatment of duodenal injury is conservative. Keep the patient 'nil by mouth', insert a nasogastric tube, and wait until the hole is sealed. Colon trauma is manageable conservatively with insertion of a double-J stent into the kidney to divert the urine, and of a nephrostomy tube into the colon tract to divert the faeces. However, trauma to the colon usually requires formal, open, surgical correction. Pneumothorax or haemothorax are conservatively treated with the insertion of a chest tube. Renal vascular puncture leads to severe bleeding, when the procedure should be stopped and close observation of the patient instituted. Operative intervention may be necessary.

♦ Sepsis presenting after kidney puncture is rare and indicates the presence of acute infection. Abandon the procedure and treat with antibiotics.

Complications related to tract dilatation

♦ Inadvertent removal of the guide-wire. Placement of a second or safety guide-wire is essential to prevent this problem.

♦ Kinking of the guide-wire necessitates its replacement.

♦ Torsion of the renal pelvis or torsion and avulsion of the ureteropelvic junction during tract dilatation must be prevented by the use of fluoroscopy. Postpone the procedure for 2–7 days to allow complete collecting system healing.

♦ Bleeding is always tamponaded by the presence of the dilator and/or the nephroscope sheath.

Complications to stone removal

♦ Bleeding is usually parenchymal in origin. If it becomes severe stop the procedure, insert a large-calibre nephrostomy tube, and reinsert the nephroscope in 48 hours.

♦ Persistent bleeding postoperatively is usually venous in origin. Treat it by clamping the nephrostomy tube for 1 hour. Give mannitol intravenously.

♦ Marked amounts of postoperative bleeding may be due to arteriovenous fistula or pseudoaneurysm formation. The degree of bleeding usually demands transfusion and treatment. Arteriography with embolization is the treatment of choice.

• Fluid extravasation may be into the vascular system or into the retroperitoneum. Stop the procedure, leave a nephrostomy tube in place, and treat fluid overload.

• Retained fragments. These stones become a complication if their size is such that spontaneous passage could not be expected, or if they are residual infected stones. ESWL or another PCNL may be needed.

• Sepsis may occur following PCNL. Treat immediately and vigorously with antibiotics.

Endopyelotomy

Percutaneous management of ureteropelvic junction obstruction is a well-established treatment option.

Postoperative complications

• Bleeding may occur from injuring an aberrant vessel, which frequently passes adjacent to ureteropelvic junction. Surgical exploration or arteriography and embolization may be needed.

• Urinary extravasation to the retroperitoneum is an indication of a successful procedure, but causes pain. Insert a ureteric stent for 6–8 weeks.

• Failure of the procedure and recurrent stricture is minimized by the use of stents 6–8 weeks postprocedure.

Ureteroscopy

Ureteroscopy permits visualization of the interior of the ureter, biopsy of ureteric lesions, treatment of ureteric strictures, and removal or destruction of ureteric stones and tumours.

Postoperative complications

• A false ureteric passage is common. Although it is not a contraindication to proceed with the ureteroscopy, as long as the true lumen can be identified, it is wise to leave a double-J stent in place for a few days before the procedure is repeated.

• Inadequate ureteral dilatation, as seen in fluoroscopy, may need insertion of a double-J stent for a few days. Do not try to force the area with the ureteroscope.

• Perforation in the process of passage or during the procedure requires the operation to be stopped. Insert a stent retrogradely or antegradely for several days.

• Stricture of the ureter may occur and usually requires balloon dilatation and stenting for a month.

• Ureteric avulsion is a serious complication and requires prompt surgical correction.

Transurethral resection (TUR) of the prostate (TURP)

Transurethral resection of the prostate is the 'gold standard' surgical treatment for symptomatic benign prostatic hyperplasia.

Postoperative complications

- Bleeding. It is crucial to achieve good haemostasis during the operation. Assess the patient while he is still in the operating or recovery room. Apply gentle traction to the catheter. Rarely, reinserting the resectoscope and coagulating the bleeding points is required.
- Blocked catheter. Empty the drainage bag if it is too full. Flush with sterile water to remove a clot or a prostatic chip from the eye of the catheter. Change the catheter.
- TUR syndrome may occur.
- Overabsorption of irrigation fluid during TURP can lead to the so-called post-TUR syndrome. The manifestations of this syndrome include hypertension, bradycardia, restlessness, muscle twitching, disorientation, visual alterations, seizures, and vascular collapse. Monitor serum osmolality, serum electrolytes (severe hyponatraemia is the rule), CVP, and vital signs. Reduce water absorption and administer hypertonic saline (250–500 ml of a 3–5% solution) and furosemide (frusemide) (40–100 mg).
- Failure to void following removal of the catheter can be due to pain, insufficient resection, or longstanding chronic retention and failure of the detrusor muscle. Replace the catheter for 1 or 2 weeks. Repeat resection to remove residual tissue.
- Urinary tract infection, epididymitis, and sepsis are rare and respond to antibiotic therapy.
- Bladder neck contracture and urethral strictures need surgical correction.
- Incontinence and impotence following TURP are rare. They need careful evaluation and treatment.

Endoscopic procedures within the bladder

Transurethral resection of bladder tumour and removal of bladder stones are common endoscopic procedures.

Postoperative complications

- **Bleeding**—haemostasis must be complete before the patient goes back to the ward. Severe bleeding may necessitate re-operation.
- **Bladder perforation**—extraperitoneal perforations are mostly managed by leaving the catheter for 1 week. Intraperitoneal perforation may need abdominal exploration to correct bowel injury, drainage of the intraperitoneal cavity, and closure of the bladder defect. The patient needs antibiotic cover.

Extracorporeal shock-wave lithotripsy (ESWL)

ESWL for urinary stone disease has become one of the most common procedures urologists perform.

Postoperative complications

- Inadequate stone disintegration is probably the most common complication of ESWL. Identify and offer alternative treatment for stones resistant to ESWL (cystine and calcium oxalate monohydrate stones). Repeat the treatment if needed.
- Haematuria is common but usually resolves spontaneously.
- Subcapsular haematoma is rare. Suspect it if the patient complains of an unusual amount of pain after the treatment or if there is an unusual drop in serum haemoglobin. No treatment is usually necessary as these eventually resolve spontaneously.
- Sepsis is the result of ESWL treatment in the presence of an uncontrolled urinary tract infection (UTI). Cover with antibiotics and drain an obstructive kidney by inserting a nephrostomy tube or a double-J ureteric stent prior to treatment.
- Skin petechiae are most likely to be found in thin people. They disappear readily, and are of little significance.
- Pain usually disappears after a few days. If it persists suspect subcapsular haematoma.
- Renal colic secondary to stone fragments impacting down the ureter is common. Occasionally the fragments collect in the ureter and form a column of stone referred to as a 'steinstrasse' or 'stone street'. Further ESWL or ureteroscopic stone extraction is the treatment of choice.

Chapter 20
Complications after head and neck surgery

Cervical lymph node biopsy

The main complications associated with lymph node biopsy happen at the time of surgery and therefore can be avoided by careful selection and preparation, understanding of the local anatomy, and a meticulous technique. As a rule, it is not a procedure to be undertaken by an inexperienced, unsupervised practitioner and this will reduce many of the more significant postoperative complications. For added security, selecting a representative node that is easily accessible and superficial will avoid deep dissection and decrease the danger to adjacent structures.

Complications

Haemorrhage

Lymph nodes have an extensive blood supply derived from arteries that enter at the hilum, branch within the medulla, and drain back to the hilum via thin-walled veins. Venous haemorrhage can be a significant problem and great care should be taken to identify, ligate, and individually divide vessels as they are encountered. Bipolar diathermy can be used with caution in the neck, as long as nerve tissue has been identified and not accidentally caught within the beaks of the forceps.

When rapid bleeding occurs, the temptation to blindly apply artery forceps must be resisted as this is the main cause of damage to adjacent structures (and will rarely control the bleeding). Direct pressure and adequate suction will create a clear field, allowing time to continue exposing the area and to identify the vessel under direct vision. This is important when dissecting on the deep surface of a node because of the close proximity to the internal jugular vein.

Nerve damage

Motor and sensory nerve trauma is an avoidable, but common, complication. Depending on the area of the neck being dissected, damage can occur to the facial nerve (marginal mandibular branch), accessory nerve, or brachial plexus. These are often traction injuries and recovery can be expected.

Thoracic duct fistula

Trauma to the thoracic duct can occur when dissecting lymph nodes on the medial aspect of the left supraclavicular fossa. Most fistulas close spontaneously, although prolonged drainage has significant biochemical and nutritional implications; protein loss leading to hypoproteinaemia can be troublesome. Conservative management with accurate fluid-volume replacement and a low-fat diet is recommended until drainage stops.

Local tumour spread

This remains one of the persisting controversies. Failure to excise a discrete node because several glands have enlarged and matted into a fixed group may necessitate an incisional biopsy. There is a small, but significant, risk of fungation and infiltration of the overlying skin, compromising treatment and survival. In this situation fine-needle aspiration cytology (FNAC) or cone biopsy is recommended.

Tonsillectomy

Tonsillectomy is a routine procedure with several potential postoperative complications.

Complications

Haemorrhage

Primary, reactionary, and secondary haemorrhage can be frightening conditions and remain a cause of mortality. Primary haemorrhage occurs at the time of surgery due to exposure of capillaries and the external palatine vein in the tonsillar bed, which must be controlled before the patient leaves theatre. Reactionary haemorrhage, occurring within hours of the operation, is more serious. Insidious and frequently unnoticed because the blood is swallowed, the first indication of continuing blood loss is a tachycardia and symptomatic fall in blood pressure, characteristic of hypovolaemic shock, or a dramatic large-volume vomit of altered blood, due to gastric irritation from swallowed blood.

Secondary haemorrhage occurs between the fifth and tenth postoperative day. It is associated with local infection, which allows premature separation of the protective slough covering the tonsillar bed. It should be suspected (and anticipated) if the patient has a persistent low-grade pyrexia without chest signs or symptoms.

Immediate management remains ABC (airways, breathing, circulation). Patients with minor oozes require removal of the clot, re-admission, and close observation. For more significant bleeding, placing in the recovery position with 10 degree Trendelenberg tilt, intravenous access, fluid resuscitation and transfer to theatre to identify and control bleeding points is necessary. Severe haemorrhage requires transfusion.

Otitis media

Commonly seen after tonsillectomy, possibly due to endonasal intubation.

Referred otalgia

Earache after tonsillectomy is usually referred pain via the auricular branch of the vagus.

Lower respiratory tract infections

Pneumonia and lung abscess secondary to inhalation of blood and mucus are rare. These present with chest symptoms and persistent postoperative pyrexia: usually respond to appropriate systemic antibiotics.

Dental trauma

Displacement of the Boyle–Davis mouth gag can fracture tooth edges or avulse anterior teeth, causing postoperative discomfort from exposed pulp tissue. This may require the attention of a dental practitioner in the early postoperative period.

Adenoidectomy

Surgical removal of nasopharyngeal lymphoid tissue is performed either separately or at the time of tonsillectomy. While some complications are therefore similar, others are unique to the area.

Complications

Haemorrhage

Reactionary haemorrhage can be troublesome. Posterior nasal packing may be required.

Rhinolalia aperta

Excision of grossly hypertrophied adenoids, especially if the soft palate is short, can create scarring and eventual stenosis. The resulting palatal incompetence can produce pronounced hypernasal speech.

Lymphoid regrowth

Recurrence of symptoms can occur following hypertrophy of residual adenoidal tissue.

Tracheostomy

Placement of a tracheostomy, either as a semi-emergency or elective procedure, for bypassing actual or anticipated airway obstruction is not without complications and does have a distinct morbidity. The complication rate is similar for surgical and percutaneous methods.

Immediate complications

Haemorrhage

Troublesome bleeding may be encountered from the anterior jugular veins, thyroid isthmus, terminal branches of the superior thyroid artery, or skin edges. This must be arrested by meticulous use of diathermy before entering the trachea. Secondary haemorrhage may occur in the postoperative period due to poor haemostasis at the time of surgery or late erosion of a large vessel, especially the innominate artery, due to pressure necrosis from an incorrectly fitted tube.

Trauma to adjacent structures

Injury to paratracheal structures can occur but should be avoided by careful technique and ensuring that a midline approach is maintained. Reports of trauma to the recurrent laryngeal nerve, oesophagus, and left brachiocephalic vein (particularly in children) are commonly cited. The potential to create a pneumothorax should be remembered and eliminated by a semi-erect anteroposterior plain chest radiograph taken during recovery.

Intermediate complications

Subcutaneous emphysema

Occurs due to unnecessary wide dissection of the tissue planes of the anterior neck. Resolves spontaneously.

Tube displacement

Dislodgement can be complete or partial. Partial dislodgement, commonly into the pretracheal space, is particularly dangerous and if unrecognized can lead to asphyxiation. This can be avoided by correct siting of the tracheostomy to prevent unnecessary forces on the tube, using an appropriately sized tube and secure fixation, either by direct suture to the skin or by tapes tied with a square knot (avoiding bows which can become loose).

Tube obstruction

Bypassing the natural warming and humidifying mechanisms of the upper airway allows inspired air to directly enter the lower airway, thereby drying secretions and promoting metaplasia of tracheal mucosa. The retained tenacious secretions can occlude the tube lumen. This can be avoided by attentive nursing care, adequate humidification (by heated water-bath or nebulizer), warming inspired gases, and regular physiotherapy to encourage coughing.

Lower respiratory infection

Tracheostomy sites are always colonized by bacteria, the longer the tube remains *in situ* the greater the risk of colonization by *Pseudomonas* spp. Together with retained secretions, there is a high chance of developing chest complications. Regular physiotherapy, early mobilization, and tracheobronchial toilet using sterile suction catheters reduce this risk. Prophylactic antibiotics have no role in preventing chest infections.

Dysphagia

This is common with a tracheostomy and, in the period immediately following decannulation, due to compression of the oesophagus by the tube.

Apnoea

This complicates the management of patients with chronic obstructive pulmonary disease (COPD), who rely on a high carbon dioxide content to stimulate a respiratory effort. The abrupt decrease in arterial PCO_2 may lead to apnoea. Administration of 5% carbon dioxide in the inspired oxygen will compensate during the initial postoperative period.

Late complications

Tracheal stenosis

Subglottic stricture can occur with an ill-fitting tube, after incision through the cricoid ring, or following long-term ischaemia from cuff pressure. Usually this does not cause major symptoms unless narrowing under 5 mm occurs.

Tracheo-oesophageal fistula

This follows pressure-induced necrosis of the tracheal cartilage and can lead to aspiration pneumonia. Initially managed conservatively with parenteral or enteral nutrition via gastrostomy, if spontaneous closure does not occur the neck is explored and the tract excised. The incidence has been significantly reduced with modern low-pressure cuffs.

Tracheoinnominate artery fistula

This is a rare complication of displacement of the tube into the pretracheal space.

Thyroidectomy

Successful surgical management of thyroid disease is based on a detailed knowledge of the normal and pathological anatomy combined with a meticulous operative technique. The complications after thyroid surgery have huge litigation implications (4% of all general surgical claims settled by the defence organizations). It is mandatory that the potential complications are discussed at the preoperative counselling session and that this should be clearly documented in the patient's case notes.

Immediate complications

Haemorrhage

Postoperative haemorrhage into the thyroid bed is an acute, life-threatening emergency. The aim of successful thyroidectomy is to maintain a near bloodless field, so preventing accumulation of blood in the pretracheal space postoperatively and allowing the accurate intraoperative identification of important structures. Prominent vessels should be clipped, ligated, and divided under direct vision, whereas smaller vessels can be coagulated with bipolar diathermy before closure over a small-calibre closed suction drain to remove residual blood and serum. Accumulation of blood within the anterior neck compartment can potentially produce tracheal compression and respiratory embarrassment, although laryngeal oedema secondary to venous obstruction by the expanding haematoma is the commonest cause of airway compromise and stridor. Immediate management requires protection and maintenance of the airway with endotracheal intubation, evacuation of any haematoma, and identification of bleeding points, either at the bedside, or preferably if time allows, in the operating theatre.

Recurrent laryngeal nerve injury

The recurrent laryngeal nerve is a mixed nerve; motor supply to all the intrinsic laryngeal muscles, except the cricothyroid and sensory, supply to the mucosa below the vocal cords. It is an anatomically consistent structure found within the tracheo-oesophageal groove. Damage can be caused by traction, haematoma, ligation, diathermy, or sectioning at the time of surgery. Carefully identifying the course of the nerve is the best way to avoid injury. Injury to one nerve results in a weak, hoarse voice. Bilateral incomplete nerve injury produces respiratory distress and airway obstruction due to cord adduction by the unopposed cricothyroid muscles, necessitating re-intubation and tracheostomy. In bilateral complete injuries, the cords adopt the cadaveric position, the voice is absent, but dyspnoea is not pronounced.

The ineffective cough predisposes to respiratory infections and may necessitate a cuffed tracheostomy.

Superior laryngeal nerve injury

The external branch supplies the cricothyroid, which adducts and tenses the cords. It is most at risk during dissection of the superior pole of the thyroid. The resulting ipsilateral cord weakness produces subtle changes in voice quality and projection.

Injury to the internal branch is uncommon, but the loss of supraglottic sensation can result in aspiration.

Thyroid crisis

Thyroid crisis is an extreme exacerbation of thyrotoxicosis that can be precipitated in patients with Graves' disease who have been inadequately prepared for surgery. Diagnosis is clinical and the warning signs of tachycardia, hyperpyrexia, arrhythmias, and extreme agitation require urgent attention. The patient should be immediately transferred to the intensive therapy unit (ITU) and intravenous fluids and supplemental oxygen administered. Symptom control is achieved with propranolol, propylthiouracil, potassium iodide, and dexamethasone.

Tracheomalacia

Long-standing tracheal compression from a large multinodular goitre can produce softening and collapse of the cartilage rings. This is a rare cause of immediate postoperative respiratory obstruction.

Intermediate complications

Hypocalcaemia

Hypoparathyroidism is rare after lobectomy and uncommon after subtotal thyroidectomy. It is commonly due to devascularization or the inadvertent excision of parathyroid tissue, and avoided by careful surgical exploration and avoiding ligation of the main trunk of the inferior thyroid artery. Symptoms are related to the serum calcium level, determined from the adjusted ionized calcium assay. Mild hypocalcaemia (>2 mmol/l) is usually transient but may require oral calcium supplements. Symptomatic hypocalcaemia (<2 mmol/l) is managed medically with intravenous calcium gluconate, oral calcium, and vitamin D derivatives (1α-hydroxycholecalciferol).

Late complications

Hypothyroidism

All patients undergoing total thyroidectomy and, to a lesser extent, bilateral subtotal thyroidectomy develop hypothyroidism. Thyroid hormonal replacement is usually required.

Recurrent hyperthyroidism

Can present many years after primary surgery, emphasizing the need for clinical and biochemical follow-up.

Hypertrophic or keloid scarring (see Chapter 22)

Numbness of the upper skin flap

Parathyroidectomy

Exploration of the neck for primary hyperparathyroidism carries similar risks to thyroid surgery. Postoperative complications are due to technical or localization errors.

Immediate complications

Haemorrhage

Avoided by meticulous attention to haemostasis.

Nerve damage

Injury to the recurrent and superior laryngeal nerves create the same problems seen in thyroid surgery.

Horner's syndrome

Damage to the cervical sympathetic trunk gives rise to the characteristic signs of miosis, enophthalmos, ptosis, and anhidrosis.

Hypocalcaemia

Usually transient, due to negative feedback suppression of the remaining parathyroid tissue. If severe, then temporary oral calcium supplements are required.

Intermediate complications

Persistent hyperparathyroidism

Persistent hypercalcaemia after parathyroidectomy is a difficult problem to manage. The diagnosis should be reconfirmed and other causes of hypercalcaemia excluded. Radioisotope or magnetic resonance imaging (MRI) localization studies are useful in identifying ectopic glands—the commonest reason for failure. Referral to an experienced surgeon is advised because the risk of permanent recurrent laryngeal nerve injury and hypoparathyroidism after re-operation is considerable.

Superficial parotidectomy

Parotid surgery is performed for the removal of neoplastic lesions, duct obstruction, chronic inflammation, or duct obstruction due to stenosis or calculi. Procedures in this area should not be considered 'minor surgery' and only be undertaken by experienced surgeons.

Immediate complications

Haemorrhage

This is a common problem. Reversal of the hypotensive effects of anaesthesia, aimed at reducing intraoperative bleeding, can produce marked reactionary haemorrhage. With adequate suction drainage this should not cause a problem. If the drain is blocked the patient has to be returned to theatre, re-anaesthetized, the wound explored, and identifiable bleeding points arrested in order to avoid a haematoma. It can be avoided by meticulous ligation or application of ligaclips to vessels—often appearing as 'strands' during dissection.

Intermediate complications

Facial nerve damage

This is the most serious complication. Trauma to the terminal branches is more common than sectioning the actual nerve trunk or major branches. The risk is reduced by a meticulous technique that exposes the nerve throughout its intraglandular course, and by avoiding enucleation in preference for formal superficial lobe excision.

Most patients show some degree of temporary facial weakness due to neuropraxia, which is more severe after 24 hours than in the immediate postoperative period. One or more branches may be affected but, provided all were anatomically intact at the end of surgery, full recovery can be anticipated.

Complications vary depending on the branch affected. The most serious is the inability to close the eye, exposing the cornea. Hypromellose eye drops help irrigate the eye and prevent conjunctivitis, but a lateral tarsorrhaphy is usually advised to protect the cornea from drying and abrasion.

Complete nerve section requires immediate repair. Microneural anastomosis or grafting from the greater auricular, sural, or medial cutaneous nerves should be undertaken.

Techniques to disguise irreversible facial paralysis include lateral and medial tarsorrhaphy, gold implants to assist upper lid closure, and fascia lata slings to elevate the angle of the mouth. Successful when at rest, the cosmetic benefit is lost when compared to the normal active facial muscles.

Salivary fistula

An external fistula can develop if Stenson's duct is not ligated intraoperatively. Spontaneous resolution occurs but the complication can be avoided by excising as much duct as possible.

Late complications

Frey's syndrome

Presents approximately 6 months postoperatively. The patient complains of gustatory sweating, often accompanied by vasodilatation of the skin innervated by the auriculotemporal nerve. It is caused by misdirected re-innervation of the sectioned parasympathetic secretomotor fibres that originally supplied the parotid and sympathetic fibres within the great auricular nerve to the skin, sebaceous glands, and blood vessels. Frey's syndrome can be demonstrated in almost every patient, but only 5–10% are symptomatic. Most treatments are ineffective but it may respond to atropine. Surgical correction has its advocates, ranging from intracranial sectioning of the glossopharyngeal nerve, auriculotemporal neurectomy, intratympanic parasympathetic neurectomy to excision of the overlying skin.

Prophylactic methods have been used to reduce this complication. Superficial musculoaponeurotic system flaps (SMAS) derived form the fascia in the periauricular region can be interposed between the skin and gland to interrupt aberrant anastomosis. Superiorly based sternocleidomastoid flaps have a similar benefit.

Interest is being shown in the use of botulinum toxin type A for the management of symptomatic Frey's syndrome. Intracutaneous injection into the affected skin area has been shown to control symptoms within 2 days and recurrence is rarely observed.

Great auricular nerve damage

A neuroma derived form the cut proximal end of the nerve presents as a tender, palpable, subcutaneous nodule at the anterior border of sternomastoid muscle. No treatment is required unless there is a suspicion of recurrent tumour. Avoid by placing the cut end into the sternomastoid muscle. The loss of cutaneous sensation to the ear lobe is not a significant problem to most patients.

Submandibular gland excision

Submandibular gland excision is commonly performed for sialolithiasis, chronic sialadenitis, or as part of a neck dissection. As with all neck surgery the main postoperative complications relate to poor haemostasis and nerve injuries (which should not be underestimated as three individual nerves have to be considered).

Immediate complications

Haemorrhage

An uncommon complication, but seen when a chronically inflamed gland has been removed. Can cause a large haematoma if low-volume closed drains are not used, but rarely requires re-exploration.

Intermediate complications

Facial nerve paralysis

A common complication that produces an unsightly deformity. The marginal mandibular branch is most vulnerable to traction, compression, and diathermy injuries and, while commonly only a neuropraxia (92% of cases in one reported series), it can be permanent. The incidence of nerve injury can be minimized by making a low and generous skin-crease approach, careful dissection in the subplatysmal plane, controlled retraction, and avoiding wide exposure of the nerve.

Lingual nerve injury

Produces temporary or permanent paraesthesia on the ipsilateral half of the tongue. The patient must exercise care when eating and drinking hot fluids to avoid local trauma.

Hypoglossal nerve injury

An uncommon complication. The tongue deviates toward the affected side and eventually wastes and shows fasciculation. No treatment is advised for unilateral wasting.

Scar

A prominent, aesthetically unacceptable scar can be produced by inappropriate siting of the incision. Can be avoided by careful planning and placement in a suitable skin crease.

Residual stones

Inconvenient for the patient and embarrassing to the surgeon. One series found 18% of patients undergoing submandibular gland excision for sialolithiasis had residual stones within Wharton's duct. Removal via an intraoral approach is recommended if accessible and symptomatic.

Sublingual gland excision

Excision is normally undertaken for the treatment of a ranula or for stone disease. Rarely, they are removed for malignancy. The procedure is performed via an intraoral floor-of-mouth approach and the main problems encountered relate to the local anatomy.

Immediate complications

Haemorrhage

The floor of the mouth has a rich blood supply. Bleeding can be encountered from the sublingual veins, sublingual artery, and smaller vessels supplying the gland from branches of the sublingual and submandibular arteries. Vessels can be controlled by careful use of bipolar diathermy.

Intermediate complications

Submandibular duct trauma

The duct is the first structure encountered deep to the oral mucosa. It must be identified and isolated to avoid damage. Duct obstruction secondary to traumatic section or stenosis cause chronic submandibular sialadenitis, which may require subsequent submandibular excision.

Lingual nerve damage

The lingual nerve is intimately associated with the gland and submandibular duct. Damage produces either temporary or permanent paraesthesia on the ipsilateral half of the tongue.

Neck dissection

Dissection of the cervical lymph nodes and interfascial fat with combined resection of a primary tumour is a standard surgical oncological procedure for managing cancer of the mouth, pharynx, thyroid, or larynx. Lymphatic drainage of the entire head and neck region is ultimately into the deep jugular chain alongside the internal jugular vein. Removal of this chain and adjacent tissue has been shown to have therapeutic and prognostic advantages, but with the unnecessary sacrifice of important structures such as the external and internal jugular veins, sternocleidomastoid muscle, and the accessory nerve. Technical modifications to this radical neck dissection (e.g. functional, selective) aim to preserve these structures, but they can still be damaged as a consequence of surgery.

Immediate complications

Haemorrhage

Haemorrhage after major head and neck surgery is revealed either by bleeding into the mouth or pharynx or haematoma formation under the skin flaps. Potential sites are skin edges, superior or inferior ends of the divided jugular veins, superior or inferior thyroid pedicles, and branches of the external carotid artery. While drain volume is normally unreliable for assessing blood loss, rapid accumulation within the suction bottle suggests ongoing bleeding. The principle of management is the same as that after any operation: protect the airway; maintain breathing; and replace lost circulatory volume before identifying and ligating the bleeding vessel. Trying to arrest haemorrhage by pressure dressings or packing cavities is futile and dangerous.

Airway obstruction

Extensive resection of oral, pharyngeal, or laryngeal tissue causes inevitable oedema and potentially compromises the airway. This is even more pronounced after bilateral radical neck dissection because ligation of both internal jugular veins causes considerable soft tissue oedema. Prevention by elective tracheostomy reduces the incidence of this problem.

Facial oedema

Often subsides within a month if precautions are taken (e.g. avoid neck dressings, nurse in the upright position). Once established it is untreatable and leaves the patient disfigured.

Raised intracranial pressure

A rare, but potential, complication. Ligation and division of the internal jugular vein temporarily raises the intracranial pressure (over 5 times for bilateral ligation). Normally asymptomatic, some patients may complain of headache, facial swelling and congestion, and agitation. This can be minimized by recovering the patient in an upright position, avoiding constricting neck dressings, and preventing neck hyperextension. Rapid symptomatic relief can be achieved by inducing diuresis with intravenous mannitol. The intracranial pressure can be expected to return to normal values within 24 hours and therefore long-term treatment is not required.

Pneumothorax

Damage to the cervical pleura when operating low in the neck can produce a pneumothorax. This may be overlooked in the ventilated patient and only become apparent in the recovery area. A portable plain chest radiograph should be taken of all patients before returning them to the ward.

Intermediate complications

Chylous fistula

Damage to the thoracic duct is common and often a necessary procedure when performing a thorough neck dissection. This has no significant sequelae unless the surgeon fails to recognize that the injury has occurred. Although the complication is not initially apparent because the starved patient has little lymphatic circulation, it becomes apparent when enteral tube feeding is started (2nd–5th postoperative day). The volume in the suction drains dramatically increases and the consistency changes to a thick creamy fluid. The diagnosis should be obvious but it can be confirmed by assaying the lipid level within the exudate. As the drains are unable to cope with the volume, chyle will accumulate under the skin flaps leading to the disastrous situation of an external fistula. The patient loses protein and fluid (up to 4 litres a day), leading to dehydration and emaciation during the most critical phase after major surgery. Management is controversial and protracted. It has been suggested that exploration of the lower neck and ligation of the duct should be performed when the leak has been detected, although this is technically difficult and usually unsuccessful if 24 hours have elapsed. Conservative management has traditionally consisted of a low-fat diet, which reduces the volume of chyle produced and facilitates spontaneous closure of the fistula. Unfortunately, this reduces the caloric intake during a time of maximum catabolism and tends to compound the problem. Intravenous parenteral nutrition has a limited role and does not reduce chyle volume. Replacing normal dietary fat with medium-chain triglycerides is the only technique shown to be effective in reducing chyle volume and is the accepted current practice.

Seroma

Although suction drainage reduces the risk of a collection of serum under the skin flaps, it can still occur after removal of the drains. Failure to recognize this problem compromises the skin and leads to wound breakdown. Managed by regular aspiration and pressure dressings until dry.

Carotid artery rupture

Rupture of a major neck vessel is the culmination of a number of serious complications. Wound breakdown secondary to infection, irradiated tissue, inadequate tissue cover for the vessel, or erosion of the artery wall by residual tumour are all implicated. It can be prevented by protecting all arteries at risk by an interposed levator scapulae muscle graft at the time of surgery. Vigilance can anticipate the problem as there is nearly always a preceding herald bleed 48 hours before rupture. At this stage rupture can be avoided by returning the patient to theatre, debriding the area, and covering the exposed vessel with a levator scapulae graft.

Massive rupture should be controlled with finger pressure, the airway secured by re-inflating the tracheostomy tube (if still *in situ*), and fluid replacement (ideally with blood). Cerebral blood flow is maintained by head-down tilt, maintaining a high systolic blood pressure and normocarbia to avoid cerebral vasodilatation. The artery should be isolated, clamped, transfixed, and divided. No attempts should be made to suture or graft the defect as further rupture becomes inevitable. Unfortunately one-third of patients will die and over half of those who do survive will be hemiplegic.

Fistula

Orocutaneous or pharyngocutaneous fistulas result from pre- (prior radiotherapy, poorly controlled diabetes, anaemia), peri- (inadequate suturing), and postoperative factors (untreated seroma or haematoma). If caused by suture failure, spontaneous closure can be expected as long as epithelialization of the tract is avoided. Infected skin with areas of necrosis requires debridement and control of local infection by dressings, with eventual formal excision of the fistula and closure of the defect by providing a lining for the inside of the mouth and the skin defect.

Nerve damage

The potential to damage the phrenic, hypoglossal, lingual, vagus, accessory, brachial plexus, and lower branches of the facial nerve are always present during a radical neck dissection. Injuries to the sympathetic trunk produce a postoperative Horner's syndrome.

Late complications

Recurrent tumour

Recurrence at the primary site or contralateral lymph glands can occur. The neck nodes can be treated by neck dissection but may risk the potential complications of facial oedema and raised intracranial pressure due to ligation of the internal jugular veins.

Laryngectomy

The problems after laryngectomy should be anticipated and therefore prevented.

Immediate complications

Haemorrhage

Reactionary haemorrhage is the commonest cause. If severe, the wound may need re-exploring and the bleeding vessel ligated.

Intermediate complications

Infection

Wound infection is common. Perioperative prophylactic antibiotics have reduced the incidence.

Pharyngocutaneous fistula

Commonly seen in patients who have been previously irradiated. Occurs in the second postoperative week. Managed conservatively with nasogastric feeding until closure, which can take many weeks.

Stomal crusting

Inadequate attention to tracheal toilet and humidification can allow crusts to form in the upper trachea, restricting the airway. It can be prevented by diligent nursing care.

Excision of pharyngeal pouch

The aim of surgery is to close the neck of the diverticulum—either by excision of the sac and ligation of the neck, or by diathermy ablation (Dohlman's procedure). Surgical access via a cervical incision carries all the risks associated with neck operations. It may be accompanied by a myotomy. Endoscopic stapling techniques may suffer similar complications.

Immediate complications

Surgical emphysema

This is due to the escape of air from the pharynx into the soft tissues of the neck.

Mendelsohn's syndrome

Stagnant saliva and foodstuff retained within the pouch can be inhaled during anaesthesia. It is recognized by the characteristic features of bronchospasm, tachycardia, cyanosis, and pulmonary oedema during induction. Emergency management involves bronchoscopy and lavage, broad-spectrum antibiotics, intravenous aminophylline, and intravenous hydrocortisone. In extreme cases admission to ITU for elective ventilation is required. Regular physiotherapy should be given during convalescence.

Intermediate complications

Recurrent laryngeal nerve injury

The presence of the nerve within the tracheo-oesophageal groove increases its vulnerability. Damage may be temporary or permanent.

Salivary fistula

Due to leakage from the ligated pouch neck. Responds to conservative management, e.g. nil by mouth and nasogastric feeding.

Mediastinitis

Fistulous leakage can introduce infection into the mediastinum. The risk is reduced by prophylactic antibiotics. Higher incidence with Dohlman's procedure.

Chest infection

Inhalation of pouch contents at the time of surgery can cause lower tract infections. The incidence can be reduced by prophylactic antibiotics and careful observation for the symptoms and signs of infection.

Late complications

Oesophageal stricture

Iatrogenic postcricoid stricture can be created at the site of closure. The patient presents with dysphagia to solids and the sensation of food 'sticking' in their throat. It occurs less commonly if a cricopharyngeal myotomy is performed, although this remains controversial because of the increased risk of oesophageal reflux.

Recurrence

Similar presentation to a stricture and is less common after cricopharyngeal myotomy.

Zygomatic complex fractures

Most complications arise as a direct result of the injury. Periorbital oedema, ecchymosis, subconjunctival haemorrhage, and paraesthesia in the distribution of the infraorbital nerve are common and resolve within 2–4 weeks of the injury. Retrobulbar haemorrhage is the serious complication that must be remembered after elevation of a fractured zygoma.

Immediate complications

Retrobulbar haemorrhage

This is an unpredictable, rare, but serious complication that can be seen immediately after elevation of a fractured zygoma. Arterial bleeding into the enclosed intraconal and extraconal spaces produces a substantial rise in orbital pressure. The ciliary arteries do not withstand high pressures and occlusion leads to irreversible retinal ischaemia. Pain aggravated by movement, decreasing visual acuity, sudden onset of proptosis, and a unilateral dilating pupil are cardinal features. Immediate action is indicated.

Surgical decompression, under local or general anaesthesia, by an approach along the orbital floor or through the maxillary antrum, allows a suction catheter to be passed into the intraconal space.

Medical treatment has been advocated, especially if there is a delay while preparing for surgery. Reducing the intraocular volume with osmotic diuretics will decrease the intraocular pressure, hence increasing the retrobulbar space (and reducing the pressure). Intravenous mannitol and acetazolamide induce a renal diuresis and high-dose dexamethasone reduces neural oedema.

Bradycardia

Parasympathetic stimulation during the elevation of a fractured zygoma can produce a profound bradycardia. The anaesthetist can reduce the effect by administering intravenous atropine. The major concern in a medically compromised patient is cardiac hypoperfusion and risk of cardiac arrest.

Third-molar surgery

While most basic surgical trainees will not be experienced in the removal of impacted wisdom teeth it is one of the commonest procedures performed in district general hospitals. Patients commonly present to accident and emergency departments with complications and therefore most doctors will encounter these problems.

Immediate complications

Haemorrhage

Generalized oozing from the gingival margin is commonly experienced and easily controlled by local pressure with a gauze pad. Brisker bleeding may occur if the inferior alveolar artery in the base of the socket has been damaged, but this responds to packing the socket with an absorbable haemostatic agent, e.g. surgicel. Continuing haemorrhage can be controlled by apposing the gingival edges with absorbable sutures under local infiltration. This places tension on the vessels in the gingival margin and controls bleeding by local ischaemia.

Pain

Very common. Requires adequate analgesia.

Swelling

Related to local trauma and the accumulation of a haematoma under the gingival flaps. Resolves spontaneously. No value in steroids unless given at the time of surgery.

Intermediate complications

Nerve damage

This is an important complication because it can be permanent, cause the patient considerable distress, and has a high litigation potential. The inferior alveolar and lingual nerves are at significant risk because of their anatomical proximity to wisdom teeth.

Inferior alveolar nerve damage produces paraesthesia of the skin and vermilion of the ipsilateral lower lip. Lingual nerve damage affects sensation to the ipsilateral half of the tongue.

Any sensation loss that persists after 6 months is likely to be permanent. All patients undergoing third-molar removal should be warned preoperatively of this risk.

The potential for soft tissue trauma due to this disability is significant and patients have to be educated appropriately.

Dry socket

This is a painful condition that may follow the extraction of any tooth, but is more prevalent after lower third-molar surgery (incidence is approximately 10%), with a peak occurrence at days 3–5. Aetiology is poorly understood, but there is an intense inflammation within the socket wall which leads to loss of the blood clot. Patients present with severe localized pain, difficulty eating, and halitosis. A self-limiting condition, symptomatic treatment is required. Adequate analgesia, treatment of obvious infection, and irrigation with or without packing of the socket may provide relief. There is no evidence that antibiotics improve symptoms.

Trismus

This transient complication is precipitated by swelling and pain and resolves when these factors are addressed.

Temporomandibular joint pain

Caused by local trauma at the time of extraction. Discomfort may affect eating but is managed conservatively with rest, analgesia, soft diet, and physiotherapy.

Pathological mandible fracture

Deeply impacted teeth weaken the mandible at a natural point of stress. The void that remains after extracting the tooth can predispose to fracture, especially if the patient is edentulous.

Chapter 21
Complications after breast surgery

Introduction

Complications after breast surgery may be considered after local excision or biopsy, mastectomy, axillary surgery, or reconstruction using the time-scales shown in the table below. Complications after biopsy can be substantial and include haematoma, infection, and, rarely, pneumothorax, all of which may occur after fine-needle aspiration for cytology in a small breast. Core (Trucut) biopsy needs a local anaesthetic and carries a higher risk of haematoma. It is safer to undertake this as a day-case type procedure, where a long enough observation period can reduce the risk or allow the recognition of continued bleeding with action taken, if necessary.

Time-scales of complications after breast surgery

Immediate	Haemorrhage
	Damage to skin flaps
	Damage to axillary structures
Intermediate	*Breast*:
	seroma
	haematoma
	wound infection
	wound breakdown
	Axilla:
	lymphocele and lymphoedema of arm
	numbness
	paraesthesia
	reduced shoulder movement
Late	*Breast*:
	recurrence
	deformity
	hypertrophic, keloid, or widened scar
	Axilla:
	frozen shoulder (worsened by radiotherapy

Local complications

Bleeding from the wound

Skin flap necrosis

Wound infection

Serous discharge

Local complications

Bleeding from the wound

Although this is easily recognized and rectified, bleeding into the cavity left after excision of a fibroadenoma, for example, or under the skin flaps after mastectomy may not be obvious. If the collection is small and symptomatic it can be left to resolve spontaneously. However, large haematomas need evacuation and attention paid to any bleeding vessel, which may necessitate a general anaesthetic. If bleeding is excessive, it may lead to anaemia, e.g. after bilateral mastectomy. There is little evidence that placing drains postoperatively avoids this complication. Their purpose is the control of lymph from divided lymphatics following axillary lymph node sampling or clearance.

Skin flap necrosis

Skin flap necrosis may follow mastectomy if the flaps are made too thin or sutured under tension. Incisions must be made at right angles to skin to avoid this. Excessive diathermy may damage the skin edges. Early recognition may avoid superadded infection and a worsening of the complication. Dead tissue needs excision and any defect closed with help from a plastic surgeon, as a flap may be required. Hypertrophic or spread scars may follow tight sutures. Nipple necrosis after Hadfield's operation or after reconstruction may require excision. Cosmetically acceptable, plastic surgery can remedy this problem. The patient may accept simple excision, and prosthetic adhesive nipples are available.

Wound infection

After breast surgery, wound infection occurs in over 10% of patients, depending on the definition. There is little evidence that antibiotic prophylaxis is of any use, with the possible exception for some procedures, e.g. axillary lymph node sampling or cavity re-excision at 2 weeks. Most infections are minor and settle spontaneously. Major 'purulent' infections may reflect a failure of fatty tissues to heal, with or without fat necrosis, rather than a true infection. Incision and drainage may be needed and there may be a delay in starting chemotherapy or radiotherapy.

Serous collections

Serous collections are common. Suturing skin flaps to the pectoralis fascia after mastectomy or the placement of drains for several days postoperatively do not avoid the complication. It probably relates to the two large raw areas under the skin flaps and the muscle fascia rather than poor technique. There may also be a lymphatic element. Although seromas usually respond to simple painless aspiration through the wound suture line, this often need repeating. Formal drainage is occasionally needed for persistent collections.

Neurovascular injury

Damage to axillary structures may either present early or be recognized and rectified during surgery, e.g. axillary vein. Damage to nerves may only be realized postoperatively, such as anaesthesia of the medial skin of the upper arm (intercasto brachial), or motor effects involving the subcapsular nerves or the nerve to the latissimus dorsi. Very rarely, there may be brachial plexus damage, most likely due to traction on the arm during surgery.

Other paraesthesia

Paraesthesiae or numbness are intermediate complications. Although most resolve, they can be distressing and persistent. Reduced shoulder movements can be avoided by early physiotherapy, but frozen shoulder is a late and difficult complication to control. It is more common after radiotherapy.

Lymphoedema

Lymphoedema is more likely after high axillary dissection followed by radiotherapy. It is avoidable by only undertaking level I axillary dissection when radiotherapy is part of treatment. Specialized lymphoedema clinics may be able to control this complication with compression garments. A very rare complication of lymphoedema is angiosarcoma (Stuart–Treves syndrome).

Breast deformity

Postsurgical breast deformity can be avoided by the use of appropriate incisions. Defects after wide biopsy lessen over time, but 'dimpling' caused by sutures placed deep to close cavities does not. Fat stitches can be avoided. Severe deformity may require reconstruction.

Carcinoma recurrence

All local complications are distressing after breast surgery but recurrence of carcinoma in the wound is particularly so and reflects a failure of local control. Excision may need restorative surgery with the help of a plastic surgeon, and a response can be expected after radiotherapy, if it has not already been used, a change in hormonal adjuvant therapy (e.g. megestrol for tamoxifen) or chemotherapy. The chances of a putative cure are reduced.

Pain

Breast pain, or wound pain, can be worsened after surgical procedures, particularly those undertaken for benign diseases. Management can be difficult; gamma-linoleic acid (evening primrose oil), bromocriptine, or danazol may be helpful in cyclical mastalgia, but the mainstay in simple analgesia with non-steroidal anti-inflammatory drugs (NSAIDs) and breast support.

General complications

These can occur after breast surgery, but more specifically chest complications may relate to inadequate analgesia and the pain of a chest scar. Advice from the physiotherapist is helpful. Shoulder stiffness may be ameliorated by early graduated exercises.

There is always a high degree of anxiety and depression associated with breast surgery, particularly when undertaken for cancer. Much can be avoided by appropriate discussion and counselling from breast-care nursing support. The advent of multidisciplinary teams, the 2-week cancer rules, and one-stop clinics has done much to ensure speedy, accurate diagnosis.

Chapter 22
Complications of plastic surgery

Skin incisions

Complications occur in all branches of surgery. However, these may be minimized by meticulous attention to surgical principles and to the physiology of wound healing.

The ideal scar is flat, fine, lies within or parallel to the natural skin line (relaxed skin tension lines, RSTL), and does not affect function or appearance.

Surgical principles

- **Skin incision**—incisions are normally made at right angles to the skin. Avoid shelving incisions on the skin, as they heal leaving thick unsightly scars. However, in special areas, e.g. eyebrows and scalp, the incision is made parallel to the hair follicles.

- **Direction**—scars placed within natural wrinkles or parallel to RSTL are less conspicuous. They may require Z-plasty or W-plasty techniques to reorientate or break up the direction of the scar.

- **Tissue handling**—gentle handling and avoiding crushing of soft tissues is basic to all aspects of surgery. Consider using skin hooks or fine-toothed forceps to hold deeper tissues and avoid damaging the dermal and epidermal layers of the skin.

- **Haemostasis**—careful haemostasis prior to wound closure reduces the risks of haematomas postoperatively. These may become sites of wound infection, discomfort, scar distortion, and increased wound tension.

- **Wound evaluation**—dirty, devitalized tissue or foreign matter must be excised, otherwise these will be a nidus for future wound infection and unsightly scars. Wounds which contain foreign material may become permanent 'tattoos'. This unsightly complication can be minimized by thorough wound cleansing at the time of injury and may need scrubbing debridement with copious irrigation.

- **Wound tension**—excessive tension results in a widespread scar. Consider deep dermal sutures to reduce tissue tension and review scar alignment.

- **Tissue perfusion**—areas of the body with a good blood supply heal better than those areas with a poor blood supply. Ensure good perfusion (including optimal correction of shock) and nutrition to patients following surgery to reduce risks of delayed wound healing and infection.

- **Age/comorbid factors**—older patients produce less conspicuous scars, although their healing rates are slower. Comorbid factors may affect wound healing due to nutritional, vascular insufficiency, or iatrogenic causes, e.g. chemotherapy.

- **Closure**—sutures should be placed so that the skin edges are everted and just touching. Postoperative oedema will appose the edges; excessive tension in the area surrounded by the suture may cause tissue necrosis or visible suture marks.
- **Wound care**—wounds heal better in a moist environment, occlusive dressings allow rapid epithelialization of an incision. After 48–72 hours the incision may be gently cleaned without disrupting wound integrity. Prolonged occlusion under opaque dressings does not allow identification of potential deterioration of the wound. Wound support, e.g. Steri-strips, may be used to prevent wound edges shearing and gaping during healing, and for a limited period following suture removal.

Unsightly scars

Scars are considered disfiguring. However, in some societies intentional scarring has been used for decorative purposes.

Hypertrophic scar

Raised red scar limited to the area of the incision. These are more common in young children and may occur at any site; they tend to resolve with time. They are possibly due to wound-edge shearing, subclinical infection, excessive tissue tension, or prolonged inflammation.

Treatment

Expectant, silicone gel ± pressure, steroid injection. Remember the complications of steroid injections: local hypopigmentation, dermal atrophy, widening of the scar, and telangiectasia. Intralesional calcium antagonists may be tried. Vascular specific lasers (585 nm pulse-tuneable dye or 532 nm) have shown beneficial effects on erythematous hypertrophic scars.

Keloid scars

Raised scar extending beyond the initial incision often shows a progressive increase in size. They are commonly associated with darker skin pigmentation, family history or Celtic ancestry, and tend to occur at high-risk sites, e.g. earlobe and chest. Histology reveals an abnormally high concentration of type III collagen with a disorganized collagen pattern.

Treatment

This is difficult as surgery can make it worse. Combined therapy with surgical excision and non-surgical options, e.g. steroid injections, pressure, radiotherapy, and/or calcium antagonists.

Widespread scars

Flat or recessed scar. These are usually caused by tissue tension pulling the wound edges apart, e.g. removal of sutures too early or not using buried sutures to support the wound, and are seen in areas of increased tissue tension, e.g. limbs. The scar does not contain excessive collagen.

Treatment

Either accept the scar or consider revisional surgery with prolonged wound support or a 'plasty' procedure.

'Morse code' (• — •) scar ('stitch marks')

Seen when skin sutures are left in place for longer than 5–6 days, or if the initial wound closure is so tight that tissue oedema causes dermal necrosis under the suture. Suture abscesses occur at each point of skin entry.

Treatment

Avoid the cause and consider using buried dermal suture technique, e.g. subcuticular closure.

Erythematous scars

Flat pink or red scar in the incision line. Note that all scars are erythematous during the initial stages of wound healing, and particularly following curettage or dermal shaving. They are caused by prolonged angiogenesis and decreased capillary regression and tend to resolve with time. Persistence beyond 12 months indicates a lack of resolution.

Treatment

They respond well to vascular specific lasers—used early to hasten resolution or in later stage to lighten colour.

Pigmented scars

Flat tan/dark scar in the incision line. Associated with darker skin tones and are due to increased melanogenesis or postinflammatory hyperpigmentation with deposition of pigment into the dermis.

Treatment

These tend to resolve with time. Prolonged hyperpigmentation may be treated with topical hydroquinone.

Contractures

Wound contraction is a normal part of wound healing; however, a short thick scar results in a scar contracture. This causes functional effects if the contraction crosses joints or is near the eyelids, and it may also have cosmetic effects by distorting soft tissues.

Treatment

Using techniques to lengthen or break up the contracture, e.g. Z-plasty or Y–V-plasty.

Skin grafts

A graft is a tissue that lacks its own intravascular blood supply and is dependent on the blood supply at the recipient site for its survival. A split-thickness skin graft (SSG) contains epidermis and a variable thickness of dermis; a full-thickness skin graft (FTSG) contains the whole dermis and adnexal structures, e.g. hair follicles. The graft bed must be vascularized, clean, and free of necrotic tissue. Skin grafts will not take on bone, cartilage, or tendon without the presence of periosteum, perichondrium, or paratenon. They are used to repair areas of skin loss or close wounds that cannot be closed by primary suture.

Initial graft adherence to a wound bed is effected by fibrin deposition, lasting 72 h. This is followed by graft revascularization ('take'): the process of serum inhibition (24–48 h), inosculation (alignment of graft and donor capillaries), and capillary ingrowth and revascularization.

Complications

These are mainly failure of skin grafts and late complications. The partial loss of a skin graft may require regrafting or leaving the wound to heal by secondary intention; total loss may require regrafting or another surgical approach, e.g. flaps.

Failure of skin grafts

Haematoma

This is the most common reason for skin graft failure. Careful haemostasis of the graft bed and removal of any residual clot prior to skin graft application with close contact between graft and bed is essential. Firm dressings, fenestrating the graft, and quilting sutures will allow close contact and the escape of any accumulated fluid. If detected early, incise the skin graft over the haematoma and evacuate, redress with firm pressure.

Infection

Infection is the second most common reason for skin graft failure. Avoid by attention to the preparation of the wound bed. Early signs of infection (cellulitis or suppuration) should be treated with systemic antibiotics and frequent antiseptic dressing changes.

Graft movement

Shearing forces between the graft bed and graft may dislodge the graft from the bed. Grafts should be firmly fixed to the recipient site bed and, if dressed, use a non-shearing dressing technique with relative immobilization of the grafted area. Prolonged immobilization of the patient is not recommended.

Seroma

Collections under the skin graft may result in skin graft necrosis. Using firm dressings, fenestrating the graft, and quilting sutures allows close contact and the escape of any fluid. If detected early, incise the skin graft over the seroma and evacuate, redress with firm pressure.

Congestion

Venous congestion or lymphatic stasis by prolonged early dependency or proximal constricting dressings will result in localized oedema preventing perfusion of the graft and resulting in failure. FTSG may show superficial desquamation and may manage to survive if congestion is relieved.

Pressure

Excessive pressure (>30 mmHg) on the surface of a skin graft will cause necrosis.

Late complications

Contraction

Primary contraction is the immediate shrinkage of a graft as it is harvested, due to recoil of the elastic fibres within the dermis. Therefore, a FTSG loses approximately 40% of its original area, and an SSG contracts by about 10–20%.

Secondary contraction is clinically more significant and occurs as the graft wound heals. SSG exhibit secondary contracture more than FTSG. After wound healing, FTSG continue growing with the surrounding tissues. SSG remain in a fixed state and grow minimally compared to the surrounding tissues and therefore may cause future contractures. This may result in a functional problem, e.g. across flexor or extensor areas, or aesthetic problems due to soft tissue distortion which may require revisional surgical procedures.

Aesthetic appearance

+ **Pigmentation**—initially a graft appears erythematous, but this gradually fades. Hyperpigmentation may occur in SSG.
+ **Elasticity**—SSG lacks elasticity of normal skin, appearing thin, shiny, and darker; FTSG gives a better colour match and preserves skin elasticity. FTSG harvested from above the clavicular areas are a good colour match for the face, SSG are best avoided in the face.
+ **Aesthetic units**—must be considered when using skin grafts particularly in the face, avoiding 'patch' appearance of graft.

Skin function

As FTSG contain adnexal structures they take on the characteristics of the recipient area, e.g. sweating. SSG lack these structures and remain dry, so requiring long-term moisturization to prevent them drying and becoming keratotic.

Reinnervation

FTSG have a greater chance of reinnervation compared to SSG, with a slow recovery starting after 4–5 weeks and completed by 12–24 months. Sensory recovery of pain, light touch, cold, warm, and heat occur in that order, hence the patient needs to be aware of thermal insensitivity to avoid injury.

Flaps

A flap is a unit of tissue containing its own intravascular blood supply transferred from a donor site to a recipient site.

Classification of flaps

- Type (vascularity):
  - random (cutaneous)
  - pedicled/axial
- Technique (movement):
  - advancement
  - V–Y, Y–V
  - single pedicle
  - bipedicle
  - pivot
  - rotation
  - transposition
  - interpolation/island
  - distant
  - direct
  - tubed
  - free (microvascular anastomosis)
- Tissue (composition):
  - cutaneous
  - fasciocutaneous
  - musculocutaneous
  - muscle
  - osseocutaneous
  - sensory

Complications

Flap loss

Survival of a flap is dependent on the blood supply incorporated in its design. Clinical monitoring of flaps enables the early detection of problems, sophisticated monitors (laser Doppler) are also available. Ensure patient is physiologically stable at all times postoperatively: well hydrated, warm, and pain-free. Reasons for flap loss are mainly:

- **Flap design**—partial (distal) flap loss is the most common complication with flaps. The flap designed may be too large for the intrinsic blood supply. Other causes of vascular pedicle compromise due to extrinsic compression from dressings, sutures, adjacent haematoma, or mechanical trauma may lead to more extensive total flap loss. A delay procedure to divide part of the vascular supply to a flap, prior to transfer, allows an increase in the surviving length of the flap. Proper flap design, avoiding pedicle compression, tight wound closure, and venous congestion reduces the incidence of pedicled flap loss. Early stages of distal ischaemia may be reversed by correcting the underlying cause, e.g. evacuation of a haematoma or the release of a tight suture.

- **Arterial insufficiency**—clinical examination of free flaps in particular reveals pale, mottled skin. Capillary refill is sluggish (>2 s) and demonstrated by pressing the scissors' handle on skin. Pricking the dermis with a sterile needle reveals scant dark blood or serum. Ensure adequate perfusion, circulatory blood-volume replacement, and temperature. Explore pedicle or anastomosis for intrinsic or extrinsic occlusion, which may be relieved.

- **Venous occlusion**—skin appears cyanotic or dusky. Capillary refill is brisker than normal, dermal blood is dark with rapid bleeding on pricking. Relieve venous occlusion, reduce congestion by elevation, and reduce tissue tension by releasing tight sutures. Venous engorgement may be relieved by the use of medicinal leeches—ask for help in their use.

- **Ischaemia–reperfusion injury**—following ischaemia and the establishment of vascular perfusion, direct cytotoxic injury may result from free radicals. This is greater than the damage from the ischaemia itself. Hence, it is important to limit the period of ischaemia to the flap.

- **No-reflow phenomenon**—following prolonged ischaemia (>12 h), vascular obstruction within the microcirculation becomes irreversible and it is not possible to re-establish perfusion; this precedes flap death.

- **Infection**—this is associated with initial necrosis of the flap and may lead to further flap loss. Flaps are generally resistant to infection. Treat with systemic antibiotics and wound excision.

- **Tissue contour**—following flap inset and healing, tissue contour irregularities may require flap debulking/thinning to match the surrounding tissue.

- **Donor site**—wound and closure problems may occur at the donor site.

Total loss of large pedicled or free flaps are a complex problem to deal with and require an expert opinion regarding reconstruction, therefore seek help early.

Chapter 23
Wound complications (after laparotomy and surgery in general)

Laparotomy wound failure

Wound dehiscence

Wound dehiscence (*burst abdomen*) is a serious complication which carries a mortality of 15–30%. It usually occurs 6–10 days postoperatively, and is often heralded by the 'pink' sign—a discharge of serosanguinous fluid on to or beneath the wound dressing. The patient is often aware of something 'giving way', but usually has little in the way of systemic disturbance until the abdominal contents begin to protrude on to the surface. It should always be assumed that there is disruption along the full length of the deep layers of the wound. This really should be historical—the complication represents technical failure: knots slip (inexperienced surgeon), tissues tear (musculofacial bites are not large enough), suture material breaks (inadequate choice of suture). Continuous mass closure using a synthetic monofilament polymer (polypropylene is the best) with wide bites, that achieve the theoretical 'gold standard' of 1:4 wound length:suture length, should minimize the complication to less than 1%.

Management involves resuscitation with establishment of venous access, administration of suitable analgesia (and an anxiolytic if necessary), and covering of the exposed viscera with a sterile, saline-moistened dressing. Antibiotics have no proven effect. Passing a nasogastric tube may be dangerous because the patient has probably already started dietary intake and it risks the induction of vomiting. Induced retching may cause further protrusion of viscera from the wound with the risk of inhalation. After careful induction of anaesthesia, a nasogastric tube can be passed more safely if considered necessary.

The technique of resuture is similar to the placement of all-layers, deep tension sutures (which have no place in elective primary suture). With muscle relaxation and general anaesthesia, all remaining suture material can be removed and the fibrinous adhesions between the bowel and abdominal wall gently separated to allow suture placement. Sutures should be 1 cm apart and incorporate a 2-cm bite. Protruding viscera must be protected from the needle when taking bites and not be allowed to slip in between the sutures. A number 2 BP prolene with a rubber stent is probably the best suture, with some interrupted skin sutures between to tidy the wound edges. A second attempt at mass closure may be made if the tissues are deemed capable of holding sutures.

Incisional hernias

When incisional hernias are full length, they probably represent a covert dehiscence where the skin is the only layer to heal. Smaller incisional hernias may follow deep wound infections, but they can keep presenting over 5 years postoperatively. It is possible that sutures have an ischaemic or 'cheese-wire' effect to allow the defect to appear. It is the smaller necked hernias that are most likely to be symptomatic and be at risk of irreducibility, bowel obstruction, and strangulation. The cosmetic appearance is another indication for surgery. The skin over large incisional hernias may ulcerate. Approximately 10–15% of laparotomy wounds are followed by an incisional hernia and one-third will need repair. Recurrence rates after repair are even higher, 20–40%.

The most successful repairs follow the use of a permanent mesh; prolene is the most popular. This may be supplemented with fascial repair. Mass closure and the keel repairs have the worst results. Mesh repairs can be an onlay graft, the most popular, or as an interposition subfascial extraperitoneal placement (or both with large hernias). Tension-free repair is important.

Suture sinuses, knots, and wound pain

These may occur after laparotomy closure and require wound exploration, usually with a local anaesthetic (but a general anaesthetic may be needed), to excise the offending suture or knot. There is no clear risk of wound failure following this. All complications are less common with the introduction of effective antibiotic prophylaxis and the avoidance of braided materials, particularly silk which is biodegradable and causes an intense tissue reaction. After laparotomy, closure with continuous polymeric monofilaments such as polypropylene (non-absorbable) or polydioxanone suture (absorbable) give the least complications.

Wound pain is complex and may be the cause of litigation. After hernia repair it has been attributed to neuroma formation or chronic inflammation (osteitis pubis). The cause may not be clear and may need the involvement of a pain clinic. Post-herniorrhaphy wound pain is less common after mesh or endoscopic repair, although the latter rarely has been associated with nerve injury (e.g. femoral nerve).

Numbness or paraesthesia are common complications. They occur under hernia and upper abdominal roof-top scars and should be considered when taking consent.

Wounds that involve undercutting the skin, rather than ensuring an incision is made at right angles to the skin surface, may develop necrosis at the edge. Care should be made when making long incisions in the leg for saphenous vein harvest, for coronary artery bypass, and around the umbilicus prior to paraumbilical repair. Healing can be delayed and there is a risk of exogenous infection.

Chapter 24
Complications of neurosurgery and spinal surgery

Craniotomy

Craniotomy is the access to the skull contents, and therefore the basis of intracranial neurosurgery. Any type of brain surgery carries a risk of approximately 1% of death and a 5% risk of permanent morbidity. Most acute complications will occur within 6 hours of surgery.

Immediate complications

Haemorrhage

Bleeding can be anticipated from a number of sites: bone edges, meningeal vessels, and dural venous sinuses. Haemorrhage from the bone edges is reduced with bone wax. The meningeal vessels can be controlled with meticulous diathermy. If the venous sinuses are breached, the bleeding must be controlled and repaired with a free muscle graft. If hypotensive anaesthesia has been employed the blood pressure must be normalized before closing the skull, as it is usually a generalized oozing (rather than a single vessel) that produces extradural and intradural clots.

Air embolus

This is a rare but potential complication, particularly of posterior fossa craniotomy when the patient is placed in the sitting position. The prominent intraosseous venous channels are breached during craniotomy, with the risk of air entry into the systemic circulation. A sudden fall in end-tidal PCO_2 is usually the only warning. Emergency treatment involves manual compression of the internal jugular veins while hyperinflating the lungs. This encourages back-bleeding, allowing time to insert bone wax to the cut bone ends.

Cerebral oedema

This should not be a significant problem with modern anaesthetic techniques.

Intermediate complications

Cerebrospinal fluid fistula

If detected at the time of surgery, dural tears need careful repair either by direct closure with resorbable sutures or onlay grafting (using pericranium or fascia lata). The major threat is meningitis.

Postoperative pyrexia

An elevated temperature within the first 36–48 hours is due to blood in the subarachnoid space, or related to the area of operated brain (i.e. hyperpyrexia due to hypothalamic surgery). Pyrexia after the third day is due to infection and a full sepsis screen is required. It must be remembered that urinary tract infections are common, since these patients are catheterized perioperatively. The rate of wound infection is low (3–5%), but most studies show that prophylactic antibiotics reduce this incidence.

Meningitis

This is a constant threat. The features of meningism and a rise in temperature after surgery mandate an immediate lumbar puncture. Samples should be cultured and antibiotics commenced (broad spectrum) even before microbiological confirmation. A CSF Gram stain containing <200 white blood cells/ml can be accepted as normal, representing a reaction to blood in the subarachnoid space; a higher count is abnormal and suggests infection.

Periorbital oedema

Seen in relation to coronal, hemicoronal, and frontal flaps. More related to individual susceptibility rather than technique, it therefore varies in extent between patients. Caused by either oedema or haematoma, it is an important consideration because it obscures eye signs.

Epilepsy

All craniotomies, even burr holes, carry a small risk of triggering epilepsy. This risk is dependent on the nature of the lesion and the degree of cortical damage during surgery. There is a school of thought that prophylactic anticonvulsants should be prescribed for all patients undergoing craniotomy.

Late complications

Deformity

Craniotomy is destructive and, although the largest pieces of bone are replaced, defects can occur. This is especially prominent in the frontal region. Reconstruction with custom-made acrylic or titanium plates can be achieved.

Osteomyelitis

Osteomyelitis is suspected when a chronically discharging sinus occurs months after surgery. It is a clinical diagnosis, as radiographic findings are subtle. The sequestrum needs to be fully excised, which normally requires removal of the entire craniotomy flap. This produces a defect that requires late reconstruction (see Cranioplasty below).

Cranioplasty

This procedure is performed for cosmetic rather than clinical indications. It involves the insertion of a prefabricated plate, either acrylic or metal, to replace absent skull bone. Its complications are less than that of a craniotomy.

Immediate complications

These include haemorrhage with a similar risk as for craniotomy.

Intermediate complications

Delayed haemorrhage

Bleeding from under the plate occurs very rarely. This is strictly an extradural haematoma and is managed by surgical evacuation.

Infection

This is the most significant complication, seen in 5–10% of cases. Localized pain, swelling, cellulitis, and sinus formation all suggest plate infection. Extrusion of the plate can occur. Conservative management normally fails and it requires definitive plate removal.

Skin necrosis

Sharp edges or plate movement can cause skin-pressure ulceration.

Late complications

Residual deformity

Despite reconstruction, some patients are not content with the result.

Psychological

Surgical or traumatic deformity of the skull can have significant effects on the patient's body self-image. This may be the reason for the patient presenting for surgery, but it may also continue afterwards. This is very difficult to manage, as there are many different presentations.

Acoustic neuroma surgery

The majority of patients with an acoustic neuroma require surgery, unless they are unfit for the procedure.

Immediate complications

Haemorrhage

Postoperative haemorrhage and haematoma are the most serious complications. It is a clinical diagnosis and should be anticipated in the ITU setting, and should be suspected if the patient shows features of rising intracranial pressure (deteriorating conscious level, rising blood pressure). Re-opening the wound is mandatory.

Hearing loss

This is an unavoidable consequence of surgery in the cerebellopontine (CP) region and the patient must be warned prior to surgery. It is generally accepted that tumour resection should not be compromised to save hearing that is already affected, which may be irredeemable anyway. It occurs in all patients undergoing the translabyrinthine approach, and tends to occur despite attempted 'hearing conservation' procedures. It is normally impossible to preserve hearing if the tumour is larger than 2.5 cm. It is possible to preserve some hearing in approximately 50% of cases for tumours less than 2.5 cm.

Intermediate complications

Facial nerve damage

The facial nerve is at risk during surgery in the CP angle. Up to 30% will have temporary or partial facial weakness. Long-term recovery is anticipated for most patients, with approximately 5% having permanent weakness. This is tumour size-dependent: the larger the tumour, the greater the risk. The main concern is loss of the protective blinking reflex, which exposes the eye to the risk of corneal exposure. Eye protection is mandatory. Mechanical protection, such as lubrication (e.g. hypromellose eye drops) and eye pads, should be provided. If the weakness persists, temporary tarsorrhaphy or upper-eyelid gold weights should be considered.

Trigeminal nerve paraesthesia

Loss of corneal sensation predisposes to corneal exposure and abrasion.

Meningitis

This is an infrequent complication (5–8%), mainly due to the introduction of broad-spectrum prophylactic antibiotics. Postoperative pyrexia warrants a lumbar puncture and CSF microscopy.

Dysphagia

This is a transient but frequently observed finding. It is commonly seen in patients with profound facial nerve weakness. The risk is aspiration and subsequent aspiration pneumonia.

Raised intracranial pressure

Surgery requires opening the dura, and the risk of a temporary subdural CSF collection is possible. This has an indirect compressive effect and elevates the intracranial pressure. Managed by daily lumbar puncture unless hydrocephalus develops (very rare), which requires a ventriculoperitoneal shunt.

Cerebrospinal fluid fistula

Sudden CSF rhinorrhoea must be taken seriously. CSF may escape into the mastoid process, discharge into the middle ear, through the Eustachian tube, and drains into the posterior nasal fossa. In some cases it settles spontaneously. While conservative management (prophylactic antibiotics, repeated lumbar punctures or a lumbar drain) can be tried for a short period, it is advisable to return the patient to theatre to identify the source.

Dizziness

Imbalance and dizziness are reported due to loss of vestibular function, although it is not a significant problem as vestibular function was already reduced prior to surgery.

Late complications

Recurrence

Complete tumour resection can not be guaranteed. Recurrence is always a possibility.

Lumbar puncture

Lumbar puncture allows access to the cerebrospinal fluid for diagnostic purposes (e.g. bacterial meningitis, subarachnoid haemorrhage, demyelinating conditions) and for therapeutic reasons (e.g. drug instillation, CSF removal in benign intracranial hypertension).

Complications

These include the following.

Dry tap

Failure to enter the subarachnoid space may be related to scarring and fibrosis from previous surgery, arachnoiditis, or anatomical anomalies.

Headache

Extradural leakage of CSF, normally caused by multiple attempts at dural puncture, causes downward traction of the brainstem. This is posturally dependent, with increased symptoms when standing or sitting. The headache can be severe and is relieved by lying flat. VIth cranial nerve palsy and tinnitus have also been reported. It can be managed by a venous blood patch, with 20 ml of autologous blood being injected into the epidural space under full aseptic conditions.

Subdural haematoma

Bleeding into the subdural space should be suspected if the patient experiences severe, persistent headache, fluctuating conscious level, and new focal neurology. Requires a confirmatory CT scan and referral to a neurosurgical unit.

Cervical laminectomy

Cervical laminectomy necessitates removal of a portion of bone and stabilization of the spine with a bone graft. The complications are those of any major procedure, plus the complications specific to the procedure and the bone graft. The specific complications are increased because of the anatomical constraints encountered in gaining access to the cervical spine. Anterior, posterior, and combined anterior–posterior approaches have been described, each with their unique pattern of complications.

Immediate complications

Haemorrhage

Intraoperative haemorrhage is encountered if the dissection is performed too far laterally and the vertebral artery is damaged. Bleeding is difficult to control and necessitates wide exposure of the vessel to allow repair. Ligation should be avoided unless bleeding can not be controlled.

Damage to other vessels

The anterior approach requires dissection of the carotid sheath, with lateral retraction of the carotid artery and internal jugular vein. These structures can be damaged.

Perforation of trachea and oesophagus

This is a rare complication. The trachea and oesophagus are retracted medially to allow access to the anterior aspect of the cervical spine and can be torn by sharp edges on the retractor.

Neurological injury

Surgery at the spinal cord level naturally has an associated morbidity. Complete quadriplegia, partial paralysis, and isolated nerve root injuries are all possibilities. The commonest complication is damage to the nerve root, which produces fibrosis and persistent pain or paraesthesia. The incidence is reduced when the procedures are performed in specialist spinal units.

Anaesthetic problems

The posterior approach requires the patient to be placed in the prone or knee–chest position. This can restrict mechanical ventilation, requiring a higher ventilation pressure with a small risk of barotrauma. This is prevented by 'breaking' the operating table in appropriate places to reduce the constriction on the chest.

Intermediate complications

Wound infection

There is a small risk due to inadequate aseptic technique; prophylactic antibiotics and thorough wound irrigation should be employed at the end of the procedure. Occurs in approximately 1% of reported cases.

Haematoma

This is a potential risk that is avoided by meticulous haemostasis. Neck drains are not routinely recommended.

Dysphagia

This is a transient problem caused by retraction of the oesophagus.

Extradural haematoma

This is an uncommon (0.2%) condition from which a full recovery can be anticipated. Suspicion should be raised if the patient develops pain, paraesthesia, and a neurological palsy during the immediate postoperative period. These symptoms can be uni- or bilateral, regardless of the side of surgery. Detection requires close monitoring of all spinal patients in the initial 6 postoperative hours. Normally requires re-operation and leads to a delay in recovery.

Vocal cord paralysis

The recurrent laryngeal nerve is an anatomically consistent structure, running within the tracheo-oesophageal groove. It is susceptible to traction injury, but is also at risk of ligation and diathermy injury at the time of surgery. Injury to one nerve results in a hoarse voice and is temporary if due to traction.

Hypoglossal nerve injury

The hypoglossal nerve descends through the neck between the internal carotid artery and internal jugular vein. Upward retraction to gain access to the upper cervical vertebrae can produce a traction injury. Alternatively, as the nerve runs close to the facial vein, venous bleeding may obscure the nerve and accidental diathermy damage may arise. Paralysis of the ipsilateral tongue produces deviation towards the affected side.

Oedema

This is an unusual complication. Any neck surgery can produce oedema with potential airway compromise. There have been incidents where an emergency tracheostomy has been performed.

Blindness

A series of case reports have recorded this very unusual complication. It appears to have no known aetiology.

Bone graft

The commonest complications involving the bone graft are infections, non-union, and deformity induced by incorrect angulation on insertion. There are also the usual donor-site problems (pain, infection, and restricted mobility).

Horner's syndrome

The cardinal signs of ptosis, meiosis, enophthalmos, and ipsilateral anhydrosis can be identified in <1% of patients. Due to interruption of the sympathetic supply to the face.

Late complications

Relapse

The current vogue for pedicle screws and bone grafting, with or without metal cages, ensures a stable result. Relapse of symptoms may arise with failure of the mechanical fixation, infection, or disc degeneration at other cervical levels.

Lumbar laminectomy

Lumbar surgery is a more commonly performed procedure, which is designed to relieve nerve root pressure caused by disc herniation or spinal stenosis. The complications show similarities to those of cervical and thoracic laminectomy, but the incidence of these complications is better understood.

Immediate complications

Neurological damage

Two particular forms of injury are identified. The commonest is nerve root damage (affecting 1% of patients), which produces residual footdrop or weak plantar flexion. The second, more serious, is the cauda equina syndrome, precipitated by surgery. Compression of the cauda equina produces pain, dermatomal sensory changes (genital area particularly affected), and altered bladder and bowel function. The patients commonly retain urine and faeces. This is a neurological emergency.

Intermediate complications

Wound infection

Seen in 3.2% of cases. Reduced by aseptic technique, prophylactic antibiotics, and thorough wound irrigation before closure (some centres favour the pulse-lavage system).

Deep infection

Disc space infection is less commonly seen, but a potential hazard. Affects 1.1% of cases.

CSF fistula

Unrecognized dural tears allow the escape of CSF. The patients complain of persistent headaches.

Thromboembolic disease

The incidence of pulmonary embolism is 1%. Anticoagulation is avoided in spinal surgery and the incidence is related to postoperative immobility. The incidence of symptomatic deep vein thrombosis after lumber spinal surgery is 0.3% and this is dependent on the approach adopted, with the majority related to anterior fusion. Simple mechanical prophylaxis is adequate for posterior procedures, but is not protective for combined anterior and posterior spinal surgery. There remains a need for a well-designed, randomized controlled study to define the efficiency of thromboprophy-laxis in elective spinal surgery.

Sciatica

Chronic, persistent root pain can be seen in a small proportion of patients.

Extradural haematoma

See Cervical laminectomy above.

Late complications

Relapse

5% of patient will prolapse again at the same disc level.

Thoracic laminectomy

As the thoracic discs lie anterior to the spinal cord, surgical access is difficult and the complication rate is therefore significant. A number of approaches have been described, either anterior, thoracotomy, or costotransversectomy. The complications are similar to laminectomy at other sites.

Immediate complications

Neurological damage

Paraplegia is a disastrous complication. Commonly due to an incorrect approach, where the cord can not be safely retracted because the disc is anteriorly prolapsed.

Ventriculoperitoneal shunt insertion

Raised intracranial pressure can be managed by draining cerebrospinal fluid from the ventricular system into the peritoneal cavity. This is a neurosurgical procedure involving a skull burr hole.

Immediate complications

Haemorrhage

Bleeding from the dural vessels must be controlled at the time of burr hole preparation.

Intermediate complications

Intracerebral haemorrhage

Seen in <1% of procedures.

Infection

Early infection rates are 1–3%. Careful wound handling, prophylactic antibiotics, and an aseptic technique reduce this risk.

Shunt obstruction

Seen in 1–5% of reported series. Need to ensure the tube is not kinked when inserted. Requires replacement.

Complications of head injury

Immediate

Death

Statistics show that 0.5% of all patients with head injuries die and that 20% with head injuries are admitted to hospital, 2% of whom will die. Death is normally the result of the primary brain injury.

Cerebral oedema

Traumatic oedema increases the intracranial pressure, which in turn causes herniation and brainstem compression. Ultimately this can precipitate a respiratory arrest.

Intermediate

Epilepsy

This is the most disabling complication. The risk is greater after subdural than extradural haematoma (18% vs. 2%). Two forms are recognized: early (within the first week) and late (after the first week). Early seizures affect 5% of patients hospitalized with head injuries, they tend to be focal and predispose to post-traumatic epilepsy. The significant risk is status epilepticus (10% of patients). Late seizures have a low incidence of long-term epilepsy. The social and professional implications are obvious, restricting eligibility to hold a driving licence.

Seizures require immediate treatment because of the risk of cerebral hypoxia and venous congestion, which can aggravate primary brain injury by raising the intracranial pressure.

Cranial nerve injury

Traumatic cranial nerve injury depends on site of the skull fracture. Nerves are commonly damaged as they traverse foramina.

CSF fistula

Otorrhoea and rhinorrhoea may be difficult to detect. The major risk is ascending infection leading to meningitis. This may develop years after injury when the patient has forgotten having a CSF fistula. A proven fistula is initially managed conservatively with bed rest, lumbar drain, and prophylactic antibiotics. The majority will stop spontaneously. Persistent leak requires surgery: either endoscopic (frontal sinus) or craniotomy and dural repair.

Meningitis

Suspected meningitis is the only indication for lumbar puncture after head injury. Treat immediately with intravenous benzylpenicillin (2.4 g/every 4 h), chloramphenicol (12.5 mg/kg every 6 h), and metronidazole (500 mg/every 8 h) while awaiting microbiological culture and sensitivity testing.

Cerebral abscess

Abscesses present with the symptoms of a space-occupying lesion (focal signs, headache, decreased conscious level) or post-traumatic epilepsy. Commonest organism is *Staphylococcus aureus*. Small abscesses can be managed with antibiotics (fusidic acid and erythromycin) or drainage. Prophylactic anticonvulsants are recommended due to the high incidence of post-traumatic epilepsy.

Subdural empyema

Rare complication. Requires craniotomy and drainage. Significant risk of venous sinus thrombosis, intracerebral abscesses, and meningitis.

Fat embolism

Head injuries can be combined with other injuries, commonly orthopaedic long-bone fractures. Release of marrow tissue into the systemic circulation can produce neurological and respiratory symptoms. Confusion, agitation, decreased conscious level, and seizures may all be mistaken for raised intracranial pressure. Usually diagnosed when the characteristic truncal petechial rash appears (day 3). Managed by ventilatory support, systemic antibiotics, and diuretics.

Caroticocavernous fistula

This is an abnormal communication between the cavernous sinus and internal carotid artery. Onset occurs a few days after head injury, including a trivial blunt head trauma. The patient complains of a noise within the head that synchronizes with the carotid. A bruit is easily demonstrated by auscultation over the eye pulse because of the high-flow fistula into the ophthalmic veins. Pain and proptosis develop and the eye may show a visible pulsation. The eye shows marked chemosis and conjunctival suffusion. There is an increased risk of corneal ulceration due to lid retraction.

Diagnosis is confirmed by angiography.

Treatment is variable and depends on symptoms. Spontaneous resolution can occur, while in others the patient accepts the symptoms. Surgery is reserved for extreme symptoms (e.g. unsightly proptosis, very loud bruit). Endovascular embolization of the fistula has superseded carotid artery ligation.

Intracranial haematoma

Affects 1–2% of all admissions. Intradural haematoma predisposes to post-traumatic epilepsy.

Late

Post-traumatic hydrocephalus

Commonly associated with subarachnoid haemorrhage. Blood within the subarachnoid space can produce adhesions in the region of the tentorium or obstruct the arachnoid granulations. This disrupts CSF circulation. May require shunt insertion (see above, Ventriculoperitoneal shunt complications).

Rebleed

Continued haemorrhage produces worsening symptoms. Requires surgical management.

Psychiatric

Generalized brain injury leaves subtle personality changes. A decline in intelligence, disinhibition, loss of social status, and a reduced attention span are frequently detected.

Chronic subdural haematoma

This follows minor trauma in the elderly. Males are affected more frequently than females. Cortical atrophy permits brain mobility and the bridging veins are easily torn after minor injury. May be uni- or bilateral.

The diagnosis can be confused with dementia or stroke. Presents as headache, reduced intellect, hemiparesis, and fluctuating conscious level. Evacuation of the haematoma can lead to a full recovery.

Post-traumatic amnesia

Associated with a closed head injury.

Diabetes insipidus

Cranial diabetes insipidus is characterized by polydipsia and polyuria, leading to increased plasma osmolality and hypernatraemia. Diagnosed by the desmopressin test.

Postconcussion syndrome

This is a constellation of symptoms that persist following head injury: headache, dizziness, impaired concentration and memory, anxiety, and depression. Improves with supportive care (and after conclusion of litigation cases!).

Chapter 25
Complications after gynaecological surgery

Introduction

The majority of obstetric and gynaecological operations are performed on relatively young and healthy women. There is a low incidence of underlying medical conditions and major complications are comparatively few. Many operations lend themselves to day-case surgery, which avoids immobilization and is associated with a low risk of hospital-acquired infections. The rational use of prophylactic antibiotics and anticoagulation reduces postoperative morbidity. The commonly used transverse, suprapubic incision has a low dehisence rate and heals well.

The cervix is a natural barrier to infection. Instrumentation of the cervix predisposes to infection of the genital tract. Bladder catheterization is performed before major obstetric and gynaecological surgery and predisposes to postoperative urinary tract infection, which rapidly resolves once the catheter is removed.

Obstetrics

Caesarean section

Reduced cardiac output from compression of the inferior vena cava by the uterus is prevented by a left lateral tilt of the patient whilst supine on the operating table. A lower uterine segment incision is usually chosen because complications are fewer than with a vertical incision. If incidental pelvic pathology is found, it is left in place until the uterine arteries have shrunk to the non-pregnant state to reduce the risk of haemorrhage. Surgical intervention, if required, is undertaken on a later date.

Complications

Haemorrhage

This is the commonest complication. Blood loss is notoriously difficult to estimate, particularly when mixed with amniotic fluid. It is usual to lose 300–500 ml in a normal Caesarean section (more than 500 ml is defined as a postpartum haemorrhage).

Causes

The commonest cause of haemorrhage is failure of the uterus to contract adequately (uterine atonia) after delivery of the baby. Predisposing factors include prolonged labour, uterine overdistension (e.g. twins), or a history of postpartum haemorrhage.

Too high an incision on the uterus cuts into muscle rather than the collagenous lower segment. Low placental implantation causes large vessels, which traverse the lower segment, to bleed profusely if cut. As the baby is delivered, the incision may be extended laterally into the uterine arteries thereby causing further haemorrhage. Occasionally, a broad ligament haematoma may ensue. Bleeding from retained placental tissue is prevented by checking that the uterine cavity is empty before uterine closure.

Clinical features and management

Blood loss from the pregnant uterus can be considerable before the classical signs of haemorrhage, tachycardia, hypotension, or clamminess appear. Once these signs have occurred urgent help is needed. Blood should be taken for a full blood count, clotting, and cross-matching for a minimum of 2 units of whole blood. Intravenous fluids need to be given rapidly through two large-bore cannulas (16-gauge minimum) when haemorrhage is suspected, starting with crystalloid but with early resort to whole-blood transfusion once blood is available. Severe haemorrhage requires consultant participation: often a combination of obstetrician, anaesthetist, and haematologist (the latter especially where there are concurrent clotting disorders when specialized blood products will be required).

Central venous-pressure monitoring is advisable in cases of severe haemorrhage and requires patient transfer to the high-dependency unit (HDU). In cases of uterine atonia, the surgeon can massage the uterus to produce contractions. Oxytocin, 10 IU as an intravenous bolus may be given, followed by an infusion of 40 IU in 500 ml saline. In the presence of continuing haemorrhage, up to five intramuscular doses of 0.25 mg carboprost (a prostaglandin), a minimum of 15 min apart, are given primarily into the thigh or directly into the uterine muscle.

If bleeding persists despite surgical repair, the presence of adequate uterine contractions, and the correction of clotting disorders, life-saving procedures must then be attempted. Some obstetricians opt for ligation of the internal iliac arteries, while others proceed directly to hysterectomy, which is more likely to arrest the haemorrhage.

Bladder damage

Perforation of the bladder is a particular risk of a repeat Caesarean section because the bladder is adherent to the previous scar. Vesicovaginal fistula occurs rarely, when inadvertent damage to the bladder goes unnoticed or with severe local infection causing tissue necrosis. Ureteric damage is rarer but may still occur.

Management

The bladder is repaired in two layers, followed by 7–10 days of urethral catheter drainage. Urological assistance should be sought for ureteric damage. Fistula repair is an interval procedure and would usually be undertaken by a consultant urologist as an elective procedure.

Infection

Infection of the wound, endometrial cavity, and urinary tract are common but reduced by prophylactic antibiotics.

Thromboembolic disease

This is the leading cause of maternal mortality. Both clotting factors and the incidence of thromboembolic disease are increased in pregnancy and the puerperium. Caesarean section further increases this risk. The Royal College of Obstetricians and Gynaecologists (RCOG) has produced guidelines on the prevention of thromboembolism. It is recommended that prophylactic subcutaneous fractionated, low molecular-weight heparin is administered until the patient is discharged—e.g. tinzaparin 3500 units once daily. The first dose is given preoperatively, but not before the siting of regional anaesthesia. Graduated elasticated stockings are worn by the patient at high risk. The patient is mobilized on the first postoperative day.

Mendelsohn's syndrome

This is where regurgitated stomach contents with a low pH are inhaled during anaesthesia causing acute pneumonitis which may lead to death.

The risk is increased in pregnancy because intubation is more difficult due to neck swelling. There is increased intra-abdominal pressure on the stomach and its contents and, combined with a reduced rate of stomach emptying, the risk of regurgitation of gastric contents is appreciable.

Prevention

Use regional anaesthesia preferentially. Oral intake should be reduced during labour to sips of fluid only. Alkali (as 30 ml sodium citrate) is swallowed prior to the induction of anaesthesia, with patients undergoing elective operations receiving H_2-receptor blockers the evening and morning prior to Caesarean section. The consultant or senior obstetrics-experienced anaesthetist should be aided by a trained anaesthetic assistant; cricoid pressure is applied and intubation performed.

'Vaginal' Caesarean section

Occasionally, if a Caesarean section is performed at full dilatation, the uterine incision may be made so low that it is actually through the top of the vagina. No problems usually arise but large venous plexuses are nearby and access is difficult.

Episiotomy

+ **Haemorrhage**—this can be considerable, especially if there are perineal varicose veins. Haematomas are not common but do cause pain; if large, they need surgical evacuation with a drain left in place for 24 hours. It is unusual to be able to find the actual bleeding point.

+ **Wound breakdown**—when superficial this is frequent and heals by secondary intention, but a larger breakdown should be resutured once the wound is clean.

+ **Infection**—is also mostly superficial and does not require antibiotics.

+ **Chronic dyspareunia**—most cases resolve spontaneously. Surgical widening of the introitus (Fenton's procedure) can be performed as a day-case procedure if indicated.

Gynaecology

Day-case surgery

Hysteroscopy, dilatation of the cervix, and endometrial biopsy/curettage

Uterine perforation

If this occurs it is usually at the uterine fundus and is more common in the postmenopausal uterus. A bolus of antibiotic is required but overnight stay is unnecessary. The vast majority have no significant consequences, but immediate laparotomy may be necessary if intraperitoneal damage is suspected.

Tearing of cervix

This happens if undue force is required to dilate the cervix. Bleeding stops spontaneously and no treatment is normally necessary. Cervical dilatation can also create a false cervical passage, but is prevented if the uterine sound or smaller dilator finds the direction of the cervical canal before applying force.

Uterine bleeding

This is rarely a problem and settles spontaneously.

Suction termination of pregnancy/evacuation of retained products of conception

Similar complications to those described immediately above do occur, but they may be more serious because more cervical dilatation is required and the pregnant uterus is softer.

Haemorrhage

This occurs because of retained products; the uterus fails to contract or vessels in the myometrium are opened by the curettage. Care must be taken to ensure that the uterine cavity is empty. Oxytocin, 10 IU, should be given intramuscularly as a routine, followed by an infusion of 40 IU in 500 ml saline if necessary. Bimanual rubbing of the uterus can be performed to induce contraction and 0.25 mg carboprost given (see above) if severe bleeding continues. Transfusion may be necessary.

Infection

In addition to the standard risk of infection from uterine instrumentation, there is a high rate of *Chlamydia* sp. infection in young women undergoing termination. All should be screened preoperatively or, alternatively, all given prophylactic antibiotics (e.g. IV azithromycin 1 g) at induction of anaesthesia.

Incomplete evacuation or continuation of pregnancy

Failure is most likely if suction termination is performed at less than 7 weeks (medical management is the method of choice at less than 7 weeks). It should be confirmed, intraoperatively, that products are aspirated and that the quantity of products removed is in keeping with gestation. Retained products present with bleeding, pain, or symptoms of infection, usually within the first week following the operation, but not after the next menstrual period. Examination is often unhelpful in differentiating between retained products and infection, with a closed cervical os and bulky uterus being present in both. Retained products tend to be associated with heavier bleeding. Ultrasound scan, although frequently done, is a poor discriminator between blood clot and retained products. Endocervical and high vaginal swabs should be taken and antibiotics given, with re-evaluation after 24–48 hours. Do not rush into re-evaluation unless there is a good clinical suspicion of products remaining.

Rhesus isoimmunization

All rhesus-negative women are given 250 IU of anti-D antibodies within 72 hours of termination or miscarriage. Rarely, this is forgotten or fails; if the fetus is rhesus-positive, isoimmunization can occur.

Psychological distress

There is considerable variation in women's response to pregnancy loss. Do not underestimate the degree of distress that may be experienced after a miscarriage, and avoid insensitive management. Early-pregnancy units, which allow more time for discussion/counselling, may provide a better service than the busy general-ward staff.

Bowel damage

If the uterus is perforated, bowel is at risk of being sucked into the suction curette and uterus, with the potential for serious complications. If this goes unnoticed, severe peritonitis can lead to death. Early laparotomy is necessary to inspect the bowel and undertake repair.

Diagnostic laparoscopy

Minor complications are often seen because so many laparoscopies are performed. Occasionally the consequences of laparoscopy are serious. Inserting instruments 'blindly' into the abdominal cavity risks damaging underlying structures, e.g. an overinflated stomach or full bladder, bowel, or vessel. Gas insufflation may cause cardiorespiratory problems. Obesity increases the technical difficulty and the risk of complication.

Bowel injury

Previous abdominal surgery increases the risk of periumbilical adhesions and bowel perforation, most commonly by the Veress needle. If adhesions are suspected, visualize the full trocar length to ensure no through-and-through bowel perforation has occurred. High insufflation pressure, an offensive smell, passage of gas per rectum, or the presence of faeces on the Veress needle may indicate that a perforation has occurred, but it may go unnoticed. However, Veress-needle injuries are usually minimal and unusual. An immediate dose of broad-spectrum antibiotics is given intravenously: the patient is informed and usually allowed home.

Trocar perforation may cause leakage from the bowel or haematoma of the bowel wall or the mesentery. Rarely, there may be visualization of the intestinal mucosa. This requires laparotomy and bowel repair. Do not remove the trocar prior to abdominal opening because it maintains a seal and can identify the site of damage.

Anterior abdominal wall insufflation

This is more likely in the obese patient. The Veress needle fails to enter the peritoneal cavity and gas distends the abdominal wall reaching to the retroperitoneum. Trocar insertion becomes hazardous. Alternatives are to perform open laparoscopy; insert the Veress needle through the vaginal posterior fornix; through the left upper abdominal quadrant; or to abandon the procedure. However, some surgeons use the technique of open insertion of the trocar with subsequent insufflation (Hassan technique), arguing that Veress-needle complications are thereby completely avoided.

Vessel injury

Intra-abdominal and retroperitoneal vessel damage (most commonly iliac) is usually inflicted by the Veress needle, but presentation with collapse may be delayed until entry into the theatre recovery room. Vascular repair, performed by a vascular surgeon, is required urgently. Lesser vessels of the omentum may be coagulated with bipolar diathermy. The iliac vessels can be avoided by keeping the Veress needle in the midline during insertion.

Abdominal wall vessels

Superficial and deep epigastric arteries may be injured by lateral trocar insertion and bleeding is rapidly obvious. It can be controlled by bipolar diathermy via the peritoneal cavity, compression with an inflated Foley catheter tip, or dissection round the trocar to find the bleeding vessel ends for ligation. Transillumination of the anterior abdominal wall with the laparoscope may highlight the vessels, but it is not always reliable. Insertion of the trocars medial to the obliterated hypogastric arteries, lateral to the site where the round ligament enters the inguinal canal, or lateral and high, almost at the level of the umbilicus, minimizes this risk.

Respiratory acidosis

This is a hazard in the patient with respiratory compromise. CO_2 is rapidly absorbed into the bloodstream and raised intra-abdominal pressure reduces movement of the diaphragm. Reduced abdominal insufflation pressure may help with completion of the procedure without delay.

Gas embolism

This is rare. Theoretically, either gas is blown through the Veress needle directly into a vessel, or a large bubble of gas passes into a cut vessel. It is reduced by using an absorbable gas such as CO_2.

Laparoscopic sterilization

Occluding clips or electrocautery are applied to the Fallopian tubes and the risks of diagnostic laparoscopy apply. Risks of electrocautery are discussed in the operative laparoscopy section below.

Failure

Reported rates vary between 1:200 and 1:500. The sterilizing clips may incompletely occlude the Fallopian tube or be applied incorrectly, most frequently to the round ligament. Recanalization of the tube can occur and is usually a feature of late failures. Medicolegal litigation frequently follows failures.

Cervical ablation/cone biopsy

Haemorrhage

Bleeding is the most common complication. Usually, it occurs in the first 24 hours, or after 10 days when it is associated with infection. Vaginal packing is often all that is required, but individual bleeding points may be cauterized or oversewn.

Infection

Bleeding, discharge, or pain secondary to pelvic infection may occur. Swabs for microbiological diagnosis are taken prior to starting broad-spectrum antibiotics.

Cervical stenosis/distortion

Problems are more common with knife conization. Identification of the cervical os may be difficult and the squamocolumnar junction may be inaccessible to smear-taking. Dilatation under anaesthetic breaks down the stenosis but smear-taking may remain awkward.

Cervical incompetence

Evidence identifying cone biopsy as causative for cervical incompetence, and leading to subsequent mid-trimester miscarriage, is poor. However, avoid large-cone biopsies in nulliparous patients if possible.

Hysteroscopic endometrial resection/laser ablation

Complication rates are related to operator experience, uterine size, and concurrent uterine pathology, commonly fibroids. Inexperienced surgeons must be supervised. New techniques, e.g. microwave or balloon ablation are alternatives.

Fluid overload

To distend the uterine cavity, glycine fluid is flushed through the cavity under pressure. Some fluid will be lost into the peritoneal cavity and absorbed. This amount can be considerable and result in serious overload with heart failure and pulmonary oedema. Glycine is also hypertonic. Careful monitoring and measurement of fluid flushed in and out is essential. Stop the operation if too much fluid has been absorbed. Diuretics can be administered and urea and electrolyte levels need checking.

Perforation

This is most likely to occur at the cornu where the uterine wall is thinnest. Surrounding structures, most commonly bowel, can be damaged. Major vessel injury has been reported with compromise to the lower limb. It is essential to keep the resectoscope under direct vision when it is 'live' and to avoid undue pressure at the cornu: the rollerball may be preferable in this region.

Endometrial regeneration

Although many women are amenorrhoeic after resection, small islands of endometrium may escape destruction, gradually enlarging over months. Menstruation may return and may be heavy (menorrhagia).

Cervical stenosis/haematometra

Resection of the endocervix may result in the canal walls sticking together as they heal. Menstrual products are then retained and may cause monthly pain. Avoid removal of endocervical epithelium.

Pregnancy

A remaining island of endometrium may allow implantation and pregnancy. Women must be informed of the need for contraception.

Marsupialization of Bartholin's cyst

Recurrence

This is all too common. It is less likely with marsupialization rather than attempted removal of a cyst or abscess. Avoid leaving the marsupialized opening too narrow.

Dyspareunia

An incision on the fold between labia majora and minor is less likely to cause dyspareunia.

Inpatient surgery—abdominal

Hysterectomy with or without bilateral salpingo-oophorectomy

Complications depend on concurrent pathology. Uterine fibroids increase the blood supply and distort the anatomy. Endometriosis and pelvic inflammatory disease may cause dense adhesions. It is wise never to start a hysterectomy until normal anatomy has been restored. Less intraoperative complications, particularly of the urinary tract, arise with subtotal hysterectomy.

Haemorrhage

The blood supply to the uterus is considerable, especially if the uterus is enlarged. All the pedicles can bleed profusely and spread into the broad ligament with haematoma formation. The vaginal angles may slip out of an often bulky pedicle, and bladder-base venous plexuses ooze with reflection of the bladder. Taking smaller pedicles will reduce bleeding from pedicles.

Infection

Prophylactic antibiotics reduce the incidence of wound, vaginal vault, and urinary tract infections.

Bladder injury

This would not be expected in a simple hysterectomy. A previous Caesarean section tethers the bladder to the lower uterus and increases the risk of bladder injury.

Vesicovaginal fistulas

Such fistulas occur rarely after difficult surgery complicated by bladder damage in conjunction with haemorrhage or infection, which leads to tissue necrosis.

Ureteric injury

This may complicate difficult cases in which the anatomy is distorted by fibroids, adhesion, or ovarian cysts. It should not occur with a simple hysterectomy.

Bowel injury

Adhesions secondary to endometriosis, pelvic inflammatory disease, or previous surgery predispose to bowel injury. Restore normal anatomy before commencing the hysterectomy. Perform a subtotal hysterectomy and consult with a general surgeon if necessary, preferably preoperatively if difficulty is anticipated.

Thromboembolic disease

Pelvic surgery predisposes particularly to this late complication. Many gynaecologists use prophylactic subcutaneous heparin, commenced immediately preoperatively.

Irritable bladder

The full consequences of hysterectomy on the bladder have not been fully evaluated. The surgery produces damage to the neural plexus around the bladder. Women may notice an increase in urinary frequency, a sense of urgency, and sometimes stress incontinence. However, these symptoms are also common in women who have not undergone hysterectomy.

Emotional sequelae

These are not well studied. Feelings of regret and resentment have probably declined as paternalistic medicine has declined, because women are now more involved in the decision to have a hysterectomy. Sadness at the loss of fertility is considered normal. The giving of adequate preoperative information is essential.

Tubo-ovarian surgery

The incidence of intraoperative complications is quite low. (See below under Laparoscopic tubo-ovarian procedures.)

Inpatient surgery—vaginal

Vaginal hysterectomy

Complications are similar to those of abdominal hysterectomy. However, bowel and ureteric injury are less frequent because the vaginal route is usually not attempted in the presence of pelvic adhesions.

Pedicle loss and haemorrhage

Both may require abdominal incision and exploration. This is infrequent but is more likely when a surgeon is learning the technique or access is particularly difficult.

Vault haematoma

This is the commonest complication and presents with mild pyrexia. An oedematous induration is palpated at the vaginal vault on examination per vaginum. Antibiotics are prescribed after taking a high vaginal swab and progression to a pelvic abscess is rare. If it does, a finger may be inserted through the vaginal vault to release the pus if it is clearly pointing there; otherwise consider ultrasound-guided percutaneous drainage.

Vault prolapse/enterocele

Occurs months to years later. The true incidence is not known but has been quoted as 6%, although it is probably higher. Variations in technique have been described in an attempt to prevent it. Traditional repair of enterocele does not have good success rates. Greater success is achieved by tethering the vaginal vault to the sacrum (sacrocolpopexy) or to the ischial spines (ischiocolpopexy).

Sexual dysfunction

Vaginal hysterectomy should not give rise to dysfunction. Problems may arise if posterior or anterior vaginal repair is performed in conjunction with vaginal hysterectomy that results in overly shortening or narrowing the vagina.

Vaginal prolapse repair

Operations included are enterocele, anterior and posterior repair, with or without perineorrhaphy. Preoperative oestrogen administration for several weeks thickens vaginal tissues and possibly improves postoperative healing.

Urinary retention

Retention is particularly likely with posterior repair and perineorrhaphy. The bladder is routinely drained, either by suprapubic or urethral catheter, for 24–48 h.

Haemorrhage

Excessive electrocautery and ligation should be avoided when controlling bleeding because it may cause too much tissue necrosis. A vaginal pack may be left in place for 24 h postoperatively to control persistent oozing.

Bladder perforation

Injury is rare but the risk is increased with repeat surgery.

Rectal perforation/fistula

Care must be taken to avoid rectal damage when separating the posterior vaginal skin off the prerectal fascia. Unrecognized injury may lead to fistula formation. Whilst closing the peritoneal cavity during enterocele repair, small bowel can be ensnared and form an adhesion to the vaginal vault: some surgeons no longer close the peritoneum.

Recurrent prolapse

This is quite common and is difficult to repair in the elderly patient with thin tissues.

Recurrent incontinence

An anterior repair was originally thought to cure both prolapse and stress incontinence. However, objective evidence of an incontinence cure occurs in only 40% of patients. It is preferable to perform a suprapubic procedure in cases of genuine stress incontinence, which have success rates as high as 80–90%.

Sexual dysfunction

Posterior repair with perineorrhaphy is most likely to cause painful intercourse. Care must be taken to avoid excessive narrowing of the vagina or excessive removal of vaginal skin. As a guide, the vagina should admit two fingers at the end of the operation.

Cyst of Gartner's duct

These cysts are seen now and again and are a congenital remnant. Rarely, the cyst can be mistaken for a cystocele that extends up from the vagina under the ureter and uterine artery: it is prudent to marsupialize it in such an instance.

Inpatient surgery—operative laparoscopy

The risks of diagnostic laparoscopy also apply to these procedures, for which the complication rate is considerably greater. Common to operative laparoscopies are the risks of electrosurgery, particularly monopolar, which, although it carries most of the risk, is more flexible than bipolar electrosurgery.

Laparoscopically assisted vaginal hysterectomy

Ureteric injury

The incidence of ureteric damage is higher than for conventional hysterectomy. The ureter may be kinked, ligated, stapled, and/or have thermal damage or various degrees of laceration. Prompt recognition and repair is crucial if severe complications of renal damage and infection are to be prevented.

Detection

If damage is suspected, pass a retrograde ureteric catheter—this should slide up to the renal pelvis without resistance and more importantly, urine should pass from it. If resistance is met, a retrograde pyelogram is performed; contrast is injected via the catheter and an X-ray taken to identify the site of damage.

Treatment

Obtain urological assistance. Remove the staples or ligature causing kinking. Thermal damage may require excision with reanastomosis or reimplantation.

Bladder damage

Injury is caused by electrocautery or cutting or tearing with instruments as the bladder is dissected off the lower uterus. It may not be recognized and a high level of suspicion is necessary. Cystoscopy should be performed if there is uncertainty. Postoperative presentation may include unexplained haematuria, decreased urine output, anuria, suprapubic swelling and pain, and abdominal distension with an elevated serum urea.

Prevention

Empty the bladder prior to surgery. Insertion of dye into the bladder may highlight leakage. Secondary trocars should be inserted under direct vision with avoidance of undue electrocautery around the bladder. Sharp dissection, not blunt, should be used around the bladder and the bladder must not be in the jaws of a staple gun before firing. The bladder should be reflected via the vagina in preference to via the laparoscope.

Burns

Bowel burns or burns to other intra-abdominal structures may not be obvious at the time of surgery, but the patient develops peritonitis 3–7 days later.

Prevention

Ensure the active electrode is not in contact with other tissues or metal instruments. Regularly check the integrity of electrode insulation and use all metal, or plastic, trocar cannulas through which the electrode is to be passed.

Laparoscopic tubo-ovarian procedures

Ovarian cystectomy/diathermy/oophorectomy: ectopic pregnancy: division of adhesions

Haemorrhage

Haemorrhage of the ovary is often difficult to control and requires removal of the ovary. Other bleeding is usually light and easily controlled with bipolar diathermy.

Cyst rupture

The significance of this depends upon the contents and type of cyst. Contents may irritate the peritoneum or malignant cells may seed.

Ureteric injury

Large or inflamed ovarian cysts distort the anatomy and can become adherent, particularly to the peritoneum overlying the ureter. Adherence is common with endometriotic or inflammatory cysts.

Adhesions

Surgery to the ovary causes adhesion formation, particularly where the capsule is breached. Ovarian diathermy, which has replaced ovarian wedge resection as the treatment for polycystic ovaries, entails multiple punctures of the capsule and may lead to the omentum enveloping the ovary. Almost all ectopic pregnancies are complicated by varying degrees of adhesion formation. In tubal surgery for the treatment of infertility, use of glass rods with meticulous attention to control of bleeding and administration of steroids may be used to reduce adhesion formation. Various commercial products are marketed as reducing adhesion formation but none has a clear-cut indication.

Reduced fertility

This may be in addition to an already reduced infertility potential of some women with ectopic pregnancy. A Fallopian tube may be removed or adhesions develop as described above, particularly tubo-ovarian, which are detrimental to fertility.

Bowel damage

Both burns and tears are easily inflicted when vision through the laparoscope is limited by adhesions and palpation is not an option. The temptation to divide tissue bundles, which may involve bowel, in large bites must be avoided.

Laparoscopic incontinence procedures

See below under Bladder neck surgery.

Inpatient vulval surgery

Vulvectomy

+ **Infection**—the area should be kept as dry as realistically possible. Frequent bathing, showering, or bidet use is recommended to reduce infection but with the avoidance of talcum powder and creams.

+ **Haemorrhage/haematoma**

+ **Sexual difficulty**—scarring from the healing process may markedly narrow the vaginal introitus. Dilators and topical oestrogen will help to some degree. (It is usual to conserve the clitoris.)

+ **Recurrence of primary pathology**—chronic skin conditions frequently recur in the 'new' vulva.

+ **Psychological distress**—women may feel sexually unattractive and have difficulty coming to terms with their altered anatomy. Pre- and postoperative counselling is essential.

Bladder neck surgery for urinary incontinence

Complications after Burch colposuspension/Marshall–Marchetti–Krantz

+ **Haemorrhage/haematoma**—bleeding from the perivesical veins is common with the development of a haematoma. Many surgeons leave a drain *in situ* for a routine procedure. Surgery may be required for bleeding that is not related to a coagulopathy.

+ **Bladder/urethral injury**—methylene blue can be instilled into the bladder to aid disclosure of the site of injury. Prompt recognition and repair are necessary with urological referral.

+ **Voiding difficulties**—detrusor instability, presenting as frequency, urgency, or urge incontinence occurs in around 30% of patients. Some 3% develop urinary retention and require intermittent self-catheterization, which may be prolonged, up to 40% have no cure.

+ **Rectocele formation**—elevation of the anterior vaginal wall creates a space which may cause the posterior vaginal wall to prolapse. Some surgeons perform posterior wall buttressing at the time of colposuspension to avoid this complication.

+ **Ureteric injury**—this has been described after colposuspension and requires early recognition.

+ **Osteitis pubis**—stitches, inserted into the periosteum of the symphysis pubis as part of the Marshall–Marchetti–Krantz procedure, may become infected and the patient develops persistent localized pain. Exploration and curettage may be required or referral to a chronic pain clinic.

Stamey procedure and tension-free vaginal tape

There are fewer complications with this procedure than with colposuspension because the incisions used are small and minimal exploration is undertaken:

• **Bladder/urethral perforation**—Stamey needles are used to thread a loop of non-absorbable suture or mesh between the rectus sheath and paraurethral tissues. These needles easily perforate the bladder or urethra. Cystoscopy is performed after needle insertion to exclude perforation.

• Materials.

• **Infection** around the non-absorbable may need removal.

• **Voiding difficulties**—these are less than with colposuspension. Urinary retention is the most notable and is usually self-limiting after a period of catheterization.

• Exposure of mesh requires antibiotics and closure.

Gynaecological cancer surgery

The radical nature of gynaecological cancer surgery causes a greater incidence and severity of complications in general.

Radical hysterectomy for cancer

• Intraoperative complications include haemorrhage after vascular trauma and ureteric, bladder, bowel, and nerve damage.

• Postoperative complications are ileus, infection, thromboembolic disease, lymphocyst, and vascular, ureteric, bladder, and bowel fistulas.

• Long-term complications include lymphocyst and leg oedema, bladder dysfunction, and ureteric or bladder fistulas.

Ovarian surgery

The usual major intervention is bilateral salpingo-oophorectomy and total abdominal hysterectomy with omentectomy. Tumour frequently involves the colon and may require bowel resection with a defunctioning colostomy with its attendant risks. Complications are those of major abdominal surgery and hysterectomy.

Radical vulvectomy

Wound breakdown is the major complication. It is treated by meticulous local cleansing, dilute topical antiseptics such as chlorhexidine, povidone-iodine or hydrogen peroxide. Honey dressings and artificial sea-water baths are well known anecdotal treatments which may promote wound healing after breakdown.

Other complications include secondary haemorrhage, thromboembolic disease, femoroinguinal lymphocysts, leg oedema, and, rarely, hernias or vaginal prolapse.

Laparoscopic lymphadenectomy

Neurovascular injury is a major risk and only experienced operators should undertake lymphadenectomy. Considerable bleeding can occur from small venules which can be difficult to control.

Chapter 26
Medicolegal aspects of postoperative complications

Introduction

In the last 10 years there has been an upsurge in medical negligence litigation. This may not reflect an increase in the number of acts of negligence but rather an increased awareness of rights and a desire for accountability should things go wrong.

Standard of skill and care

Standard of skill and care

In order to determine that a doctor is negligent the claimant must establish three things:

(1) the doctor owed him a duty of care;

(2) there has been a breach of that duty;

(3) the plaintiff has suffered damage as a breach of that duty.

The standard of care required by law is expressed in the Bolam test (*Bolam v. Friern Hospital Management Committee* [1957]). This states:

> ...it is the standard of the ordinary skilled man exercising and professing to have that special skill. A man need not possess the highest expert skill; it is well-established law that it is sufficient if he exercises the ordinary skill of an ordinary competent man exercising that art.

The standard of care relates to the specialty in which the doctor practises. A lack of experience is no defence against an allegation of negligence, but a trainee surgeon may discharge his duty by seeking the help of a superior (*Wilsher v. Essex Health Authority*). The prudent trainee will not step beyond his capabilities but always seek advice when in doubt.

The Bolam test has established that a doctor will not be held negligent simply because he holds a different view to other members of his specialty, provided that he can prove that there is a reasonable body of opinion that supports his view. Every doctor has a duty to keep himself abreast of developments in his field. It is, however, probably reasonable not to be aware of a single paper that might have prevented the negligent act. It is likely, however, that not to be aware of practice that has become widespread would be unacceptable to a judge (*Crawford v. Board of Governors of Charing Cross Hospital*).

Consent

You are advised to read the General Medical Council's (GMC) document *Seeking patients' consent: the ethical considerations*.

Every touching is a potential battery and to render the contact lawful the doctor must obtain consent. How much information is given to the patient will depend on the circumstances, but the professional standard set by the Bolam test still applies. This means that the medical profession is the arbiter of how much information should be given. In the law of England and Wales there is no notion of informed consent, unlike United States where the amount and nature of information to be disclosed is dictated by what a patient would want to know. Such medical paternalism is being repeatedly challenged in this country. The doctor should realize that in *Sidaway* (*Sidaway* v. *Board of Governors of the Bethlem Royal Hospital* [1985]) when the question, 'Is informed consent a part of English law?' was put to the five law lords the answer was not unanimous, SCARMAN said 'Yes', DIPLOCK said 'No', and BRIDGE, KEITH, and TEMPLEMAN said 'Yes, with reservations'. However, the increasing use of the term 'informed consent' by surgeons in this country without fully realizing what the term means legally will probably lead to the introduction of the American standard which appears to favour the reasonable patient.

When deciding what material risks a patient should be told about, the surgeon should consider the seriousness of the possible injury and what is the likelihood of this happening. It is not appropriate to warn of risk as published in research papers, but rather the surgeon should warn of the risks pertinent to his own skill. Where a surgeon is a trainee or inexperienced in a particular procedure the wise practitioner will tend to err on a fuller explanation with an increased risk of that published by the more experienced. There is a concept often voiced that risks of less than 1% do not need to be explained to a patient. This has no basis in law and such 'old wives tales' should be stamped out. A risk, even if it is a mere possibility, should be disclosed if its occurrence would cause serious circumstances (*Hopp* v. *Lepp* [1979]).

The explanation should include the consequences of the injury. For example, it is not enough to say: 'There is a risk of a vocal cord palsy and your voice could be a bit weaker.' The prudent surgeon will say: 'There is a risk of a vocal cord palsy. This means that your voice will be weak and you will lose your place in the church choir. Furthermore, as you cannot bring your vocal cords together you will be unable to lift heavy weights. This means that you are likely to lose your job. If you lose your job then you might not be able to meet you mortgage payments and your home could be repossessed.'

The patient will require to understand the natural course of a disorder without treatment before coming to a decision on which treatment option he should opt for.

Children

A person over 16 years of age may give consent to medical treatment as though he was an adult. For those under 16, the principle laid down in *Gillick* applies (*Gillick* v. *West Norfolk and Wisbech Area Health Authority* [1986]). The parental right to determine whether a child under 16 receives or refuses medical treatment ends when the child achieves a significant understanding and intelligence to enable him to fully comprehend what is proposed. Where an apparently competent child refuses treatment, case law suggests that it may still be possible to treat the child provided that there is someone else with the capacity to consent, consents on the child's behalf (in Re *R.* [1991] and Re *W.* [1992]). The position is different in Scotland where those with parental responsibilities cannot authorize procedures a competent child has refused.

Mentally incompetent patients

The Mental Health Act 1983 does not provide the means by which a mentally ill patient may treated against their will for a physical disorder. The doctrine of necessity permits a doctor lawfully to operate on or to give other treatment to adult incompetent patients, provided that the treatment is in their best interest, either to save their lives or to ensure improvement in their physical or mental health.

Refusal of treatment

This may arise for many reasons including religious, such as the right of a Jehovah's Witness to refuse a blood transfusion. In the case of Re *T.* [1992] LORD DONALDSON said:

> *An adult who suffers from no mental incapacity has an absolute right to choose whether to consent to medical treatment, to refuse it, or choose one rather than another of the treatments being offered.*

A refusal of medical treatment does not have to be sensible, obviously rational, or well considered, and in the case of a competent patient the surgeon cannot override the patient's view. This right to decide applies equally to pregnant women as to others and includes the right to refuse treatment where the treatment is intended to benefit the unborn child.

Advance directives

If a patient has lost the capacity to consent to or refuse treatment the doctor should attempt to ascertain whether the patient has previously indicated preferences in an advance statement. The GMC guidance states that the doctor must respect any refusal of treatment given when the patient was competent, provided that the decision given in the advance statement is clearly applicable to the circumstances, and there is no reason to believe that the patient has changed his or her mind. If there is no advance statement then the patient's known wishes should be taken into account.

Proof of medical negligence

Proof of medical negligence

It is not sufficient for a plaintiff to show that a surgeon's actions were below an acceptable standard but they also must prove that the damage suffered was a result of the surgeon's poor performance. In *Barnett* v. *Chelsea and Kensington Hospital* [1968], the casualty officer failed to examine a patient who attended with signs of poisoning. Yet the case was successfully defended when it was established that the poison had no antidote.

The claimant has to show that his version of events with expert analysis is, on the balance of probabilities, more likely to be true than that of the defence. Where the issues are equally balanced then the claimant will fail.

An apparent reversal can occur when *res ipsa loquitor* is pleaded. This literally means 'the facts speak for themselves'. Good examples of this would be a retained swab following surgery or amputation of the wrong leg. In these circumstances, the onus is on the defence to provide an adequate explanation of how the injury occurred that is consistent with an acceptable standard of care.

The Criminal Law

Assault and battery

Involuntary manslaughter

The Criminal Law

Surgeons rarely face criminal proceedings as a result of medical practice, but two offences need to be covered.

Assault and battery

The courts are reluctant to consider actions in tort for battery arising out of a failure to gain consent. However, when a surgeon performs a procedure which goes far beyond that for which consent was obtained then a charge of battery may be considered. If the therapeutic procedure was an operation then the more serious charge of assault causing grievous bodily harm may be alleged.

Involuntary manslaughter

There are two forms of involuntary manslaughter: an unlawful act manslaughter; and gross negligence manslaughter. In gross negligence manslaughter, the test to be applied to determine culpability was clarified in two cases from the Court of Appeal and The House of Lords.

The first case involved two junior doctors, Prentice and Suliman. Dr Prentice injected vincristine intrathecally under the supervision of Dr Suliman. The patient died. The Court of Appeal observed that a version of what is known as the 'recklessness test' had been put to the jury resulting in the doctors' conviction. However, as there were many mitigating circumstances which could be taken in to consideration, the traditional gross negligence test which has no rigid formulation should be applied, thus enabling excuses and mitigating circumstances to be put forward in assessing overall culpability.

The second case involved an anaesthetist, Dr Adamoko. During the course of an operation the endotracheal tube had become disconnected from the anaesthetic machine. Cut off from his supply of oxygen the patient died, Dr Adamoko failing to appreciate the situation. The Court of Appeal determined that the traditional test of gross negligence should apply and so Dr Adamoko's conviction was upheld. Dr Adamoko appealed to The House of Lords, who upheld the conviction and that the traditional test of gross negligence should apply. In applying the gross negligence test a jury will consider:

(1) on the ordinary principles of the law of negligence, whether or not the defendant has been in breach of a duty of care to the deceased; and if so,

(2) if the breach of duty, which involved a risk of serious injury or death, caused the death of the victim; and if so,

(3) whether the breach of duty should be categorized as gross negligence and therefore as a crime.

The Court of Appeal in the Prentice case identified four states of mind which could be indicative of gross negligence:

(1) indifference to an obvious risk of injury to health;

(2) actual foresight of the risk coupled with the determination nevertheless to run it;

(3) an appreciation of the risk coupled with the intention to avoid it, but also coupled with such a degree of negligence in the attempted avoidance as the jury considers justifies conviction;

(4) inattention or failure to avert serious risk which goes beyond mere inadvertence in respect of an obvious and important matter which the defendant's duty demanded that he should address.

Proof of one of these states of mind alone is not indicative of guilt. A jury must also consider mitigating circumstances and excuses before agreeing a guilty verdict.

Criminal Procedure and Investigation Act 1996

Where a doctor refuses to give evidence to the police during an investigation, the police may go before a magistrate and request the doctor to be summonsed. The doctor can then be called to court on deposition and required to answer questions. Failure to give this evidence can lead to a criminal conviction. This procedure may arise, for example, where a casualty officer refuses to give evidence concerning a battery on the grounds of wishing to maintain patient confidentiality.

Expert witness

In cases of medical negligence and personal injury the court may require assistance to resolve the issues from a medical expert. From 26th April 1999 the Civil Procedure Rules 1999 replaced all previous rules governing the conduct of civil litigation in both the High Court and the County Court in England and Wales. Part 35 of these Rules set out obligations of Experts and Assessors.

The expert has an overriding duty to the court to help on the matters within his expertise.

In the case of the *Ikarian Reefer*, CRESSWELL J. laid down guidance on the duties and responsibilities of the expert.

1. Expert evidence presented to the court should be, and should be seen to be, the independent product of the expert uninfluenced as to form or content by the exigencies of litigation. (See *Whitehouse* v. *Jordan* [1981] 1 WLR 246. 256.)

2. Independent assistance should be provided to the court by way of objective unbiased opinion regarding matters within the expertise of the expert witness. (See *Polivitre Ltd* v. *Commercial Union Assurance Co. plc.* [1987] 1 Lloyds Rep. 379. 386. and Re *J.* [1990] ECR 193. An expert witness in the High Court should never assume the role of advocate.)

3. Facts or assumptions upon which the opinion was based should be stated together with material facts which could detract from the concluded opinion.

4. An expert witness should make it clear when a question or issue fell outside his expertise.

5. If the opinion was not properly researched because it was considered that insufficient data was available, then that had to be stated with an indication that the opinion was provisional (see Re *J.*) If the witness could not assert that the report contained the truth, the whole truth, and nothing but the truth then the qualification should be stated on the report. (See *Derby & Co Ltd. and Others* v. *Weldon and Others* [No. 9] *The Times* November 9th 1990.)

6. If after exchange of reports an expert witness changed his mind on a material matter, then the change of view should be communicated to the other side through legal representatives without delay and when appropriate to the court.

7. Photographs, plans, survey reports, and other documents referred to in the expert evidence had to be provided to the other side at the same time as exchange of reports.

Medicolegal reports and statements

The Civil Procedure Rules lay down certain rules that must be complied with in preparing a report. These are:

1. The report must be addressed to the Court stating which party or parties have instructed the expert.

2. The report must state the substance of all material instructions whether written or oral on the basis of which the report is written. It must summarize the material facts of the case.

3. Where there is a range of opinion on matters dealt with in the report the range must be summarized and you must make clear the reasons for your own opinion.

4. Your conclusions must be summarized.

5. The report must conclude with a statement of truth in the following form:

   '*I believe that the facts I have stated in the report are true and the opinions I have expressed are correct*'.

6. There must be a statement that the expert understands his duty to the court and has complied with that duty.

7. The expert must set out details of his qualifications, details of any literature or other material relied on in making the report and identify any person who carried out any test or experiment which the expert has used giving the qualifications of such person.

In preparing a report for the court the expert should be clear on what the court requires. If necessary guidance can be obtained from the instructing parties or directly from the Court. Reports usually refer to one or more of the following six areas:

(1) an initial statement on the possible merits of an allegation for a plaintiff before notes and other evidence are obtained

(2) liability

(3) causation

(4) current condition

(5) prognosis

(6) expert opinion on an area of medicine.

A quote should be given on the cost of a report in advance. It is also advisable to quote an hourly rate for work. This should include travel to meetings with counsel and a rate for attending court.

The report should be typed on A4-size paper. Each sheet should have the name of the claimant and the expert's name in the top left-hand corner. Each paragraph and each page should be numbered. It is useful to enclose a short curriculum vitae for use of counsel and the court. It is inadvisable to use the word 'negligent' in a report. The finding of negligence is the province of the judge. However phrases such as 'fell below a reasonable standard of care' or 'followed a course of action that could not be supported by any body of medical opinion' are useful to imply serious criticism. Phrases such as 'flagrant disregard' or 'reckless course of action' should be avoided as they may carry criminal connotations.

The court or any party can put written questions to the expert, who has to reply within 28 days. If the expert does not reply within the 28 days, then the party who instructed the expert in the first place will be unable to rely on his evidence or will be unable to recover the expert's fee.

The Pre-action Protocol

This Protocol has two essential aims. First, to maintain or restore the relationship between patient and healthcare provider. Second, to resolve as many disputes as possible without recourse to litigation. The Protocol establishes three central objectives:

(1) openness in communicating perceived problems and investigating adverse outcomes;

(2) timeliness in investigating and managing any potential dispute;

(3) awareness of the options opened to those involved in a dispute.

Disclosure of medical records

Patients or their advisors are requested to use the standard forms approved by the Law Society and the Department of Health. Sufficient information must be given about the possible claim and the patient must be as specific as possible about the records required. The records should be provided within 40 days. A fee may be charged under the Access to Health Records Act 1990. Currently this is a maximum of £10 plus photocopying and postage costs. If disclosure is not made in 40 days the patient may apply to the Court for an Order for pre-action disclosure.

Letter of claim

If there are grounds for a claim then a letter should be sent to the potential defendant as soon as practicable. The letter should contain:

(1) a clear summary of the facts, including the alleged adverse outcome;

(2) the patient's injuries and current condition and prognosis;

(3) details of any special damages, e.g. loss of earnings;

(4) a chronology of the relevant events;

(5) reference to any relevant documents with copies if the potential defendant does not already have these.

The claimant should not issue proceedings until 3 months have passed from sending of the Letter of Claim (unless there is a problem with limitation). The patient should indicate the level of any settlement offer which would be acceptable.

Letter of response

The Letter of Claim should be acknowledged within 14 days identifying the individual who will be dealing with the matter. A reasoned reply should be given within 3 months.

If the claim is admitted this should be stated in clear terms. Any elements of the claim that are denied should be clearly stated with an explanation.

If liability is accepted an attempt should be made to agree a time in which to settle the issue of quantum.

The court has the power to impose costs' penalties to punish a party who has unreasonably failed to comply with the Pre-Action Protocol when proceedings are subsequently issued. This includes a power to order a defaulting party to meet the whole costs, on an indemnity basis, of proceedings issued which might not otherwise have been commenced had the Protocol been complied with.

The new system of civil procedure

After a defence is filed to Claim Form with Statement of Case, a procedural judge will allocate the case to one of three 'tracks'.

Tracks

(1) The Small Claims Track

(2) The Fast Track

(3) The Multi-Track

The Small Claims Track

It is unlikely that clinical negligence claims will be allocated to the Small Claims Track as the total damages claimed are limited to £5000 and the damages for pain and suffering are limited to less than £1000.

The Fast Track

Claims are of a total value of £5000–£15 000. The trial should be complete in 1 day. Expert evidence is limited to one expert per party for each field of expertise. Directions in the form of a timetable are issued at the time of allocation of the case to the Fast Track. The timetable sets out when witness statements and expert reports should be disclosed. The trial is listed to take place within 30 weeks. A Listing Questionnaire is sent to all parties 8 weeks before the trial, after which the court will issue any further directions, e.g. a meeting of experts.

The Multi-Track

All other cases will be allocated to the Multi-Track. It is anticipated that the majority of clinical negligence cases will be allocated to this track. Upon allocation to the Multi-track the court will give directions for the management of the case, setting a timetable for the various steps and fixing either a case management conference or a pre-trial review. Directions can be issued at any point prior to the trial. The Directions given will be tailored to the needs of the case. A Listing Questionnaire has to be completed by the parties 8 weeks before the trial. The court may then either order a listing hearing or a pre-trial review or give further directions.

Relevance to the trainee surgeon

The new Civil Procedure Rules will place stringent time restrictions on the handling of the defence of a claim brought by a patient. Failure to comply with Court Directions and The Pre-Action Protocol can have significant cost implications on any Trust. If a trainee who is germane to a case has rotated to another hospital as part of his training, then delays can occur in tracing him.

As a result, it will be increasingly important to record adverse outcomes, especially if the patient is verbally complaining about the outcome on a hospital incident form. If there is no appropriate form to cope with potential issues of clinical negligence then it is best to report the incident to the hospital legal services department by way of a letter. A consultant should ensure that all individual staff prepare appropriate statements of fact, especially when they are fresh in people's minds. The wise trainee will not try and hide an adverse outcome but inform his consultant. This may be just a simple matter of copying in the consultant-to-outpatient letter saying, for example, that a hernia repair had been unsuccessful and the patient was dissatisfied. A trainee may be frightened to report adverse outcomes repeatedly lest it prejudice his performance assessments. The consultant, however, must put the trainee at his ease so that he feels free to discuss untoward incidents. Such disclosure within the hospital then prepares the hospital legal department for handling a Letter of Claim promptly. Speed of response to queries by the hospital legal department will become paramount, and failure to comply with such requests may lead to disciplinary action against the doctor.

Colleagues' health, conduct, or performance

The doctor has a paramount duty to protect patients when he believes that a colleague's health, conduct, or performance is a threat to them. Before taking action the doctor should make every effort to ascertain all the facts and to gather evidence of the suspected problem. Then the doctor should follow the employer's procedures. This will usually mean informing the medical director, director of public health, or chief executive of a trust. If you are not sure what to do then contact the GMC for advice. In the case of poorly performing locum doctors, it is not adequate just to terminate the doctor's contract as the doctor may move on to another position and pose a threat to patients. As standard local procedures may not be adequate to deal with a locum the GMC should be informed.

Maintaining good medical practice produced by the GMC gives detailed advice on what action to take over a poorly performing doctor. However, a doctor should always be referred to the GMC if:

(1) local action would not be practical;

(2) you have tried local action and it has failed;

(3) the problem is so serious that the GMC clearly need to be involved;

(4) the doctor has been convicted of a criminal offence.

At least one doctor has been struck off the medical register for failing to report a serious problem to the GMC, and so it is best to contact the GMC for advice whenever poor performance is suspected, especially if local action has failed.

The defence organizations

Every doctor should be a member of a defence organization. The insurance cover provided by the NHS is woefully inadequate. This cover does not cover a whole range of a doctor's requirements, including: representation at inquests; good Samaritan acts; representation at public inquiries; or representation at the General Medical Council.

The coroner

The coroner should be informed of death in the following circumstances:

1. Death following spontaneous abortion. This is so rare that illegal interference should be suspected.
2. Death thought to be due to an accident.
3. Alcoholism.
4. Death associated with an anaesthetic
5. Death due to drugs. Therapeutic, addictive, suicidal or adverse reaction.
6. Industrial disease or poisoning.
7. Medical mishaps. Deaths due to operative error such a failure to tie off blood vessels, perforation of a viscus during endoscopy, or other similar events.
8. Murder, manslaughter, or infanticide.
9. Pensioners. Those receiving a disability or war pension.
10. Poisoning in any form.
11. Stillbirths where there is doubt that the baby was born alive.
12. Death in prison or death of a prisoner in hospital even if the death is natural.

The inquest

The proceedings at an inquest shall be directed solely to ascertaining:

(1) who the deceased was;
(2) how, when, and where the deceased came by his death;
(3) the particulars for the time being required by the Registration Acts to be registered concerning the death.

If during the proceedings evidence of certain serious crimes is disclosed, the inquest must be adjourned and the matter referred to the Director of Public Prosecutions. An inquest cannot inquire into allegations of negligence or of crimes that did not affect the cause of the death. Allegations of delay in diagnosis or treating a natural illness would not necessarily make the death an unnatural one.

Actions after a medical accident

Appropriate action after an accident may avoid litigation or, if litigation does arise, lead to a speedy conclusion of the action.

1. Keep good records of the event. Do not alter any previous records, but if previous records have been inadequate write up your memory of the events and findings leading up to the mishap. Date and sign all entries.

2. Fill out an Incident Form or write a full description of the events to your hospital's legal department. Consider informing your defence organization, particularly if the patient has died.

3. Give a truthful explanation to the patient. However, be sure of your facts lest you give incorrect information. If the patient is dead or unconscious it is reasonable to inform the next of kin of the situation, unless the patient prior to losing consciousness had expressly forbade the disclosure. In most circumstances of a medical accident the consultant in charge of the case should give the explanation; however, if the consultant is unavailable then relatives or the patient should not be left waiting for an inordinate length of time.

4. An apology and expression of regret concerning the outcome is not an admission of guilt and so should not be withheld. Every attempt should be made to maintain the patient's confidence in the doctor and not to build up a feeling in the patient that the doctor has become self-centred and defensive. On no account be arrogant. Where appropriate, offer the reassurance of a second opinion or even transfer of the patient to a separate team or hospital if that is what the patient wishes.

Common pitfalls leading to litigation

It is impossible to give an account of every pitfall for each condition and every treatment in the scope of this chapter, but there are several broad areas worth mentioning.

Consent

It is rare for an action based on a failure to give adequate consent alone to be brought, for the patient has to prove that if he had known of the risk he would have not consented to the procedure. Nevertheless, it wise to note in the records when obtaining consent what risks and options were covered in the discussion.

Delay in diagnosis

This usually arises in relation to malignant disease. Often even if there has been an obvious breach of the duty of care and the diagnosis was obviously delayed, the claimant often has significant difficulty in proving damage except in major delays. Common malignant tumours in which this may arise are carcinomas of the gastrointestinal tract, prostate, thyroid, and lymphoma. Delay can also occur with infections, examples include meningitis especially unusual forms such a tubercular, syphilis, osteomyelitis, and *Helicobacter pylori*.

Poor surgical technique

This is often very difficult for the plaintiff to prove as there are often mitigating circumstances which can excuse an untoward outcome, such as scarring, excessive bleeding, gross obesity, unusual anatomy. It is therefore most important when writing the operation note that any unusual difficulties are mentioned and how they were managed.

Nevertheless, there are occasions when gross incompetence in surgical technique does arise. This occurs when a new surgical technique is being advocated. Occasionally a surgeon may wish for personal reasons of ego or vanity to be the first to introduce a new technique into his hospital. Accidents can occur when the training has been inadequate, for example pushing a trocar into the aorta when inducing a pneumoperitoneum in laparoscopic surgery.

However, some latitude has to be given for untoward events occurring during a learning curve.

Wrong patient, wrong side, wrong operation

There is usually no defence for performing the incorrect operation on a patient due to misidentification. Operating theatre procedures must be adhered to, to prevent this. Great care must be taken when an operating list order is changed or operation cancelled. Also, there is no excuse for leaving swabs, instruments, or dressings in a patient after surgery. Every attempt should be made to retrieve any fragments if an instrument breaks, but in so doing care must be taken not to damage the patient. In some cases it may be wiser to leave fragments behind, e.g. within brain tissue. It is essential that the broken instrument is retained as forensic examination may later be required to establish whether the instrument was defective.

Drugs

Litigation nearly always occurs in circumstances in which the doctor is unfamiliar with the drug, its side-effects, or method of administration. Cases of ototoxicity or nephrotoxicity still occur from aminoglycoside drugs. Other drugs which cause problems include, cytotoxic drugs, β-blockers and lack of care in prescribing drugs to fertile women who might be pregnant.

Acknowledgement: I wish to thank my friend and colleague Mr Barker for his advice and guidance in preparing this chapter.

Index